# Resilient Healthcare Internet of Things Systems:

## Architectures, Security, and Trust

Chin-Shiuh Shieh
*National Kaohsiung University of Science and Technology, Taiwan*

Pawan Kumar Goel
*Raj Kumar Goel Institute of Technology, India*

Mong-Fong Horng
*National Kaohsiung University of Science and Technology, Taiwan*

Hari Mohan Pandey
*Bournemouth University, UK*

IGI Global
Scientific Publishing
Publishing Tomorrow's Research Today

Vice President of Editorial — Melissa Wagner
Director of Acquisitions — Mikaela Felty
Director of Book Development — Jocelynn Hessler
Production Manager — Mike Brehm
Cover Design — Jose Rosado

Published in the United States of America by
IGI Global Scientific Publishing
701 East Chocolate Avenue
Hershey, PA, 17033, USA
Tel: 717-533-8845 | Fax: 717-533-7115
Website: https://www.igi-global.com E-mail: cust@igi-global.com



Library of Congress Cataloging-in-Publication Data

(CIP Data Pending)
ISBN13: 9798337376103
Isbn13Softcover: 9798337376110
EISBN13: 9798337376127
British Cataloguing in Publication Data
A Cataloguing in Publication record for this book is available from the British Library.

# Table of Contents

# Detailed Table of Contents



The use of Internet of Things (IoT) technologies in healthcare is changing the way medical services are delivered by allowing for real-time monitoring, smart automation, and patient-centered care. This chapter discusses the basic structure of IoT in healthcare and how it is changing over time. It focusses on how IoT can help with managing chronic diseases, automating hospitals caring for the elderly, and responding to emergencies. It looks closely at the complicated security and trust issues that come up when IoT devices connect to cloud-based systems. There is a lot of talk about new types of threats, the problems with old security models, and how important it is to have dynamic trust frameworks right now. The chapter also discusses the future, including blockchain, edge computing, and AI-driven threat intelligence. This chapter gives healthcare practitioners, IT architects, academics, and politicians useful information about how to develop safe and resilient IoT-enabled healthcare systems by connecting technical ideas with strategic ones.



IoT technologies connect physical objects to the internet and collect data without human intervention. The IoT is employed worldwide, but mainly in logistics, manufacturing, and healthcare. IDS use AI algorithms to quickly identify and stop a variety of threats, protecting critical data. IoT network traditions are a prominent issue in academia. ML and DL are used by many to construct intrusion detection systems. Despite its pervasiveness, the IoT remains a mystery. This implies a huge Internet change. From linking tablets, computers, and phones to transmitting every part of the actual world, the goal is to blur the lines between the real and virtual. Massive object-connected systems have security flaws. Many network attacks, especially routing protocol attacks, target them. The security of these systems cannot be assured by authentication and encryption. The proliferation of linked gadgets has made security a major issue. Web connectivity and trusted data sharing define the IoT. Therefore, most cyberattacks, including DDoS attacks, can target IoT systems.



The proliferation of Internet of Things (IoT) devices across critical sectors has intensified the adoption of lightweight security protocols designed to accommodate resource-constrained environments. However, the inherent trade-offs between computational efficiency and security robustness in these protocols have introduced significant vulnerabilities that threaten the integrity of IoT ecosystems. This chapter provides a comprehensive analysis of security weaknesses in prevalent lightweight IoT protocols, including MQTT, CoAP, LoRaWAN, and DTLS-based implementations. Through systematic vulnerability assessment and empirical security testing, this research identifies critical attack vectors, evaluates their potential impact on IoT infrastructures, and proposes a multi-layered mitigation framework.



The exponential growth of Healthcare Internet of Things (H-IoT) technologies has introduced unprecedented opportunities for patient monitoring, diagnostics, and operational efficiency. However, these advancements have also magnified the cybersecurity risks inherent in distributed, device-rich environments. Traditional perimeter-based security models have proven inadequate in addressing the evolving threat landscape, necessitating the implementation of Zero Trust Architecture (ZTA), which adheres to the principle of "never trust, always verify." In this chapter, the applicability of ZTA in H-IoT settings has been critically analyzed, with focus placed on its core principles—least privilege access, micro-segmentation, continuous monitoring, and context-aware policy enforcement. Implementation strategies such as dynamic access control, software-defined segmentation, and machine learning-based anomaly detection have been discussed to offer a comprehensive security posture.



Healthcare data contains highly sensitive information, making privacy a top priority in AI-based medical systems. Traditional centralized machine learning aggregates data from multiple sources, raising concerns about privacy breaches, data ownership, and regulatory compliance. Federated Learning (FL) offers a solution by allowing AI models to be trained across decentralized data sources without moving patient data. Only model updates are shared, preserving privacy. FL uses tools like differential privacy and secure multi-party computation to enhance security. Algorithms such as FedAvg and FedProx enable collaborative training without exposing individual data. FL also supports IoMT devices, allowing them to contribute to model training while keeping data local. This not only safeguards patient privacy but also addresses the challenge of limited, diverse medical data across institutions. Federated Learning helps build secure, compliant, and flexible AI systems in healthcare, ensuring both innovation and protection of sensitive patient information.



The advent of digitalized patient monitoring systems marks a major breakthrough in healthcare. IoT, cloud computing, and AI generate behavior-driven big data, but this integration also raises concerns about anomalies and cybersecurity threats. This chapter explores two types of anomalies: patient-centered irregular medical activity

# Preface

The global healthcare landscape is undergoing a profound digital transformation driven by the integration of Internet of Things (IoT) technologies, artificial intelligence (AI), cloud computing, blockchain, and advanced data analytics. Among these innovations, the Healthcare Internet of Things (H-IoT) stands out as a game-changer, enabling continuous patient monitoring, predictive diagnostics, smart hospital management, and personalized treatment. From wearable sensors and implantable devices to interconnected hospital systems, H-IoT promises a future of more responsive, efficient, and accessible healthcare delivery.

Yet, as healthcare becomes increasingly reliant on IoT-enabled systems, it faces unprecedented security, privacy, and trust challenges. The proliferation of connected devices creates vast and complex attack surfaces. Lightweight protocols, while efficient for resource-constrained environments, often introduce vulnerabilities. Traditional perimeter-based security approaches are inadequate for such highly distributed systems. Cyberattacks on healthcare IoT not only threaten data integrity but can also compromise patient safety directly, making resilience a paramount priority.

This book, *Resilient Healthcare Internet of Things Systems: Architectures, Security, and Trust*, is designed to address these pressing issues. It highlights the need for resilient architectures, trustworthy AI, anomaly detection, zero-trust models, and organizational culture of vigilance in ensuring that healthcare IoT ecosystems are secure, scalable, and future-ready.

## RATIONALE FOR THE BOOK

The role of IoT in healthcare is rapidly expanding, with applications in chronic disease management, elderly care, telemedicine, hospital automation, and emergency response. However, as billions of medical IoT devices communicate sensitive patient data, the consequences of breaches extend far beyond financial losses—they can directly impact patient lives.

Ensuring resilience in healthcare IoT systems involves more than securing devices or encrypting data. It requires:

- **Architectural robustness** – designing interoperable, secure, and efficient IoT systems.
- **Adaptive security mechanisms** – intrusion detection powered by machine learning, anomaly detection, and lightweight cryptographic frameworks.
- **Zero-trust strategies** – applying principles of continuous verification, least privilege, and micro-segmentation.
- **Ethical AI frameworks** – leveraging federated learning to protect privacy while enabling innovation.
- **Cultural and organizational readiness** – fostering leadership and continuous vigilance to strengthen systemic resilience.

This book integrates these dimensions to present a multidisciplinary roadmap for advancing security and trust in healthcare IoT.

## SCOPE AND STRUCTURE OF THE BOOK

The volume is organized into eight chapters, each contributing unique insights:

- **Chapter 1: Introduction to IoT in Healthcare – Trends and Applications** provides a foundational overview of how IoT is reshaping healthcare delivery. It explores applications in chronic disease management, emergency response, elderly care, and hospital automation, while highlighting the evolving security and trust challenges.
- **Chapter 2: Machine Learning-Based Intrusion Detection Systems for HIoT** investigates how machine learning and deep learning algorithms can enhance real-time anomaly detection in IoT-enabled healthcare environments. It explores threats like denial-of-service attacks and routing protocol exploits, showing why traditional encryption and authentication are insufficient.
- **Chapter 3: From Vulnerability to Resilience – Enhancing Security in Lightweight IoT Protocols** provides an in-depth analysis of protocols such as MQTT, CoAP, and LoRaWAN. It identifies vulnerabilities and proposes multi-layered frameworks to balance efficiency and robust security in resource-constrained medical IoT devices.

- **Chapter 4: Zero Trust Architecture in Healthcare IoT** introduces the principle of "never trust, always verify." It explores how zero trust can transform H-IoT security through continuous monitoring, micro-segmentation, and context-aware access control supported by ML-based anomaly detection.
- **Chapter 5: Building Trustworthy AI for Healthcare – Privacy-First Approaches with Federated Learning and IoMT** explores how federated learning enables collaborative AI without centralizing sensitive health data. By preserving privacy and compliance, it ensures secure AI-driven innovations across distributed IoT ecosystems.
- **Chapter 6: Anomaly-Resilient Digital Health – Integrating AI, IoT, and Privacy Frameworks for Secure Patient Monitoring** discusses anomaly detection in both patient health data and system operations. It presents case studies involving ECG wearables and IoT datasets, highlighting the role of federated learning and privacy-preserving frameworks.
- **Chapter 7: Machine Learning-Based Intrusion Detection Systems for Healthcare IoT** expands on IDS with healthcare-specific datasets, addressing challenges such as class imbalance and the integration of fog/edge computing for real-time threat detection. It also discusses explainable AI for improved trust in healthcare security solutions.
- **Chapter 8: Transformational Leadership Effect on IoT-Based Cybersecurity in Healthcare** investigates how organizational leadership and culture of continuous improvement influence the adoption of cybersecurity measures in H-IoT. Drawing from real-world examples, it highlights the human and institutional dimensions of resilience.

Together, these chapters provide a holistic exploration of the technical, ethical, and organizational aspects of resilient healthcare IoT security.

## TARGET AUDIENCE

This book is intended for a wide range of readers:

- **Researchers and academicians** seeking comprehensive insights into the latest security, AI, and IoT integration strategies.
- **Healthcare IT professionals and system architects** who design, implement, and manage IoT-enabled infrastructures.
- **Policymakers and regulators** aiming to develop standards and policies for secure healthcare IoT ecosystems.

- **Students and scholars** looking for foundational and advanced perspectives on IoT security, anomaly detection, and privacy-preserving AI.

## CONCLUDING REMARKS

*Resilient Healthcare Internet of Things Systems: Architectures, Security, and Trust* is more than an academic resource—it is a strategic guide for building resilient, secure, and trustworthy healthcare ecosystems in the digital era. By combining technical innovation with ethical foresight and organizational preparedness, the book offers actionable pathways to overcome the pressing challenges of healthcare IoT security.

We extend our heartfelt gratitude to all contributing authors, reviewers, and collaborators whose insights and dedication have made this volume possible. We also acknowledge the publishing team for their continued guidance and support.

It is our sincere hope that this book will inspire innovation, foster resilience, and shape the development of secure, trustworthy healthcare IoT infrastructures worldwide.

Editors

**Chin-Shiuh Shieh**
*National Kaohsiung University of Science and Technology, Taiwan*

**Pawan Kumar Goel**
*Raj Kumar Goel Institute of Technology, India*

**Mong-Fong Horng**
*National Kaohsiung University of Science and Technology, Taiwan*

**Hari Mohan Pandey**
*Bournemouth University, United Kingdom*

Chapter 1

# Introduction to IoT in Healthcare:

## Trends and Applications


**Biswajit Saha**
https://orcid.org/0000-0001-8000-6733
*Dr. B.C.Roy Engineering College, Durgapur, India*

**Dharmpal Singh**
*JIS University, India*

**Gour Sundar Mitra Thakur**
https://orcid.org/0000-0001-8907-9058
*Dr. B.C. Roy Engineering College, Durgapur, India*



## ABSTRACT

*The use of Internet of Things (IoT) technologies in healthcare is changing the way medical services are delivered by allowing for real-time monitoring, smart automation, and patient-centered care. This chapter discusses the basic structure of IoT in healthcare and how it is changing over time. It focusses on how IoT can help with managing chronic diseases, automating hospitals, caring for the elderly, and responding to emergencies. It looks closely at the complicated security and trust issues that come up when IoT devices connect to cloud-based systems. There is a lot of talk about new types of threats, the problems with old security models and how important it is to have dynamic trust frameworks right now. The chapter also discusses the future, including blockchain, edge computing, and AI-driven threat intelligence. This chapter gives healthcare practitioners, IT architects, academics, and politicians useful information about how to develop safe and resilient IoT-enabled healthcare systems by connecting technical ideas with strategic ones.*



DOI: 10.4018/979-8-3373-7610-3.ch001

# 1 INTRODUCTION

IoT is changing the way medical services are delivered, monitored, and managed in a big way. As the need for more efficient, personalised, and data-driven healthcare solutions grows, IoT technologies are making it possible to build smart, connected ecosystems that connect patients, providers, and devices. These systems use networked sensors, wearable devices, cloud computing, and real-time data analytics to make clinical outcomes better, operations run more smoothly,

and healthcare costs lower. As problems with healthcare around the world get worse, from dealing with an ageing population and chronic diseases to being ready for a pandemic, the IoT is becoming an important section of responsive and long-lasting healthcare systems.

More and more medical devices are becoming networked, which has led to more smart health monitoring systems, automated diagnostics, and remote patient care. Wearable gadgets, for instance, may constantly monitor physiological signals like heart rate, oxygen saturation, and blood glucose levels. This gives both patients and healthcare providers useful information. IoT-enabled hospital automation solutions, such as smart beds, asset tracking, and predictive main- tenance of medical equipment, are also changing how modern hospitals work. These improvements not only lead to better patient outcomes, but they also make administrative tasks easier and make better use of resources.

Even though IoT has the potential to change healthcare for the better, this change brings up new problems with data security, privacy, interoperability, and system trustworthiness. Healthcare data is very sensitive, yet IoT devices do not have a lot of resources. This makes the threat environment very complicated, and it needs to be dealt with through strong and flexible security frameworks. Trust is very important for keeping device-to-cloud connections safe, making sure that rules are followed, and protecting patients' rights. In dynamic, distributed IoT contexts, existing security measures often do not work well enough. This means that new models based on distributed trust, zero-trust architectures, and AI-driven anomaly detection need to be built.

The goal of this chapter is to give a full overview of the trends, uses, and security issues that come up when IoT is used in healthcare. It starts by giving an overview of the technology that makes up IoT and the sections of it that are relevant to healthcare. The next sections look at some of the most important areas of application, such as managing chronic diseases, caring for the elderly, automating hospital workflows, and emergency response systems. The chapter also discusses the new problems that come up when trying to make sure trust, data integrity, and compliance in cloud-integrated IoT ecosystems. Current research directions that are getting a lot of attention include using blockchain, federated learning, and edge-based threat detection to make IoT infrastructures more secure against new threats. This chapter connects technical knowledge with real-world uses, giving healthcare providers, IT architects, academics, and policymakers useful information. By knowing what IoT can and cannot do in healthcare, stakeholders can make better decisions about how to build, implement, and regulate systems that are ready for the future and are smart, efficient, ethical, secure, and strong.

To completely comprehend the present extent and significance of IoT in healthcare, it is important to know how these technologies have changed over time. Advances in sensor technology, wireless communication, cloud computing, and data analytics have all had an impact on the growth of IoT in healthcare. The next section looks at the important events in history that led to the development of modern IoT-enabled healthcare systems. This gives important background information about how they are used now and what they could be used for in the future.

## 2 HISTORICAL EVOLUTION of IoT IN HEALTHCARE

The idea of devices that can talk to each other, which is what the IoT is all about, goes back to the early days of telemedicine and remote monitoring systems. Before the word "IoT" was formally created, the healthcare industry was already looking into how to leverage networked technologies to improve patient care and make clinical labour more efficient. The history of IoT in healthcare is a story of how technology came together, how policies changed, and how public health demands grew.

Telemetry was first utilised in the 1960s and 1970s to remotely monitor physiological data, especially in critical care and space medicine. This was the first step towards IoT in healthcare. NASA was a big section of making the first bio-monitoring gadgets for astronauts, which eventually led to comparable uses in civilian healthcare. In the 1980s and 1990s, improvements in computers and telecommunications made it possible for health information systems to become more advanced and for digital technology to be added to diagnostic equipment. The late 1990s and early 2000s were important years because the internet became easier to use and cellular connectivity got better. Hospitals started using electronic health records (EHRs), and remote monitoring devices became increasingly common, especially for keeping an eye on chronic conditions like diabetes and high blood pressure. Kevin Ashton officially popularised the phrase "Internet of Things" in 1999, but it would take several more years for healthcare-

specific uses to become fully developed.

In the 2010s, the development of healthcare solutions that use the IoT sped up a lot. The rise of cellphones, wearable sensors, Bluetooth devices, and cloud computing made it easy for new ideas to grow. Fitbit and Apple Watch are examples of consumer-grade fitness trackers that made it easier to keep track of your health. Hospitals, on the other hand, started using smart beds, real- time location systems (RTLS), and automated drug dispensing systems. During this time, mobile health (mHealth) apps and telehealth platforms that used IoT designs also became popular.

At the same time, governments and global health groups started to see the promise of IoT and digital health. The FDA's Digital Health Innovation Action Plan and the European Commission's eHealth Action Plan were both meant to make regulations more friendly and encourage people to use connected health devices. The COVID-19 pandemic sped up this tendency even more, making it easier to use remote monitoring tools, contact tracing apps, and virtual consul- tation platforms.

IoT in healthcare is entering a new era today, one that includes AI, edge computing, and blockchain. These technologies make IoT systems safer, faster, and smarter, allowing for real-time analytics, predictive diagnostics, and secure data sharing. Improvements in hardware (like microcontrollers and biosensors), software (like machine learning algorithms), and network infrastructure (like 5G and LPWAN) are still changing how IoT works in healthcare.

In short, the history of IoT in healthcare shows a gradual move from basic telemetry to complex, smart ecosystems of devices and systems that work together. Every new technology has opened up new ways to provide remote care, personalised medicine, and efficient health services. Knowing how this has changed over time is important for judging existing IoT applications and predicting where connected healthcare is headed in the future.

There have been big technological advances in IoT in healthcare, from the early usage of RFID to keep track of medical equipment to the present use of AI, cloud, and edge computing in smart hospital systems. The table below shows the most important milestones along the way and how each one helped make healthcare delivery and operations more efficient.

*Table 1. Key Milestones in the Historical Evolution of IoT in Healthcare*

| Period | Milestone/Event | Technology Introduced | Impact on Healthcare |
|---|---|---|---|
| 1999–2005 | Conceptualization of IoT | RFID, early wireless communication | Enabled basic tracking of medical assets and supplies in hospitals |
| 2005–2010 | Adoption in healthcare supply chains | Wireless Sensor Networks (WSN) | Improved inventory control, cold-chain monitoring for vaccines |
| 2010–2015 | Rise of consumer health wearables | Bluetooth, smart wristbands | Promoted self-monitoring and preventive healthcare practices |

continued on following page

*Table 1. Continued*

| Period | Milestone/Event | Technology Introduced | Impact on Healthcare |
|---|---|---|---|
| 2015–2020 | Integration with mobile and cloud platforms | Mobile apps, cloud computing | Enabled remote patient monitoring and hospital automation |
| 2020–2024 | Emergence of smart hospitals | AI, Edge computing, 5G, ML | Enabled predictive diagnostics, real-time analytics, and faster decision-making |

## 3 APPLICATIONS of IoT IN HEALTHCARE

The use of IoT technologies in healthcare has created a wide range of applications that improve patient care, make clinical operations more efficient, and make the whole system more responsive. These apps go beyond the usual hospital settings and allow for ongoing monitoring, real-time diagnostics, and customised treatment regimens through smart infrastructure and connected equipment. IoT is changing the way healthcare services are offered and experienced. For example, wearable sensors that track vital signs, automated hospital work- flows, and platforms for managing patients from afar. This section looks at some of the most important ways that IoT is changing how healthcare is done, such as managing chronic diseases, caring for the elderly, automating hospitals, and emergency response systems. By looking at these examples, we may learn more about the real benefits, operational efficiency, and problems that come up when IoT solutions are used in different medical settings.

Mayani (2025) explores the many ways IoT can be used in healthcare, such as remote patient monitoring, wearables, telemedicine, and using AI to analyse data. We also talk about the problems and limitations of IoT in healthcare, especially when it comes to data security, privacy issues, and interoperability. The research ends by talking about the future of IoT in healthcare, such as how it will be used in personalised medicine, predictive healthcare, and AI-driven decision-making.

Gaikwad (2024) gives an overview of the existing IoT technology in healthcare, explain how IoT devices are making health services better, and talk about how IoT technology could change and disrupt global health care in the next ten years. IoT-based health care offers a lot of potential to make the health system work better and make people's health better.

Avaji and N (2024) investigates the ways in which IoT could change healthcare, with a focus on how it could be used for remote patient monitoring, telemedicine, and managing hospital operations. The specific issues in this area include making sure that patients get well, that operations run more smoothly, and that compliance happens on a regular basis. Existing system work shows that IoT-enabled solutions like remote patient monitor systems, telemedicine platforms, and smart hospital infrastructure can help solve these problems. Edge computing, artificial intelligence, and blockchain are some of the new trends that are shaping the future of the post-system world. These technologies open up new possibilities for improving healthcare delivery through new ideas and developments. Accepting ability of IoT to change things is the key to bet- ter health results, better patient experiences, and new ideas in the various ways healthcare is delivered.

Yogi et al. (2024) highlights about the ways IoT might help make healthcare services better, especially through telemedicine and remote patient monitoring. The suggested system also uses IoT devices to constantly and objectively send real-time data on the body, such as blood pressure, pulse rate, blood glucose levels, and physical activity. This research included persons with chronic conditions, people who were healthy, and older people who were also tested on the system. Some of the results show that it is possible to monitor the number of steps taken each day that correlate to the number of calories burned, the sleep score, which ranges from 60 to 80, and the oxygen saturation percentages, which range from 96% to 99% in different positions. The technology also shows the presence of a link between the percentage of change in the ambient temperature and the percentage of change in the pulse rate, which was quite sensitive to variations in temperature. From these data, it can be said that monitoring patients with IoT can make their conditions better as long as problems are found early and the right steps are implemented in time. The research also shows how telemedicine might make healthcare easier to get, especially for people who live in rural areas or in underdeveloped countries. The results point to a favourable direction for the system's future, but there are some major problems that need to be solved first, such as security, privacy of data, and integration.

IoT technology have made it possible for a wide range of uses in different healthcare settings. IoT is changing how care is given, managed, and experi- enced in many ways, from remote patient monitoring to emergency response systems. The table below displays some of the most important ways that IoT may be used in healthcare, along with examples of how it can be used and the benefits that come with it.

*Table 2. Applications of IoT in Healthcare*

| Application Area | IoT Use Case | Benefits |
|---|---|---|
| Remote Patient Monitoring | Wearable sensors, mobile health apps | Continuous health tracking, early detection |
| Hospital Automation | Smart beds, IoT-enabled workflows | Efficiency, reduced human error |
| Elderly Care | Ambient assisted living, fall detection devices | Improved safety, reduced hospital visits |
| Chronic Disease Management | Glucose/ECG monitors, inhaler sensors | Personalized care, better adherence |
| Emergency Response | Connected ambulances, GPS-enabled triage | Faster response, improved triage decisions |

Kelly et al. (2020) gives an overview of the existing IoT technology in healthcare, explain the ways in which IoT devices are making health care better, and talk about the various ways in which IoT technology could change and disrupt global health care in the next ten years. They discuss about how IoT could make public health services easier to get to and how it could change our existing secondary and tertiary health care system into a more proactive, continuous, and coordinated one. Lastly, this paper discusses the problems that IoT-based healthcare could cause, as well as the reasons why health care professionals and patients may not want to use it, such as lack of trust and acceptance, privacy and security concerns, interoperability, standardization and payment, data storage, and control and ownership. To make IoT work in health care today, regulations that promote it, guidelines that focus on cybersecurity, thorough strategic planning, and clear rules inside health care organizations are needed. Health care that uses IoT could make the health system work better and make people healthier.

## 4 BENEFITS OF HIoT

The use of the IoT in healthcare, which is often called Healthcare IoT (HIoT), has changed the way medical services are delivered, monitored, and managed. HIoT connects devices, sensors, systems, and people in the healthcare field to create a dynamic ecosystem that can gather data in real time, improve decision- making, and tailor care to each patient. This coming together of technologies has several benefits, such as finding diseases early and monitoring patients from afar, as well as making operations run more smoothly and lowering healthcare expenses. HIoT also helps move from reactive to proactive and preventative care, which lets healthcare providers deal with health problems before they get worse and become life-threatening. In this section, we look at the many benefits of HIoT, focussing on how it affects patients, doctors, hospitals, and the public health system as a whole.

The move from traditional healthcare systems to IoT-enabled settings has made big changes in how healthcare is given. The table below shows how tra- ditional healthcare practices and IoT-enhanced systems compare in terms of significant functional areas. It shows how care delivery, data management, and patient involvement have changed over time.

*Table 3. Comparison of Traditional vs. IoT-Enabled Healthcare*

| Aspect | Traditional Healthcare | IoT-Enabled Health- care |
|---|---|---|
| Monitoring | Periodic, in-person | Continuous, remote |
| Data Collection | Manual, low-frequency | Automated, high- frequency |
| Response Time | Reactive | Proactive and real-time |
| Cost Efficiency | Often higher long-term costs | Reduced costs through early action |
| Patient Engage- ment | Limited | High through mobile and wearable tech |

Aksenova & Gorbatov (2021) highlights the key benefits and potential uses of IoT technology in healthcare around the world and then discusses about how likely they are to be used in Russia. One of the main goals of the digital transformation of the healthcare industry in the Russian Federation is to develop IoT technology. This might have a big economic impact by making hospitals less busy. Lower costs, better treatment outcomes, and patient involvement in the treatment and preventative process are the key benefits of implementing IoT in healthcare. Using IoT in healthcare take illness diagnosis, treatment precision, and patient health tracking to a whole new level using micro- and nanodetectors and other "smart devices."

Abdulmalek et al. (2022) explains the importance of IoT-based healthcare systems and the help that these systems provide us. The report also describes IoT monitoring systems that use wireless and wearable sensors and gives a list of several types of healthcare-monitoring sensors.

Al-Shargabi and Abuarqoub (2020) explores the effects and problems that IoT designs and applications can have on healthcare. The paper discusses the main benefits and reasons for creating healthcare systems that use IoT. Next, we talk about security and privacy issues as actual problems and risks that make it hard for IoT to be used widely in healthcare. Finally, we talk about the main problems and chances, focussing on the special needs of healthcare applications.

## 4.1 Improved Patient Outcomes

The main goal of any new healthcare technology is to help patients get bet- ter, and HIoT does this very well. HIoT lets doctors make early diagnoses and respond to changes in the body in real time by constantly watching, sending alarms, and using predictive analytics. Wearable ECG monitors, glucometers, and smart inhalers are examples of devices that give doctors important informa- tion about a patient's condition so they may make changes to their treatment plans right away. This interchange of data in real time lowers the risk of prob- lems, speeds up recovery, and makes patients happier overall. Also, personalized treatment plans based on health data acquired by sensors give doctors the tools they need to customise treatments to meet each patient's needs, which leads to better health outcomes.

This report by Vatin et al. (2024) gives real-world examples of how IoT- Enhanced Healthcare has a big impact on patient care and health outcomes. Data from a wide range of patients shows how IoT technology may change things. For example, IoT devices can continuously monitor blood pressure, body temperature, heart rate, and blood glucose levels. According to statistical analyses, the use of IoT devices is closely linked to better heart health, as evidenced by consistently normal vital signs. The data also shows that patients who use IoT devices have greater control over their blood sugar levels because there are fewer incidences of high glucose levels. IoT-Enhanced Healthcare has many benefits, as shown by evaluations of the quality of patient care that reveal higher levels of satisfaction, therapy effectiveness, and communication. The results of the IoT Healthcare Test show that IoT devices are accurate and reliable for medical diagnosis. This shows how important IoT-Enhanced Healthcare is for changing how patients are cared for. These results, when taken together, show that IoT can greatly enhance patient health, treatment quality, and outcomes.

Shiny et al. (2023) highlights in their research that healthcare providers can gather more information about patients' physical and mental health by using sensors and other tools. This helps them better understand and anticipate their health. This can help find diseases earlier and make diagnoses and treatments more accurate. Healthcare providers such as doctors and nurses can utilise wearable devices, remote channels, and other remote devices to collect informa- tion about a patient's vital signs and activity levels. They one then can look for patterns and trends in that data. This can assist them find possible health problems and better manage the health of all of their patients. IoT can also help patients in remote or under served areas get care from a distance, which can make it easier for them to get the healthcare they need

## 4.2 Real-Time Monitoring and Remote Care

HIoT lets you keep an eye on patients all the time and in real time, even when they are not at a hospital. Wearable and implanted devices gather important information like heart rate, blood pressure, oxygen saturation, glucose levels, and sleep patterns. This data is then sent to healthcare providers or centralised dashboards. This makes it easier to provide care from a distance, which is especially helpful for people with long-term illnesses or those who live in rural or underserved areas. It also makes things easier for hospitals by cutting down on unneeded visits and readmissions. Real-time monitoring helps keep track of how diseases are getting worse and lets doctors make decisions before they need to, which leads to quicker treatment and greater care continuity.

This in-depth research by Kavitha et al. (2024) looks at the many ways the Internet of Things (IoT) can be used in smart healthcare infrastructure, remote patient monitoring, and managing chronic diseases. The assessment looks at how the role of IoT technology is changing in order to change healthcare models and improve patient outcomes. The remote patient monitoring section looks into how wearable gadgets and sensors can be used to track health metrics in real time, which encourages ongoing and proactive healthcare management. The research looks into how Internet of Things (IoT) solutions like smart drug dispensers and connected inhalers can be used to help people stick to their treatment plans and get the most out of their therapies when they have chronic diseases. Additionally, it also looks into ways to improve smart healthcare infrastructure by connecting hospital equipment and using IoT technologies to make healthcare processes more efficient. The main goal is to combine data analytics, machine learning, and artificial intelligence to get useful information from the data that IoT-enabled healthcare systems collect.

Shelke (2020) emphasizes that according to current estimates about 60% of healthcare organizations have used IoT in some way or another to improve pa- tient care and move from a disjointed and reactive paradigm to an interoperable and proactive service delivery model. The Internet of Medical Things (IoMT) will allow machines to talk to each other in the patient's body environment, which will make chronic disease care more effective. The research also about the ways in which technology has changed on the clinician side, detailing how IoT apps might benefit patients in different situations and the different ways in which they can be used in clinical settings.

IoT is changing healthcare by allowing for continuous, real-time monitoring of chronic conditions and improving overall patient care. This article by Algfari et al. (2020) looks at the uses, benefits, and future potential of IoT devices for real-time health monitoring for patients with chronic conditions. It covers a range of IoT-based health monitoring systems, such as wearable and implantable devices, biosensors, and remote patient monitoring systems. It also discusses the methods used by existing IoT applications, such as the UbiMon project and various ZigBee-based systems, to assess how they affect patient care. IoT technologies make it possible to monitor vital signs in real time, improve chronic disease management, and make emergency response systems better. Examples include smart inhalers, ECG monitors, and remote surgery systems. The use of IoT in healthcare has led to better patient outcomes, shorter wait times in emergencies, and better resource management in hospitals.

## 4.3 Operational Efficiency in Healthcare Facilities

HIoT helps hospitals and clinics run better in many ways, not just for individual patients. Smart devices keep an eye on how medical equipment is used and how well it works, as well as environmental factors like the temperature in pharmaceutical storage rooms. They also make sure that resources are used efficiently. For instance, RFID-based asset monitoring systems cut down on the time workers spend looking for important tools, and automated inventory management systems stop important supplies from running out or going to waste. IoT-enabled scheduling solutions make it easier to plan personnel and appointments, which cuts down on wait times and improves patient flow. These economies cut down on expenditures and make more resources available for improved patient care.

Avaji and N (2024) emphasizes the fact that IoT could change healthcare, focusing on how it could be used for remote patient monitoring, telemedicine, and managing hospital operations. The domain-specific difficulties, such as making sure that patients get well, operations run more smoothly, and compli- ance happens on a regular basis, are looked at. Existing system work shows that IoT-enabled solutions like remote patient monitoring systems, telemedicine plat- forms, and smart hospital infrastructure can help solve these problems. Emerg- ing trends like edge computing, artificial intelligence, and blockchain provide us a glimpse of what the post-system world may look like. These technologies open up new possibilities for improving and innovating healthcare delivery.

IoT and AI could bring a lot of good things to healthcare, even while there are problems like privacy issues and the need to spend money on infrastructure. This article by Ahmad (2024) gives an exhaustive strategy on the ways to use these technologies in hospitals, focusing on how they will improve patient care and efficiency. The results show that IoT and AI can greatly improve how hospitals work, making room for a better healthcare system.

## 4.4 Data-Driven Clinical Decision-Making

Adding HIoT to clinical workflows makes it easier to make medical decisions based on evidence. IoT devices collect a lot of real-time, patient-specific data that healthcare providers can use to look for patterns, find problems, and pre- dict future health occurrences. Advanced analytics platforms and AI models use this data to give useful information that helps with diagnosis, treatment plan- ning, and risk stratification. HIoT-powered decision support systems can warn doctors about possible drug interactions, suggest treatments, or flag important health occurrences. This makes diagnoses more accurate and treatments safer.

N. Kumar et al. (2022) discusses about using the Internet of Things (IoT) and the clinical decision support system (CDSS), which are two of the newest technologies, to fix difficulties in healthcare. They suggest an IoT-based solution with CDSS that doctors and carers can use to keep an eye on the patient's physiological characteristics, especially when the patient is far away (at a remote location). A five-parameter vital sign monitor sends real-time vital signs to the cloud so that one may see information about patients.

This research by Saroja et al. (2021) gives the impression of automated decision-making methods that have been recommended for looking at data from healthcare systems that use the Internet of Things. In this day and age, IoT data analytics is very important since it helps us understand the future better by showing us useful outcomes from linked devices. It discusses the different ways to make a decision-making system that gets data from IoT-based healthcare systems, processes and analyses it, and makes thorough reports that help doctors make better diagnoses. One may use the IoT data that one collects, such as pulse rate, temperature, oxygen level, and heart rate from linked devices, to figure out how bad the problem is and what has to be done about it right away with the right machine learning methods. The main goal of healthcare data is to help businesses make better decisions by using data analytics to choose the best IoT strategy. The outcomes of the next-generation expert systems can be used for more diagnosis and therapy analysis.

## 4.5 Enhanced Medication Management

Not taking medications as prescribed is a big problem for people with chronic diseases and makes treatment less effective. HIoT solves this problem with smart medication dispensers, sensors that can be swallowed, and connected pillboxes that remind patients to take their meds and let carers know if they miss a dosage. These tools keep an eye on compliance, watch how the drugs work, and change the dosages if necessary. These kinds of changes not only make people more likely to stick to their medications, but they also lower the chances of making mistakes with medications, having bad drug reactions, and going to the hospital because they did not take their medications as directed.

## 4.6 Emergency Response and Alerts

HIoT devices are very useful in emergencies when quick action is needed. Sensors can pick up on unexpected changes in the body, including falls, seizures, or heart attacks, and immediately send alarms to carers or emergency services. Devices with GPS help find patients in emergencies so that help can get to them quickly. IoT devices in hospitals can let medical staff know when equipment breaks down, the power goes out, or the environment becomes dangerous. These instant alerts let people take quick action that can save lives and keep data and equipment safe.

## 4.7 Cost Reduction and Resource Optimization

One of the best things about HIoT is that it could save healthcare expenditures while keeping or even improving the quality of care. Finding health problems early on eliminates the need for costly emergency care or hospital stays. Remote monitoring means doctors do not have to see patients as often, and they can take care of more patients at once. Automated data collection makes it easier to do your job by reducing the amount of work you have to do and the number of mistakes you make. Also, using IoT devices for predictive maintenance on medical equipment keeps it from going down and needing costly repairs. Overall, HIoT helps health systems use their resources better and makes sure they can keep going.

The current research by S. Kumar et al. (2025) looks at the various ways IoT might help the healthcare and transportation industries make better use of their resources. IoT-enabled healthcare systems need to be able to analyse and store a lot of data in a smart way. The integration has been made much easier with the addition of wireless sensor networks (WSNs) and the Internet of Things (IoT).

Using IoT technology in hospital infrastructure could help make better use of resources and improve the overall quality of care. The goal of the research by Mishra et al. (2023) is to look into how the Internet of Things (IoT) works in hospital infrastructure and how it affects the best use of resources.

There is no doubt that HIoT has the potential to change things, but there are some problems that will make it hard for it to become widely used. Putting IoT technologies into use and making them work together in healthcare settings is difficult because of a number of technological, ethical, infrastructural, and legal issues. To develop healthcare systems that are strong and open to everyone and can use the full power of HIoT, we need to understand these barriers. The next section goes into more detail about the main problems and obstacles that make it hard to use and deploy HIoT solutions to their full potential.

## 5 BARRIERS AND CHALLENGES

The IoT in healthcare systems, also known as HIoT, has many benefits, but there are also several big problems that make it hard for people to use it and make a difference. These problems affect many areas, including technology, organizations, rules, and society, and they often overlap in complicated ways. Concerns about data privacy, problems with interoperability, poor infrastructure, high costs of implementation, and opposition to technical change are all major problems. Also, the fact that healthcare data is sensitive and that people depend on services that are always available makes the hazards of HIoT systems much higher. To construct safe, scalable, and fair digital health ecosystems, we need to deal with these problems. This section discusses the many problems that healthcare providers, policymakers, and technologists must deal with in order to fully realize the potential of HIoT.

This article by Jamaluddin et al. (2024) detects and examines 14 possible problems that could make it hard for the Saudi Arabian healthcare supply chain to use the Internet of Things. The findings of the research indicate that the two main obstacles to IoT implementation in the Saudi healthcare supply chain are the non-existence of IT infrastructure and an inadequate legal and regulatory framework. Other serious issues are (1) the workforce's lack of sufficient educa- tion about the IoT; (2) the workforce's lack of sufficient resources to implement the IoT; and (3) the workforce's lack of sufficient motivation to change. The results of this research will shed light on the obstacles IoT implementation in the Saudi healthcare supply chain encounters and, thereby, serve the supply chain's top decision-makers. Even though IoT possesses the capacity to revolutionize healthcare systems for the better, several issues must be resolved before the technology can see widespread use. These include concerns about the cost of healthcare IoT, liability, and interoperability. To formulate effective strategies for increasing adoption of the technology, the healthcare IoT team must un- derstand these issues. The table below lists some of the biggest problems that might discourage HIoT from being used and some ways to fix them.

*Table 4. Key Barriers to HIoT Adoption and Potential Solutions*

| Barrier | Description | Possible Solutions |
|---|---|---|
| High Implementa- tion Costs | Expensive infrastructure, device costs, and mainte- nance | Government funding, modular deployment |
| Security & Privacy Concerns | Risk of data breaches and unauthorized access | End-to-end encryption, zero-trust architectures |
| Interoperability Is- sues | Devices from different vendors may not integrate | Use of standardized proto- cols (e.g., HL7, FHIR) |
| Ethical & Legal Concerns | Issues with consent, liabil- ity, data ownership | Clear policies, GDPR/HIPAA com- pliance, ethical design |
| Limited Digital Lit- eracy | Lack of training among healthcare providers and patients | Training programs, user- friendly interfaces |

Desingh and R (2021) attempts to identify and analyze the potential problems that could impede the adoption of IoT in the healthcare business. After reviewing the literature and consulting with experts from both business and academia, 14 obstacles to IoT adoption were identified. These experts used in- terpretive structural modeling to understand how the identified barriers relate to one another contextually. They then used fuzzy MICMAC analysis to deter- mine the strength of the barriers and their interdependence. The results indicate that legal and regulatory norms and insufficient IT infrastructure are two of the foremost obstacles to the IoT's being adopted in the healthcare supply chain.

Ramanathan et al. (2021) discusses about the strides healthcare sector is making toward digitization and the fact that IoT is being part of this transition. It identifies what stands in the way of using the IoT within an otherwise- receptive healthcare system and sorts these obstacles into distinguishable groups. The research helps pinpoint the most important challenges and enablers to effect the sort of smooth transitioning that the above description suggests is possible when moving to e-healthcare.

## 5.1 Data Privacy and Security Concerns

The most significant challenge in the use of Healthcare IoT (HIoT) devices is ensuring that delicate patient data remains confidential and secure. HIoT de- vices are in a constant state of capturing, sending, and storing copious amounts of per- sonal health information, making them prime targets for cyberattacks. The dangers of such attacks go well beyond the health violations of individ- ual breaches. They potentially expose healthcare organizations to a plethora of costly, messy situations that could seriously undermine their ongoing trust relationships with patients. And while most people in the U.S. healthcare sys- tem have probably never heard of the HITRUST Alliance, they should have. Because HITRUST, which is a bridge between the HIPAA privacy and security rules and the 21st Century Cures Act, has done a lot to ensure that encrypted personal health information (PHI) remains safe and sound.

Pathuri (2025) examines the security and privacy holes in IoT medical de- vices that are available for sale. It does this by looking at the ways in which data is sent from four popular devices: (a) the 1byOne Digital Smart Wireless Scale, (b) the iHealth Ease Wireless Blood Pressure Monitor, (c) the Withings Smart Scale, and (d) the Withings Smart Blood Pressure Monitor. Setting up a custom Wi-Fi access point to record network traffic shows that many devices provide sensitive health data in cleartext, even when they use encryption pro- tocols like SSL/TLS. Also, exposing metadata lets enemies guess sensitive user behaviours and medical conditions. They suggest a monitoring interface that is easy to use, shows how data flows, and warns users about any privacy prob- lems. The findings shows that medical IoT devices need to have stricter security standards and more openness in their development.

A systems approach is taken by Charyyev et al. (2021) toward modeling and re-searching the use of the IoT in health. This presents a clearer picture of the dynamics shaping it, the key players, subsystems, and the ways in which they work together. Subsume under this health IoT is much smart device technology. The smart devices living within the healthcare system impact the way the IoT works in health. It is thus worth researching them in the subsystems of the health IoT.

## 5.2 Interoperability and Standardization Issues

A major issue with utilizing HIoT devices and systems is their interoperability, or rather their lack of it. Healthcare environments are frequently populated with a plethora of HIoT devices and systems, most of which are not in any meaningful way integrated with each other. They often belong to multiple different and incompatible platforms, communicate in a variety of non-standard ways, and use all sorts of different (and often proprietary) data formats. This absence of cohesion, or of any standardization, not only prevents devices and systems from working together in a timely way—if at all—but also creates the sorts of information silos that are the bane of any connected system. For the HIoT to function as intended, its constituent parts have to behave in accordance with some basic, common engineering principles. This is to say that they have to at least share the sorts of standards that allow for real-time transmission of the kinds of information essential to maintaining a person's health. HL7 FHIR (Fast Healthcare Interoperability Resources) and IEEE standards are good strides forward, but not all regions and organizations use them equally. HIoT's ability to provide coordinated, patient-centered care is greatly constrained without a unified framework. This is because clinicians may not have access to all the information they need to make informed decisions

The research by Madanian et al. (2024) finda that there are three key levels of security holes in IoT in healthcare: (a) perception, (b) network, and (c) ap- plication. They looked at all the privacy and security concerns to IoT on each tier. Different technical improvements were proposed to fix the problems found in healthcare. There is a need to apply a full, multi-layered security approach, security-by-design principles, and training for both staff and end users. Reg- ulators and policymakers must also set and enforce rules and standards that protect the privacy and security of healthcare IoT. This research shows the im- portance to keep healthcare IoT safe and private, and the importance of all stakeholders to work together to deal with the many and changing security and privacy concerns in this area.

Nanayakkara et al. (2019) discusses about the different types of sensors used in IoT healthcare and the possible security and privacy problems that can come up at different levels of IoT. The primary purpose of this research is to highlight the potential risks associated with the IoT healthcare applications for the ap- plication's designers, developers, and users, which include not only the patients but also the healthcare professionals that attend to them. The results indicate that the layer most susceptible to an attack that threatens the privacy and security of the user is the network layer. The applications layer is the second most vulnerable layer, and the majority of IoT-based healthcare applications that were studied utilize wearable sensors. China and the United States are the countries that pay the most attention to the security and privacy of IoMT-based healthcare applications.

## 5.3 High Implementation and Maintenance Costs

The expense is a principal factor hampering the widespread adoption of HIoT technologies, particularly in low-resource settings. The initial outlay for an as- sortment of smart devices, infrastructure upgrades, and the education necessary for a workforce to operate these devices can be prohibitive, especially for small and medium-sized businesses. And as we noted in our first chapter, the operat- ing costs can be substantial too. Continuous maintenance, software upgrades,and cybersecurity measures (these last two are particularly urgent and vital given the current state of the digital world) are essential for keeping the HIoT up and running. And the system's ability to scale (which is really just part of the overall operating cost) is also vital for the kind of efficiencies that make the HIoT worth adopting in the first place.

Experts claim that the expansion of the Internet of Things (IoT) will confer considerable economic benefits, lead to markedly improved business efficiency. and offer a range of enhancements that will substantially upgrade the personal and professional lives of its users. Despite its purported imminent arrival, in- sufficient research has been conducted into this new mode of human-technology interaction, with even less effort put into examining the specifics of eHealth. The research carried out by Arfi et al. (2020) is an attempt to remedy this situation by exploring the contours of customer interaction with IoT in eHealthcare and, crucially, by situating this interaction within a framework that also allows for an exploration of the financial costs tied to such interaction. Using the extended UTAUT as a research framework, the research checked its model against data from a random sample of 268 individuals in France who are potential users of IoT-based healthcare equipment. Age is a big factor in whether or not people want to use IoT in eHealthcare, which led to the creation of two new groups: IoT natives and IoT immigrants. The results can be useful for IoT developers, politicians, and maybe even marketers.

## 5.4 Infrastructure and Connectivity Limitations

A healthy HIoT ecosystem relies on a robust digital infrastructure. Yet many of the nation's healthcare institutions, particularly those in rural and underserved areas, lack such an infrastructure. They may have unreliable internet access; insufficient bandwidth; or outdated, unstable IT systems. IoT devices demand stable, always-on network connections through which they can send data inces- santly and, if need be, in real time. When those devices can't connect, the data can't get sent; thus, the system loses all coughing-out-on-two-parts-its-chassis potential that makes the HIoT so cool and can put patient safety at risk. Also, power disruptions and not enough space to store data can make IoT-based healthcare systems less effective. Building strong infrastructure needs a lot of money for broadband networks, cloud services, and edge computing systems. Governments and healthcare providers need to work together to establish the digital infrastructure needed to support scalable and reliable HIoT networks. This is especially important if they want to close the gap between urban and rural healthcare.

## 5.5 Ethical and Legal Concerns

HIoT brings up numerous moral and legal problems that need to be solved to protect patients' rights and make sure everyone is held responsible. Informed permission is one of the most important ethical issues. Patients need to know exactly what data is being gathered, how it will be used, and who will be able to see it. But because HIoT systems have so many different data flows, it is hard to make this information clear. There are also worries about algorithmic bias, especially when AI and IoT are used together for diagnosis and decision-making. The algorithm might give biassed results if the training data isn't representative, which could lead to differences in care. Questions of who owns the data, who is responsible if a gadget breaks, and who has control over data that moves across borders are all legal issues. International healthcare companies and technology vendors find it increasingly difficult to comply with regulatory requirements as they navigate a convoluted global landscape. The problem is most apparent in Europe, where the new GDPR rules have added to an already complex patch- work of privacy regulations that vary from country to country. And as the so-called "privacy paradox" demonstrates, much of the new compliance work is wasted. At bottom, these moral and legal headaches have a single, human cause: the collapse of common regulatory mores. Applying IoT technologies in the healthcare sector raises many ethical and legal concerns.

These concern the fundamental human elements of our society when we talk about health and well-being. They are consent, privacy, and data owner- ship—who owns the data, and who has the right to access, use, and share it? There are also important matters of rule following, of complying with laws and regulations that govern the (many) fundamental human concerns we just listed. Deploying the Health Internet of Things (HIoT) comes with many important ethical and legal concerns. We have to navigate them if we want to move for- ward in a way that is responsible, and that is compliant with our (many) laws and (too few) regulations. Following is a table of some important issues, with our way of "dealing with them" constituting a way of "working through" these many (concerns) for you, the reader.

*Table 5. Ethical and Legal Considerations in HIoT Deployment*

| Concern | Explanation | Mitigation Strategy |
|---|---|---|
| Informed Consent | Patients may not fully un- derstand data usage | Transparent data poli- cies, user-friendly con- sent |
| Data Ownership | Ambiguity over who con- trols health data | Legal clarity and patient data access rights |
| Liability | Unclear accountability for device/system failures | Shared responsibility agreements |
| Privacy Invasion | Continuous monitoring can feel intrusive | Privacy-by-design, opt- out options |
| Regulatory Compli- ance | Varying international standards | Alignment with GDPR, HIPAA, local laws |

Kushwaha et al. (2025) discusses about certain ethical issues with IoT (IoT), such as worries about data privacy and autonomy, data quality, intellectual property, algorithmic bias, unprotected consumer gadgets, hackable cars, and the accountability of IoT systems. Some further worries are the possible loss of trust, privacy intrusions, misuse of data, inconsistent copyright, the digital divide, identity theft, problems with control and access to information, and free- dom of speech and expression. Addressing these ethical challenges requires more than good intentions. They emphasizes that there is an urgent need for things like algorithmic social contracts and programs that ensure moral behavior; addi- tionally there is also a need of guidelines and codes of ethics for developers of the Internet of Things. Solving these problems is not just a matter of programming; it's a matter of using ethics to direct the algorithms.

The IoTs connect several items and devices that exchange data to pursue a common goal. This technology is improving all the time, and with its advance- ment come a host of problems and limitations—costs, legalities, and ethics, plus connectivity, compatibility, and standards—that vie for our attention. Most consider the ethical stuff the most significant and hardest to handle in the IoT. Zakerabasali and Ayyoubzadeh (2022) does a fine job pointing out the major ethical concerns in the IoT and even sorts them into a handy grouping scheme based on the different stages the IoT is in regarding healthcare.

## 5.6 Resistance to Change and Technological Adoption

HIoT systems, require humans in addition to technology to function. This encompasses not just patients but also a wide range of healthcare professionals and paraprofessionals—doctors, nurses, and even the often-invisible but cru- cial health IT workers—who together make up an almost industrial workgroup. That workgroup is tasked with ensuring that the HIoT systems can serve their primary life-and-death function: providing healthcare to humans. Yet for all the human effort behind the HIoT, skepticism abounds among its supposed end users, those patients yanked from the everyday world into one that increasingly resembles a high-tech laboratory. To get beyond this opposition, there has to be targeted training programs, easy-to-use design, ongoing support, and clear information about how HIoT may help both clinicians and patients.

## 5.7 Skill Gaps and Workforce Challenges

As HIoT systems get more complicated, they need workers with skills in several areas, including healthcare, information technology, cybersecurity, and data an- alytics. However, there are not enough professionals with the right abilities to design, build, and keep up HIoT systems. Healthcare organizations generally do not have IT teams on staff who are experts in IoT networking, system inte- gration, or compliance audits. Also, doctors and nurses may not have enough training to understand data from IoT devices or fix simple technical problems. This lack of skills not only slows down adoption, but it also makes system breakdowns and bad use more likely. To close this gap, healthcare workers and technical staff need to work together to increase their skills through academic programs, certification courses, and ongoing professional development programs that are designed for both groups.

The research by Wang et al. (2024) shows that the Internet of Things (IoT) greatly improves the quality and efficiency of care, especially when it comes to real-time health monitoring, illness management, and supervising patients from a distance. However, there are also problems with data quality, consumer ap- proval, and making money. IoT development is anticipated to focus on making things smarter, more accurate, and more personalised in the future. However, for IoT to be used in healthcare around the world, countries need to work together and support policies. This review gives healthcare policymakers, aca- demics, and practitioners useful information and ideas for future research and technology progress.

Alkan (2023) looks at how managing the healthcare internet, also often known as the "internet of things" (IoT), affects healthcare services and the peo- ple who work in them. The way healthcare services are delivered has changed a lot because more and more IoT devices are being used in healthcare. This arti- cle discusses the goals, methods, and new results that are shown in this context. The goal is to find out how much IoT has changed healthcare services and how it has affected the workforce. The article also stresses the importance of spend- ing money on training and developing their workers for healthcare companies so that they have the skills which they need to do their jobs well in the changing healthcare environment. In general, this article gives us a fresh way of looking at how IoT affects healthcare services and the workforce. It can be used as a starting point for more research in this field.

There are a lot of problems that make it hard to use Healthcare 4.0 technol- ogy, and these problems have been talked about more and more in the literature. One of the problems is that there aren't enough trained experts who have the skills needed. These skills might be technical, methodological, social, or per- sonal, and they help healthcare workers deal with and adapt to advances in technology. The goal of this research by Jose et al. (2022) is to look at the research that has already been done on the skills needed to use Healthcare 4.0 technologies. The results reveal that the skills needed to use Healthcare 4.0 are often talked about in non-clinical uses of Industry 4.0 (I 4.0) applications. Healthcare organizations are going through a technology transition and use a lot of different technologies. It looks like companies are putting more value on technologies that can be used for "sensing" and "communication."

## 6 CONCLUSION

The Internet of Things (IoT) has changed the way medical services are delivered, monitored, and managed in a big way. HIoT technologies make healthcare much better by allowing for constant monitoring, real-time diagnostics, and remote patient care. They also make clinical operations run more smoothly. IoT can be used in a wide range of healthcare settings, from managing chronic diseases and caring for the elderly to automating hospitals and responding to emergencies. Also, smart wearables, sensor networks, and cloud-based platforms have given patients more influence over their health and made it easier for doctors to make decisions based on data.

But there are problems with the broad use of HIoT. High costs of imple- mentation and maintenance, problems with interoperability, security holes, and ethical and legal challenges make it hard to embrace, especially in places with limited resources. For HIoT systems to be used in a way that lasts, it is im- portant to protect data privacy, follow the rules, and build trust among stake- holders. Also, both patients and healthcare practitioners need to be trained in digital literacy, and the system should be designed in a way that makes it easy to use.

Edge computing, blockchain, artificial intelligence, and federated learning are all technologies that could help solve these problems by making systems smarter, speeding up processes, and protecting data privacy. The success of HIoT will depend on the creation of frameworks that are scalable, secure, and based on ethics that allow for innovation without putting patient safety or fair- ness at risk.

In conclusion, HIoT is a big step towards making healthcare systems smarter, more connected, and focused on the needs of patients, both now and in the future.

## REFERENCES


Abdulmalek, S., Nasir, A., Jabbar, W. A., Almuhaya, M. A. M., Bairagi, A. K., Khan, M. A.-M., & Kee, S.-H. (2022). Iot-based healthcare-monitoring system towards improving quality of life: A review. *Health Care, 10*, •••. https://api.semanticscholar.org/CorpusID:252892699 PMID: 36292441

Ahmad, A. (2024). Enhancing hospital efficiency through iot and ai: A smart healthcare system. *Journal of Computer Science Application and En- gineering (JOSAPEN)*. https: // api . semanticscholar . org / CorpusID: 272607805

Aksenova, E. I., & Gorbatov, S. Y. (2021). Application of iot technologies in healthcare. *City Healthcare*. https://api.semanticscholar.org/CorpusID: 251473335

Al-Shargabi, B., & Abuarqoub, S. (2020). Iot-enabled healthcare: Benefits, is- sues and challenges. *Proceedings of the 4th International Conference on Future Networks and Distributed Systems*. https://api.semanticscholar. org/CorpusID:234487349

Algfari, S. M., Alghamdi, A. S., Ali, E. I. A., Almuhaylib, A. M., Alzaher, M. A., Alshammry, M. M., Alharbi, A. T., Alharbi, S. H., & Alanazi, H. Al- waked, M. H., Alrashidi, A. A. M., Alrasheed, B. B., Alsarimi, F. A. H., Alotaibi, M. S. M., Alanazi, A. A., & Alumtairi, A. Z. (2020). Real-time health monitoring using iot devices for patients with chronic conditions. *International journal of health sciences*. https://api.semanticscholar. org/CorpusID:272628347

Alkan, G. O. (2023). The governance of healthcare internet: Understanding the impact on the workforce. *The European Proceedings of Social and Behavioural Sciences*. https: / / api . semanticscholar . org / CorpusID: 265230296

Arfi, W. B., Nasr, I. B., Khvatova, T., & Zaied, Y. B. (2020). Understanding ac- ceptance of ehealthcare by iot natives and iot immigrants: An inte- grated model of utaut, perceived risk, and financial cost. *Technological Forecasting and Social Change, 120437*, •••. https://api. semanticscholar. org/CorpusID:228829702

Avaji, G. M., & N, D. G. (2024). Iot innovations in healthcare: Enhancing pa- tient care and operational efficiency. *International Journal of Research Publication and Reviews*. https://api.semanticscholar.org/CorpusID: 270529020

Charyyev, B., Mansouri, M., & Gunes, M. H. (2021). Modeling the adoption of internet of things in healthcare: A systems approach. *2021 IEEE International Symposium on Systems Engineering (ISSE)*, 1–8. https //api.semanticscholar.org/ CorpusID:240156807

Desingh, V., & R, B. (2021). Internet of things adoption barriers in the in- dian healthcare supply chain: An ism-fuzzy micmac approach. *The In- ternational journal of health planning and management*. https://api. semanticscholar.org/CorpusID: 238218586

Gaikwad, P. S. V. (2024). Iot in healthcare domain. *International Journal for Research in Applied Science and Engineering Technology*. https://api. semanticscholar .org/CorpusID:267764216

Jamaluddin, A. A., Alkathiri, I. A., Alghmadi, W. A., Khadawardi, H. A., & Alqahtani, A. Y. (2024). Overcoming iot implementation challenges in the saudi healthcare supply chain: An integrated ism-micmac analysis. *Proceedings of the International Conference on Industrial Engineer- ing and Operations Management*. https: // api . semanticscholar . org / CorpusID:270321417

Jose, A., Tortorella, G. L., Vassolo, R. S., Kumar, M. I., & Cawley, A. F. M. (2022). Professional competence and its effect on the implementation of healthcare 4.0 technologies: Scoping review and future research di- rections. *International Journal of Environmental Research and Public Health, 20*(1), 478. https://api.semanticscholar .org/CorpusID:255252668. DOI: 10.3390/ijerph20010478 PMID: 36612799

Kavitha, V. P., Theivanathan, G., Magesh, V., & G, J. (2024). A comprehen- sive survey of iot applications in remote patient monitoring, chronic disease management, and smart healthcare infrastructure. *2024 3rd In- ternational Conference on Sentiment Analysis and Deep Learning (IC- SADL)*, 689–696. https://api.semanticscholar .org/CorpusID:271463694

Kelly, J. T., Campbell, K. L., Gong, E., & Scuffham, P. A. (2020). The internet of things: Impact and implications for health care delivery. *Journal of Medical Internet Research, 22*. https: // api . semanticscholar . org / CorpusID:226298256

Kumar, N., Kaushal, R. K., Panda, S. N., & Bhardwaj, S. (2022). Impact of the internet of things and clinical decision support system in healthcare. *IoT and WSN based Smart Cities*. https://api. semanticscholar. org/ CorpusID:249283542

Kumar, S., Pragya, e Fatima, S., & Nigam, R. (2025). Iot assisted optimization of resources for healthcare, mining and transportation industry. *Asian Journal of Research in Computer Science*. https://api.semanticscholar. org/CorpusID:277766059

Kushwaha, N., Kushwaha, S. K. S., & Khare, S. (2025). An overview of artificial intelligence in healthcare system. *Current Artificial Intelligence*. https: //api .semanticscholar.org/CorpusID:276926641

Madanian, S., Chinbat, T., Subasinghage, M., Airehrour, D., Hassandoust, F., & Yongchareon, S. (2024). Health iot threats: Survey of risks and vul- nerabilities. *Future Internet, 16*, 389. https://api.semanticscholar.org/ CorpusID:273582195

Mayani, M. B. (2025). The role of internet of things (iot) in healthcare: A rev- olutionary transformation. *International Scientific Journal of Engineering and Management, 277863219*(4), 1–8. https://api.semanticscholar.org/CorpusID. DOI: 10.55041/ISJEM00077

Mishra, T. K., Chinmay, A., & Pattanaik, A. (2023). Iot-enhanced healthcare in- frastructure: Towards efficient resource management. *2023 2nd Inter- national Conference on Ambient Intelligence in Health Care (ICAIHC)*, 01–06. https://api .semanticscholar.org/CorpusID:267701212

Nanayakkara, N. K. V., Halgamuge, M. N., & Syed, A. (2019). Security and pri- vacy of internet of medical things (iomt) based healthcare applications: A review. https://api.semanticscholar.org/CorpusID:213987655

Pathuri, K. (2025). Security and privacy vulnerabilities in iot-enabled medi- cal devices: Analyzing cleartext data leakage and metadata exposure. *World Journal of Advanced Engineering Technology and Sciences*. https: //api.semanticscholar .org/CorpusID:279386619

Ramanathan, K. M., N., & P., A. S. (2021). Mitigating risks and barriers for promo- tion and implementation of technologies in e-healthcare. https: //api.semanticscholar .org/CorpusID:236696827

Saroja, S., Haseena, S., & Blessa, B. P. M. (2021). Data-driven decision making in iot healthcare systems—covid-19: A case study. *Smart Healthcare System Design*. https://api.semanticscholar.org/CorpusID:242668972

Shelke, Y. (2020). Iomt and healthcare delivery in chronic diseases. https://api. semanticscholar.org/CorpusID:225941374

Shiny, M. L., Ramrao, N., & Murugan, K. (2023). A review on ongoing medical care observing framework for cardiovascular patients utilizing iot. *2023 7th Inter- national Conference on Computing Methodologies and Com- munication (ICCMC)*, 1310–1318. https: // api. semanticscholar. org / CorpusID:257959059

Vatin, N. I., Pant, R., Mohan, C., Kumar, A., & Rajasekhar, N. (2024). Iot- enhanced healthcare: A patient care evaluation using the iot health- care test. *BIO Web of Conferences*. https://api.semanticscholar.org/ CorpusID:267186827

Wang, B., Shi, X., Han, X., & Xiao, G. (2024). The digital transformation of nursing practice: An analysis of advanced iot technologies and smart nursing systems. *Frontiers in Medicine*, *11*, 1471527. https://api.semanticscholar. org/CorpusID:274404316. DOI: 10.3389/fmed.2024.1471527 PMID: 39678028

Yogi, K. S. V, D. G., B, M. K. S., R.Nithya, Begum, A., & Suganthi.N. (2024). Enhancing healthcare delivery through iot applications in remote pa- tient monitoring and telemedicine. *2024 IEEE North Karnataka Sub- section Flagship International Conference (NKCon)*, 1–8. https://api. semanticscholar.org/CorpusID:274641142

Zakerabasali, S., & Ayyoubzadeh, S. M. (2022). Internet of things and healthcare system: A systematic review of ethical issues. *Health Science Reports*, *5*(6), e863. https://api.semanticscholar.org/CorpusID:252709937. DOI: 10.1002/hsr2.863 PMID: 36210869

Chapter 2

# Machine Learning-Based Intrusion Detection Systems for HIoT

**K. Jyothsna**
*SRM Institute of Science and Technology, India*

**Malige Gangappa**
*VNR Vignana Jyothi Institute of Engineering and Technology, India*

**Love Kumar**
*Mangalayatan University, India*

**Dler Salih Hasan**
https://orcid.org/0009-0008-3212-5509
*University of Salahaddin, Erbil, Iraq*

**Amarnath Reddy**
https://orcid.org/0009-0002-9540-0586
*Vignana Jyothi Institute of Management, India*

**Bharti**
*MMIM, Maharishi Markandeshwar, India*

**V. Bhoopathy**
https://orcid.org/0000-0003-2175-6328
*Sree Rama Engineering College, India*

## ABSTRACT

*IoT technologies connect physical objects to the internet and collect data without human intervention. The IoT is employed worldwide, but mainly in logistics, manufacturing, and healthcare. IDS use AI algorithms to quickly identify and stop a variety of threats, protecting critical data. IoT network traditions are a prominent issue in academia. ML and DL are used by many to construct intrusion detection systems. Despite its pervasiveness, the IoT remains a mystery. This implies a huge Internet change. From linking tablets, computers, and phones to transmitting every part of the actual world, the goal is to blur the lines between the real and virtual. Massive object-connected systems have security flaws. Many network attacks, especially routing protocol attacks, target them. The security of these systems cannot be*

DOI: 10.4018/979-8-3373-7610-3.ch002

*assured by authentication and encryption. The proliferation of linked gadgets has made security a major issue. Web connectivity and trusted data sharing define the IoT. Therefore, most cyberattacks, including DDoS attacks, can target IoT systems.*

## 1. INTRODUCTION

An entirely new way of thinking about computers has started with the advent of the IoT, and it is already changing the way we live. Internet of Things devices have a wide variety of applications. Some areas that utilise Blockchain technology include transportation, healthcare, industrial production, smart homes, supply-chain management, security, and monitoring (Hasan et al., 2022). Based on their projections, Zhao and Lian estimate that there will be 30.9 billion IoT devices in use by the year 2025(Menon et al., 2025). According to this research, there were 13.8 billion Internet of Things devices in use in 2021. It shows that the growth rate of this industry is over 55%. Cybercriminals, entrepreneurs, researchers, inventors, and entrepreneurs have all taken notice of this fast expansion, reliance on IoT devices, and business possibilities (Hizal et al., 2024). There is a great deal of interest in the market for IoT devices due to the many benefits they offer. Investors are taking notice of this demand(Soldatos et al., 2016). Entrepreneurs and innovators are adding to the field's allure by developing and selling new uses for Internet of Things (IoT) devices that improve and simplify our daily lives .

Nevertheless, it has opened the door for cybercriminals to take advantage of the security holes in IoT devices(Rondon et al., 2022). Cybercriminals have found the IoT to be a lucrative target because to its potential for rapid company expansion. The exponential rise in cyberattacks against IoT devices can be attributed(Williams et al., 2017). Manufacturing Internet of Things devices with little to no focus on cyber security. According to research by R. Williams et al., there are a lot of IoT devices out there, and a lot of them are fully functional in various services, leaving them open to cyber assaults (Wyss, 2024). IoT devices are not immune to attacks (Baich et al., 2022). In most cases, other appliances and systems can be linked to IoT devices. This means that attackers can use them as entry points to get access to anything linked to them. An internet outage was experienced by Amazon, Twitter, and Netflix in 2016 as a consequence of the disastrous impact of an attack on Dyn through imaging IoT devices. Medical IoT is increasing at a faster rate than any other sector of the IoT. Because of its close relationship to medical treatment, MIoT are delicate. Cyberattack trends in the past few years, however, reveal an alarming increase in the rate of infiltration on MIoT devices(Husnain et al., 2022). The many security holes in the Internet of Things poses a serious threat. Multiple attack vectors exist for IoT devices (Zheng et al., 2022). Any cyberattack involving network connectivity is considered a cyberattack; however, cyber-physical attacks are not covered in this research. There are computational constraints on the systems that Internet of Things devices employ.

Why it's not possible to apply existing cyber-security techniques to secure vulnerable IoT settings. Due to the vast range of possible vulnerabilities in the IoT context, standard rule-based security approaches are also inadequate. (Al-Garadi et al., 2020). Setups for the Internet of Things constantly produce massive amounts of data. It is not a simple task to find outliers in different data streams. Furthermore, DL-based approaches are effective in these contexts. Data sorting according to given attributes, pattern and association identification, and huge data analysis are areas where deep neural networks truly shine.

# 2. CHARACTERISTICS OF HIOT AND SECURITY CHALLENGES

## 2.1 Computer Science

In order for HIOT technologies to be developed and put into use, computer scientists are necessary. A number of critical issues and opportunities in this area require their knowledge and experience.

### 2.1.1 Obstacles

Assuring the interoperability of various HIoT devices and systems is a major challenge. In order for various devices to communicate with one another without any hitches, standardised protocols and interfaces are necessary(Malhotra et al., 2021). Furthermore, sophisticated data processing methods are required to handle the massive volumes of data produced by HIOT devices. Another major obstacle is cybersecurity, since protecting patients' personal health information is of the utmost importance(Ali et al., 2025).

### 2.1.2 Opportunities

Possibilities to improve the performance of HIOT systems are presented by developments in big data analytics and machine learning(N. Mishra & Pandya, 2021) The implementation of HIOT technology in healthcare is a multi-faceted process that gains substantial advantages from the combined knowledge and expertise of many fields. If we want to fully grasp the possibilities and threats posed by HIOT, we need to draw on knowledge from computer science, healthcare, healthcare administration, and lawmakers. The perspectives of different disciplines on the use of HIOT in healthcare are shown in Figure 4.

*Figure 1. Interdisciplinary Viewpoints on HIOT Adoption in Healthcare*

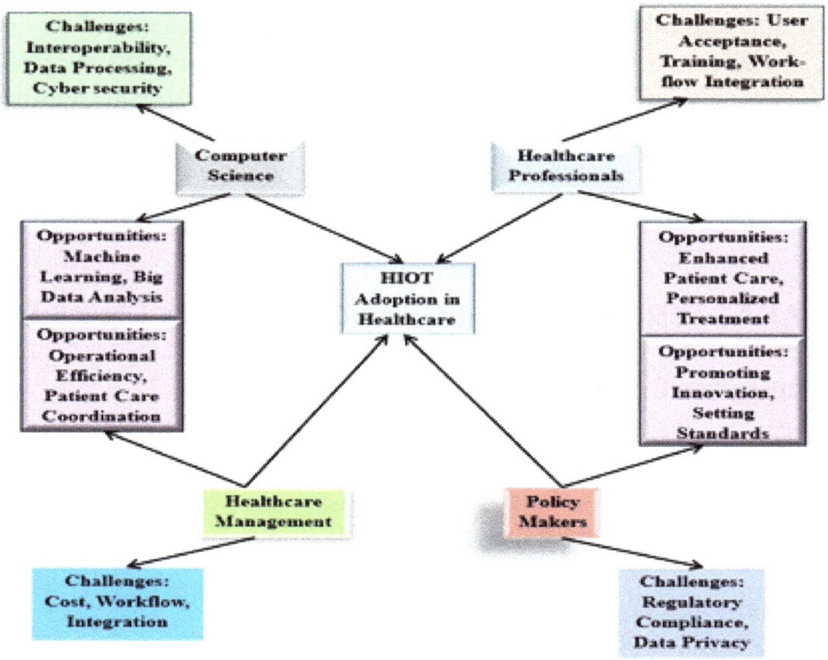


By analysing massive databases, these technologies can improve operational efficiency and patient care. Patients will have more faith in HIOT systems if strong cybersecurity safeguards are developed to safeguard their data(Qadri, Ali, et al., 2020).

## 2.2 Medical Practitioners

Adopting HIOT technologies successfully relies heavily on healthcare personnel, such as physicians, nurses, and medical researchers. If we want to solve real problems and make the most of real possibilities, we need their advice and expertise(Alamri et al., 2024).

### 2.2.1 Challenge

A major obstacle to the widespread use of HIOT technology is their level of user acceptance. Medical practitioners should be open to using these tools in their daily work. For healthcare providers to be comfortable and effective users of HIOT devices, training and education are essential. It is not always easy to incorporate HIOT data into healthcare workflows either.

### 2.2.2 Opportunities

There is a plethora of potential for HIOT technologies to improve healthcare for patients. Patients benefit from earlier intervention and better health outcomes when health problems are detected through continuous monitoring. The data gathered by HIOT devices can be used to create personalised treatment regimens, guaranteeing that patients receive care that is specifically designed for their needs.

## 2.3 Healthcare Administration

When it comes to installing HIOT systems in healthcare facilities, administrators play a crucial role. When it comes to handling the operational and financial components of HIOT adoption, their knowledge is invaluable.

### 2.3.1 Challenges

One major obstacle to adoption of HIOT devices and infrastructure, especially for smaller healthcare facilities, is their cost(Bovenzi et al., 2020). If we want the advantages of HIOT to surpass the original expenditure, we need cost management solutions that work. Also, existing procedures may be complicated, therefore it's important to plan and execute well when integrating HIOT technologies.

### 2.3.2 Opportunities

The use of HIOT technologies may lead to more streamlined processes in healthcare facilities. Administrative processes can be made more efficient, with fewer mistakes and better use of resources, through the use of automated data gathering and processing. Through enhanced data exchange and communication made possible by HIOT systems, patient care can also be better coordinated.

## 2.4 Policy makers

Developing the rules and regulations that control the implementation of HIOT technology is the job of policymakers. They play an essential role in encouraging innovation while also resolving legal and ethical concerns.

### 2.4.1 Challenges

An enormous hurdle for HIOT adoption is navigating the intricate terrain of healthcare compliance standards and laws. To avoid legal consequences and guarantee patient safety, it is vital that HIOT devices and systems meet regulatory criteria. Additional important issues that need strong regulatory actions to resolve include data privacy and security.

### 2.4.2 Opportunities

By passing laws and regulations that encourage innovation in the HIOT, policymakers may help propel the industry forward. The broad adoption of HIOT technologies can be facilitated by their promotion of standards that guarantee interoperability and security. Innovations in HIOT's technical, clinical, and regulatory domains can be propelled by joint efforts by academics, business leaders, and government officials.

## 3.MACHINE LEARNING FOR INTRUSION DETECTION

Our lives have been impacted by a wide array of problems brought about by the proliferation of the IoT, as highlighted in the preceding section's discussion of vulnerabilities, attacks(Oyelade et al., 2019). In addition, developments in computing power and large data have fostered an atmosphere where enemies can carry out unforeseen operations. The integration of ML and DL techniques with IDS is the result of ML professionals perceiving learning approaches as a practical means of tackling IoT security issues(Malhotra et al., 2021). A categorisation of current learning approaches is shown in Figure 2. Here, we'll go over the different learning approaches, the kinds of approaches, and the numerous solutions for IoT security that stem from these approaches. We can categorise existing methods according to the manner and approach that they employ(Elbir et al., 2022).

- **Based on the Mode:** Both an online and an offline mode are available. Online, data is handled piece by piece serially (kappa learning), in contrast to offline, where input is processed in batches (lambda learning).
- **Based on the approach:** The three approaches are supervised, unsupervised, and reinforced learning.

## 3.1 Supervised Learning

Functionality is learnt from the training dataset by this process(Ullah et al., 2019). Estimating the mapping function to the point where it accurately predicts the output labels given new data is the main goal. According on the core of the intended labels, it can be classified as either regression or classification. There is a vast array of events, malfunctions, (P. Mishra et al., 2019). For the purpose of attack detection in the Internet of Things, several supervised learning methods are employed, such as KNN, DT, SVM, NB, and LSTM . Even if they have good detection rates, they aren't useful in this age of many Zero-Day assaults because they consume too much resources and don't detect several attack footprints.

*Figure 2. Various Learning approaches.*

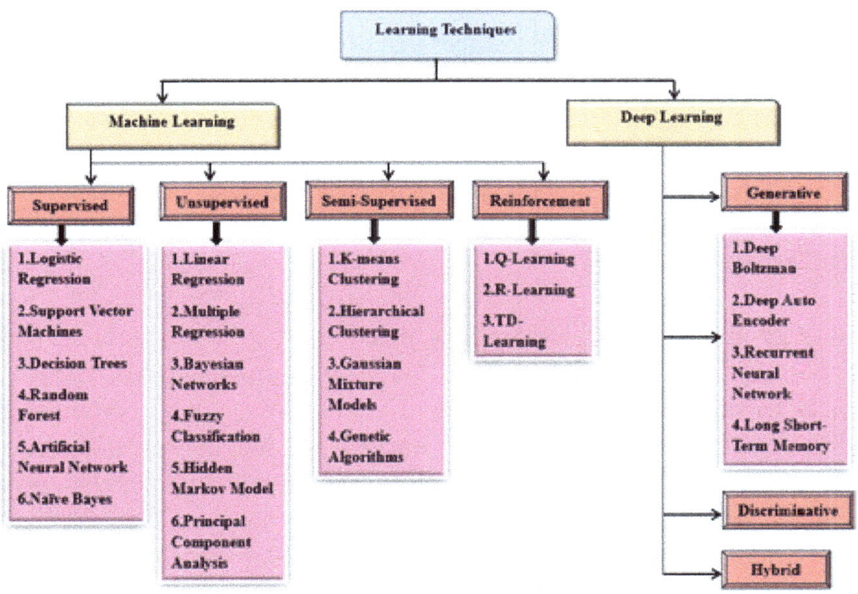


## 3.2 Unsupervised Learning

Since the labelled dataset is unavailable, it is highly beneficial for modelling the data's secret or fundamental structure(Liu & Lang, 2019). A thorough review of the data is encouraged because it differs from the supervised approach due to the labelled dataset not being available. The three main branches are clustering, dimensionality reduction (McDermott et al., 2018).Therefore, you can't miss outliers and new anomalies when you use these methods. Furthermore, features that do not contribute to class separability can be eliminated with the use of dimensionality reduction techniques such as PCA (Baraneetharan, 2020).

## 3.3 Reinforcement Learning:

Software agents can be programmed to optimise their cumulative reward in a certain environment using the reinforcement learning technique. These days, the expression "learning from the environment" is more widely used.(Gupta et al., 2022). Reinforcement learning primarily employs two strategies: policy search and value function approximation. As a whole, Q-learning, TD-learning, and R-learning cover most bases. Software agents can be taught to optimise their cumulative reward in a certain environment through Reinforcement Learning. This motto could also be used to learn from one's environment(Saranya et al., 2020). Two of RL's primary uses are in policy search and RL. It is evident that no one ML classification algorithm can handle every possible circumstance, given the strengths and downsides of the techniques mentioned(Sultana et al., 2019). As the number of IoT devices continues to grow and zero-day attacks continue to evolve, numerous fused models have been created to overcome the shortcomings of separate classifiers.

## 3.4 Federated learning

One such effective machine learning paradigm that can address IoT device security issues is FL (Ahmad et al., 2021). This cutting-edge ML method can achieve distributed model training. Updates used to entail a large communication cost when transferred from the centrally managed server to the networked devices. Network overhead has a detrimental effect on data throughput, reliability, privacy, and resource management. But the security of smart systems has been substantially improved with the advent of FL methods. Learning models that use FL make use of the distributed nature of learning to communicate just learnable parameters instead of complete datasets. In smart transport systems, FL has been a godsend for securing critical data.(Sarker et al., 2020).

## 3.5 Autoencoders

These deep learning models are based on the idea of using encoders and decoders to reconstruct the input following proper compression. The main goal is to achieve dimensionality reduction so that the data can be visualised and suitable projections can be made from it, because the input features are not totally independent and do show some relationship. Multilayer, regularised, vanilla and convolutional autoencoders are just a few of the many varieties. N-Balot, which stands for network-based detection of IoT botnet attacks utilising deep autoencoders was designed to identify botnet assaults that use autoencoders.

*Table 1. Conclusions about learning approaches.*

| MI and DI Techniques | Advantages | Disadvantages |
|---|---|---|
| DT | Inherent feature selection reduces processing time in misuse-based detection, requires less preprocessing, is straightforward and fast to implement, and can manage missing values. | Significant changes are caused by modest modifications, large complexity, and lengthy training times. |
| KNN | There is a quick training period and it produces | The dimensionality curse affects it, and it is costly, needs a lot of storage space, and is dependent on the value of K. |
| RF | The best accuracy is typically achieved without feature selection and overfitting. | Tedious due to the need to construct decision trees |
| NB | Simple, easy to execute, and robust against noise | The assumption of independence among the traits prevents it from capturing important information. |
| LSTM | Saves time on feature engineering, works with unstructured data, and remembers attack patterns in sequences | Training is a pain due to the massive memory bandwidth needs. |

Their focus was on DDOS attack detection, and they compared it to standalone Machine learning techniques. Based on bidirectional long short-term memory was presented by (McDermott et al., 2018)for the purpose of sensing botnet activities among consumer IoT devices. We additionally employed word embedding for text recognition in order to convert packets into integer format and carry out packet level detection.

## 4. ML AND DL-BASED IDS FRAMEWORK for HIOT

To aid in the detection and security of the IoT, machine learning has grown in prominence in recent years. Similarly, deep learning has been all the rage as of late. (Mehmood & Rais, 2016). This technique for predicting intrusions in networks is now considered useful. The IoT presents both opportunities and threats, according to a recent study by (Conti et al., 2018). According to the authors, detecting infected nodes, gathering proof of attacks, and storing that proof of a hostile attack is crucial for an effective IoT network. Research mainly intended to highlight major difficulties linked to IoT(Fadel et al., 2022). Because these technologies are inherently silent and self-sufficient, the authors argue that it is difficult to detect their presence. (Diro & Chilamkurti, 2018) offer new deep learning-based intrusion detection approaches for the IoT environment, and they show promise. With the inclusion of so many protocols, most of which originate from the Internet of Things, the authors also point out that thousands of zero-day attacks have been discovered. A significant portion of these assaults are slightly altered versions of cyberattacks that have been recorded earlier. These subtle changes in assaults over time may be difficult to detect, even using standard machine learning algorithms.(Lopez-Martin et al., 2017)created a novel technique for locating intrusions in Internet of Things networks. Utilising an architecture that incorporates intrusion labels into the decoding stages, it employs a CVAE(Berguiga et al., 2025). NIDS and other network monitoring systems, as well as IoT networks, could benefit from the proposed model's ability to reconstruct characteristics and other features.

The computation required is reduced by the proposed method's usage of a single training step. Although 5G networks will incorporate the IoT in due time,(Racherla et al., 2024) contend that it has drawbacks because it is challenging to implement numerous security measures on IoT for the future 5G network to be safe. The automata theory is used to propose a novel method for managing large heterogeneous IoT networks. The approach extends Labelled Transition Systems to universally define IoT systems in order to identify the incursion (Gunupudi et al., 2017). The comparison of action flows serves as the foundation for the descriptions. Gunupudi et al. showed that unlike the old methods of privacy and intrusion detection, the Internet of Things has significantly more complex implicit concerns. This study aims to represent each high-dimensional sample in the global dataset in a way that is equivalent to a reduction in dimension by iteratively clustering characteristics using a membership function. A dimensionality reduction technique was used to construct a reduced representation that was used for training classifiers. (El Houda et al., 2022).

Talked about a SDN based security architecture for the Internet of Things. In this case, SDN-based architecture, often referred to as SDN-Domain, can operate with or without infrastructure. The paper goes into great detail on the suggested architecture and explores how SDN might be used to improve network security, flexibility, and efficiency. Several architectural design considerations based on OpenFlow that affect performance were discussed in this article. These decisions included things like global traffic monitoring for ad hoc networks and network access control.(Article, 2024) Claim that because Internet of Things devices typically have limited resources, an Internet of Things middleware is required. By using such middleware, intelligently based decision-making procedures could be processed.

## 5. EMERGING TECHNOLOGIES

- **5 G and Up:** HIOT device connectivity, speed, and dependability will all be much improved with the rollout of 5 G network(Qadri, Nauman, et al., 2020). Future studies can concentrate on combining 5 G with HIOT to facilitate remote surgeries, real-time data transfer, and augmented reality applications in the medical field(Ali et al., 2025).
- **Machine learning and artificial intelligence:** Predictive analytics, individualised treatment programs, and smart monitoring systems are just a few ways in which AI and ML can revolutionise the HIOT(Qadri, Nauman, et al., 2020). Improving patient outcomes can be the focus of research into creating complex algorithms to sift through the mountains of healthcare data produced by IoT devices.
- **Block Chain Technology:** Blockchain technology provides a trustworthy and open way to handle medical records. In order to guarantee data integrity, improve privacy, and enable safe data sharing across healthcare providers, future research can investigate the use of blockchain technology(Dang et al., 2023).
- **Quantum Computing:** The future of computing may lie in quantum computation, which, as it develops, could outperform traditional computers at solving complicated computational tasks. More precise diagnoses and treatment plans can be the result of research into its potential use in processing massive datasets produced by HIOT devices.

## 6. RESULT AND DISCUSSION

### Metrics

The performance of five different models was assessed using the following metrics: accuracy, precision, recall, and F score. A model's accuracy can be described as the ratio of its true forecasts to its overall predictions. The term "precision" refers to the ratio of correct positive predictions to the entire number of positive predictions, regardless of how accurate they were. The recall is the proportion of correctly predicted positive samples to the total number of positive samples. Finally, as a measure of the validity of the test, the F-score is calculated using the recall and precision scores. These metrics are measured using the following equations: In the given equation, we can see that TP stands for True Positive, TN for True Negative, FP for False Positive, and FN for False Negative.(1) – (4).

$$Accuracy = \frac{TP + TN}{TP + TN + FP + FN} \quad (1)$$

$$\text{Precison} = \frac{\text{TP}}{\text{TP} + FP} \quad (2)$$

$$Recall = \frac{TP}{TP + FN} \quad (3)$$

$$\text{F score} = 2 * \frac{\text{Precision} * \text{Recall}}{\text{Precision} + \text{Recall}} \quad (4)$$

## Metrics Continuity

This study seeks to examine the effectiveness of supervised machine learning in learning to profile networked IoT devices, identify wireless attacks, and categorise the type of attack. It does this by training and evaluating a classification model using the corresponding network activity data. Classification tests compared to the training dataset yield four outputs that help decide whether a packet is malicious or not: True Positives (TP) - Occur when harmful packets are mistakenly projected to be malicious.

- True Negatives (TN) - Packages that aren't dangerous are mistakenly marked as such.
- False Positives (FP) - Reportedly dangerous packets that are actually harmless.
- False Negatives (FN) - where in dangerous packets are mistakenly believed to be safe.

The efficiency of a classifier can be assessed using a variety of metrics. All metrics, which can take on values between 0 and 1, should be maximised. Consequently, better classification performance is associated with higher values. A few of the most used metrics are accuracy, precision, recall, and F-measure. The proportion of successfully recognised harmful packets is measured by recall (*R*), whereas precision (*P*) is used to quantify the proportion of incorrect packets. A common combination of the two metrics is F-measure (*F*), It computes the harmonic mean of precision and recall to provide a single weighted measure for assessing classification performance. Formula (5). gives the equations that are utilised to ascertain these.

$$\text{P} = \frac{\text{TP}}{\text{TP} + \text{FP}} \; R = \frac{TP}{TP + FN} \; F = 2 * \frac{P * R}{P + R} \quad (5)$$

For some, precision is the gold standard in evaluation. One way to quantify accuracy is by counting the number of correctly classified packets. Using accuracy as a metric to evaluate a classifier's performance has its limitations, as it might lead to misleading results if the classifier is trained to consistently predict the same class. There may not be a single optimal learning algorithm because of the no free lunch theorem. What this means is that data qualities that define a problem should be considered with the algorithm's performance when making a selection. Several classifiers included in the Weka package were tested here. We selected classifiers based on their speed in classifying unknown data, high dimensional feature space support, and ability to handle multi-class classification. Doing so was necessary to guarantee conformity with standards that use machine learning methods to identify cyber-attacks in both legacy and Internet of Things networks. models that attempt to maximize information gain by using conditional independence and discriminative assumptions, or models that quickly classify data correctly without taking the data's underlying structure or probability into account. The algorithms stated earlier were chosen for their ability to provide interpretable classification models. This allows for better understanding of the classification results.

One way to evaluate a classification model's performance is to compare its predictions to the actual values in the dataset. This can be done using a confusion matrix, which is a table, as shown in Figure 3. It gives a summary of the number of right and wrong predictions for each class, which helps to understand the model's mistake kind. The confusion matrix shows the value of (98.91%).

*Figure 3. Confusion Matrix*

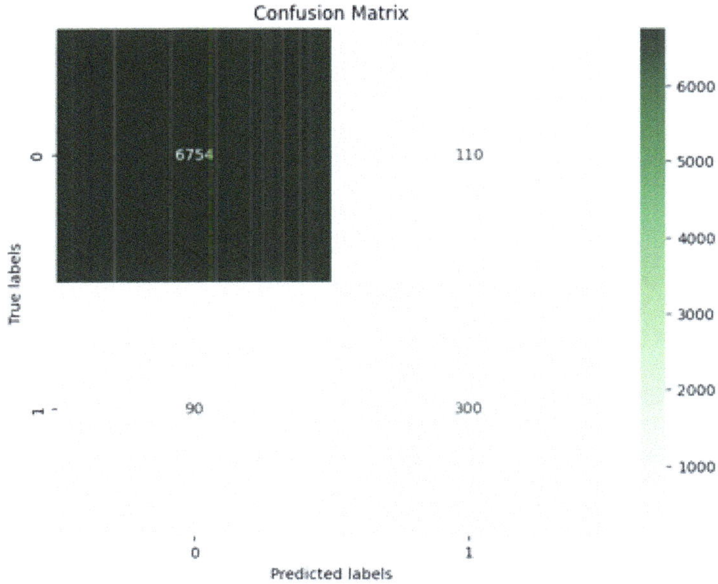

In Table 2, they can see how the suggested methods stack up against other algorithms' base hyperparameter. These other algorithms include RF, LSTM, NB, KNN, and DT. The suggested LSTM method outperformed the alternatives with respect to Accuracy (98.91%), Precision (96.06%), Recall (94.01%), F1-score (98.98%) and Time (1.12).

*Table 2. Performance of Models*

| Models | ROC | Accuracy | Precision | Recall | F1-Score | Time |
|---|---|---|---|---|---|---|
| **RF** | 94.23 | 92.41 | 90.12 | 88.10 | 92.63 | 06.48 |
| **LSTM** | **1.0** | **98.91** | **96.06** | **94.01** | **98.98** | **01.12** |
| **NB** | 91.45 | 89.23 | 87.47 | 85.39 | 89.71 | 08.30 |
| **KNN** | 76.89 | 74.64 | 72.59 | 70.17 | 74.82 | 11.20 |
| **DT** | 84.66 | 82.31 | 80.67 | 78.32 | 82.68 | 03.40 |

Figure 4 shows that when comparing the suggested model to RF, NB, KNN, DT in terms of Accuracy Loss, it performs better. The LSTM model consistently achieves the best training loss rate.

*Figure 4. Accuracy Loss*

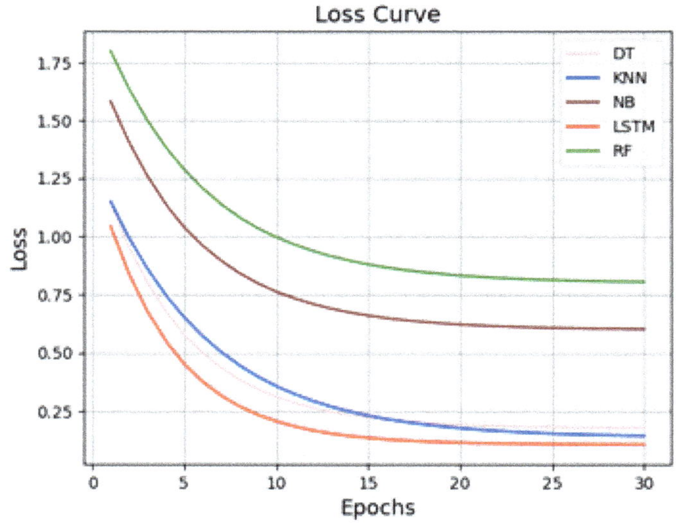

Figure 5 shows the time required to execute several ML models like RF, LSTM, NB, KNN, and DT. The least amount of time to process data is approximately 1 minute with LSTM.

*Figure 5. Computation Time*

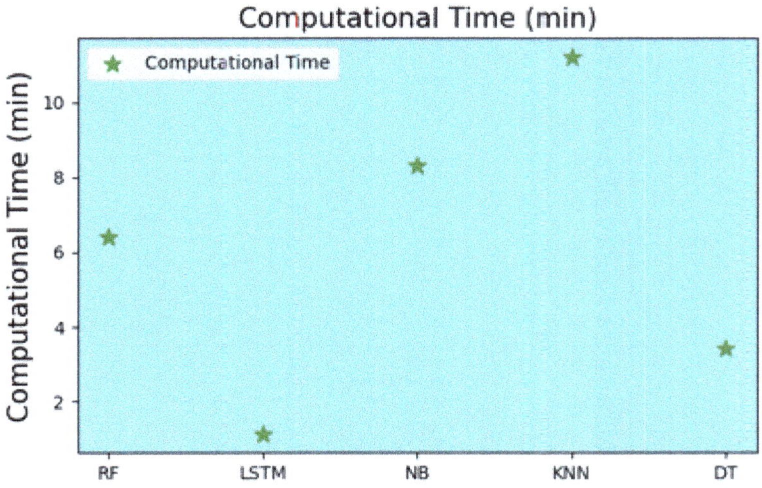


As demonstrated in Figure 6, the ROC curve which includes the model of RF, LSTM, NB, KNN and DT. LSTM has performed better than other models and our proposed LSTM model achieved high AUC value is 1.0%.

*Figure 6. Receiver Operating Characteristics*

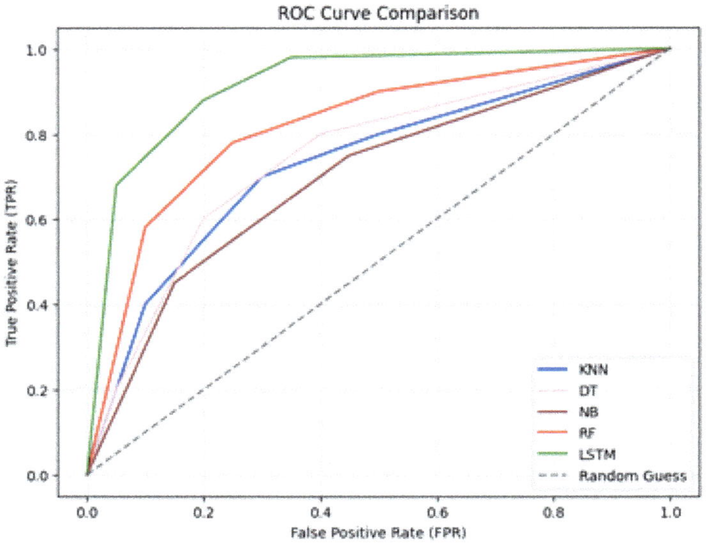


The figure 7 shows how well Five models RF, LSTM, NB, KNN and DT .All of the models exhibit some changes, but LSTM always has the highest accuracy, reaching about 98.91% in most folds. KNN, on the other hand, has the lowest accuracy.

*Figure 7. Accuracy Models*

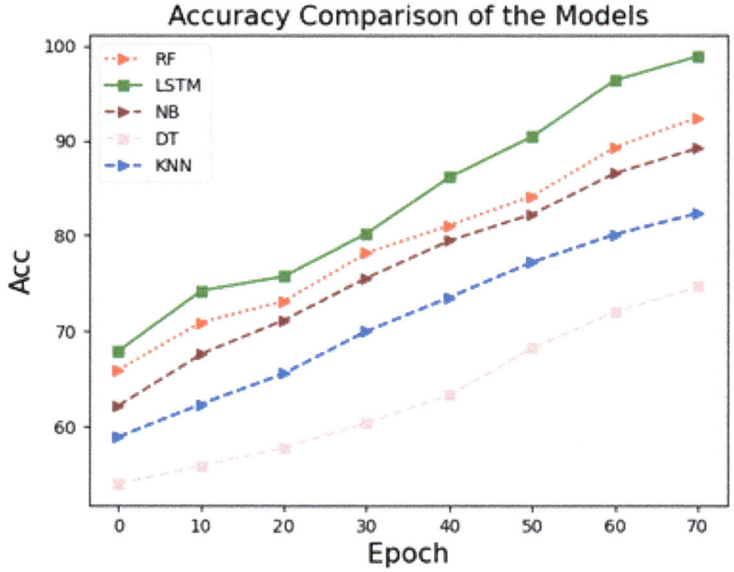

# 7. DISCUSSION AND CHALLENGES

## 7.1 Discussion

We aimed to make a significant contribution to IDS research by studying different algorithms, with a focus on bio-inspired algorithms(Ranjan & Sahana, 2024) We think that existing methods can be improved by mimicking what nature does. To make our IDSs more effective, we require other approaches. We still think ACA can't tell the difference between harmless and malicious cases. So, we upgraded to deep learning, the latest bio-inspired technique that is a neural network advancement. It will be difficult to implement deep learning algorithms as a classifier that works in real-time(Karunarathne et al., 2021). The vast majority of prior work that has used deep learning techniques in an IDS setting has limited itself to feature extraction or dimensionality reduction(Kim & Aminanto, 2017). On the other hand, we demonstrate that deep learning techniques can also complete clustering tasks. To sum up, SAE is highly beneficial for the following activities:

- Feature extraction
- Clustering
- Classification

## 7.2 Further Challenges

Future efforts to improve IDS will face more obstacles.We propose the following avenues for further investigation on IDS based on our prior work.

- Intruder detection systems have been greatly enhanced by deep learning. However, in order for it to work in IoT settings, such the CAN utilised by unmanned vehicles, we need to make it lighter.
- Due to the difficulty in obtaining massive amounts of labelled data, an improved unsupervised technique is required. Hence, it is preferable to have an IDS that uses an unsupervised technique.
- Construct an intrusion detection system with sufficient sensitivity to identify zero-day assaults while simultaneously minimising false positives.
- Future efforts will require a holistic approach that addresses both detection and prevention. Consequently, it is anticipated that an IPS or similar device will be built with both detection and prevention capabilities.

## 8.FUTURE DIRECTIONS

Internet of Things intrusion detection systems have been the subject of numerous academic studies. The IoT intrusion and anomaly detection utilizing ML and DL approaches still has many unanswered questions.(Qadri, Nauman, et al., 2020). The problem is that there isn't a tried-and-true way for ensuring that the suggested systems or methods are valid. The majority of the research papers show how their suggested systems perform on synthetic datasets and solve a single problem; however, this approach might not work when faced with real data and other real-world challenges(Asharf et al., 2020). This study, along with others like it that have examined the current state IDS for the internet of things, has shown that designing an IDS that meets the needs of all stakeholders while simultaneously being deployable, online, scalable, and effective on real data is extremely challenging(Rashad et al., 2022). On the flip side, the majority of published works rely on biassed parameters, only cover a small portion of the system, and provide evaluation results using faked datasets. In addition, it is not a simple process to define and achieve confirmation of completeness and correctness for any proposed IDS. The difficulty of developing an IDS capable of detecting and preventing every possible threat is, hence, one takeaway from this study..(Patel et al., 2022). Some of the most pressing problems that scientists are currently or will soon be confronting include the ones listed below. Future research in this area, especially in anomaly and intrusion detection using ML and DL algorithms, has great promise as the security mechanisms for the IoT are still in the development stages. Newer problems have been associated with:

- A vital component for testing and validating any NIDS is a high-quality dataset pertaining to IoT IDS(Chakraborty et al., 2020). For this kind of dataset, it is crucial to have sufficient tagged network traffic data that differentiates between malicious and benign activity. In addition to attack data needed to test the NIDS, ordinary traffic data from numerous types of IoT devices is also necessary for capturing usual behavior.(Aledhari et al., 2022). However, as indicated before, most datasets that are available to the public do not have all the required attributes. Raw pcap files that are either lacking labels or are incomplete or contain incorrect information, raw csv files that are either difficult to comprehend or contain incorrect information, and so on. In addition, the present datasets can only record the usual behaviors of a limited number of IoT devices, which restricts the range of devices that may be trained for intrusion detection systems. Making a dataset that can deal with these problems in the actual world is one example of a research subject.(Patel et al., 2022).
- Building an anomaly-based IDS for IoT networks that operates online and in real-time is no easy feat. This is due to the fact that in order for such an IDS

to identify malicious or abnormal behavior, it would have to learn typical behavior first. During this time, the learning phase presupposes but does not prove—that there will be no attack traffic or background noise(Pakrooh et al., 2024). Fake alarms could be caused by such an IDS if these problems aren't fixed.

- According to this research, most anomaly-based NIDS try to construct a model that includes every possible pattern of normal traffic behavior. The problem is that these models tend to give a lot of false positives as they favor the dominant class, the normal class, which makes things very tough. An further factor contributing to false-negative rates is the impossibility of recording every potential typical observation in a network, which is particularly true in the diversified context of IoT networks. Finding a solution to the problem of NIDS's high false-positive and false-negative rates is another area that requires more research. Building models that are customized to certain gadgets would be fascinating. Other companies' IDSs that use the same kind of device can benefit from these models as well. Other organization can benefit from this since they can implement these models without having to spend time collecting data and training IDSs. Additionally, it will aid in the detection of compromised IoT devices that are malevolent, as their behavior would deviate from the typical patterns collected by trained models. It will be difficult to develop such models, but this might be a good topic for future studies.
- Processing data, reducing features, training models, and deploying NIDS all add computational complexity to the design and implementation process. This is particularly true for ML and DL based NIDS. Constructing an efficient NIDS with low computational needs is, then, another challenge and possible area for new research. While dimensionality reduction and feature selection may be effective in a static environment, they may fail to identify certain types of assaults or normal traffic if used with some of the suggested intrusion detection systems. The dynamic nature of the Internet of Things makes this point more salient than ever. As a result, one possible area of study could be developing a feature selection system that can adapt to different kinds of normal and attack traffic while being computationally efficient. Models trained on large datasets are increasingly using DL and ML based algorithms and methodologies. The management of cyber-attacks has been made possible thanks to this. Researchers still face several obstacles, even though DL and ML algorithms show great promise for detecting threats in IoT networks. One reason why DL and ML algorithms for network security aren't always completely utilized is because of the processing power limitations of IoT devices..(Xiao et al., 2018). When applying ML/DL techniques

to large and distributed networks, such the ones used by the IoT, scalability issues emerge. This is especially true when there are multiple scenarios and choices for IDS deployment. To address the limitations of both ML and DL algorithms, some writers have suggested combining them into an ensemble. Problems with network latency and processing expense rendered this method unsuitable for systems handling potentially life-threatening data or information, such as healthcare and IoV systems.

- Research in the future could center on developing an IDS for IoT security by utilizing RL, transfer learning, and semi-supervised learning. Important goals like real-time training, quick anomaly detection in IoT, and unified models can be achieved using these approaches, which have not yet been thoroughly verified or examined. The advantages that can be realized in scenarios involving IoT networks, which have extremely high data dimensionality and non-stationary environments, make the combination of RL with DL an intriguing subject for research.

## CONCLUSION

More and more security holes and attacks are appearing in the IoT as its user base expands. The objective of this research was to present HIOT, a method for intrusion detection that utilizes machine learning. Our approach begins with a novel, lightweight anomaly detection based on M2-DAE that may be implemented on-device. After that, we need to look for known and undiscovered attacks in the suspicious traffic. We can then take precautions and, with any luck, contribute to our assault knowledge base. We used the newly-released Bot-IoT dataset to test our HIOT. Anomaly detection and unknown threat recognition, especially for DoS and DDoS attacks, are areas where our H2ID excels when compared to the top-performing multi-class abuse detector. Along with supporting distributed deployments that leverage IoT networks' hierarchical structure, HIOT is compliant with the scalability and privacy limitations that are inherent to such networks. By means of the Internet of Things, it is not necessary to divide up operational traffic among numerous remote parties. With the availability of new data sets, researchers will look into how to improve the number and granularity of attack classifications, as well as how to construct criteria for specific use cases. Furthermore, we will explore decentralized solutions that safeguard privacy by leveraging the hierarchical design of HIOT. A 98.91% accuracy rate was attained by the proposed LSTM model in comparison to more traditional methods.

## REFERENCES


Ahmad, Z., Shahid Khan, A., Wai Shiang, C., Abdullah, J., & Ahmad, F. (2021). Network intrusion detection system: A systematic study of machine learning and deep learning approaches. *Transactions on Emerging Telecommunications Technologies*, *32*(1), 1–29. DOI: 10.1002/ett.4150

Al-Garadi, M. A., Mohamed, A., Al-Ali, A. K., Du, X., Ali, I., & Guizani, M. (2020). A Survey of Machine and Deep Learning Methods for Internet of Things (IoT) Security. *IEEE Communications Surveys and Tutorials*, *22*(3), 1646–1685. DOI: 10.1109/COMST.2020.2988293

Alamri, B., Richardson, I., & Crowley, K. (2024). Cybersecuriy Risk Management and Evaluation Framework of Blockchain Identity Management Systems in HIoT: Experts Evaluation. *IEEE Access : Practical Innovations, Open Solutions*, *12*(September), 144652–144683. DOI: 10.1109/ACCESS.2024.3468379

Aledhari, M., Razzak, R., Qolomany, B., Al-Fuqaha, A., & Saeed, F. (2022). Biomedical IoT: Enabling Technologies, Architectural Elements, Challenges, and Future Directions. *IEEE Access : Practical Innovations, Open Solutions*, *10*, 31306–31339. DOI: 10.1109/ACCESS.2022.3159235

Ali, T. E., Ali, F. I., Dakić, P., & Zoltan, A. D. (2025). Trends, prospects, challenges, and security in the healthcare internet of things. *Computing*, *107*(1), 1–29. DOI: 10.1007/s00607-024-01352-4

Article, O. (2024).. . *Hybrid AI Models in Network Security : Combining ML, DL, and Rule-Based Systems*, *5*(4), 109–121.

Asharf, J., Moustafa, N., Khurshid, H., Debie, E., Haider, W., & Wahab, A. (2020). A review of intrusion detection systems using machine and deep learning in internet of things: Challenges, solutions and future directions. *Electronics (Basel)*, *9*(7), 1177. Advance online publication. DOI: 10.3390/electronics9071177

Baich, M., Hamim, T., Sael, N., & Chemlal, Y. (2022). Machine Learning for IoT based networks intrusion detection: A comparative study. *Procedia Computer Science*, *215*, 742–751. DOI: 10.1016/j.procs.2022.12.076

Baraneetharan, E. (2020). Role of Machine Learning Algorithms Intrusion Detection in WSNs: A Survey. *Journal of Information Technology and Digital World*, *02*(03), 161–173. DOI: 10.36548/jitdw.2020.3.004

Berguiga, A., Harchay, A., & Massaoudi, A. (2025). HIDS-RPL: A Hybrid Deep Learning-Based Intrusion Detection System for RPL in Internet of Medical Things Network. *IEEE Access : Practical Innovations, Open Solutions*, *13*(February), 38404–38429. DOI: 10.1109/ACCESS.2025.3545918

Bovenzi, G., Aceto, G., Ciuonzo, D., Persico, V., & Pescape, A. (2020). A hierarchical hybrid intrusion detection approach in IoT scenarios. *Proceedings - IEEE Global Communications Conference, GLOBECOM, 2020-Janua*. DOI: 10.1109/GLOBECOM42002.2020.9348167

Chakraborty, C., Banerjee, A., Garg, L., & Editors, • Joel J. P. C. Rodrigues. (2020). Cognitive Internet of Medical Things for Smart Healthcare. In *Springer* (Issue June). DOI: 10.1007/978-3-030-55833-8

Conti, M., Dehghantanha, A., Franke, K., & Watson, S. (2018). Internet of Things security and forensics: Challenges and opportunities. *Future Generation Computer Systems*, *78*, 544–546. DOI: 10.1016/j.future.2017.07.060

Dang, V. A., Khanh, Q. V., Nguyen, V., Nguyen, T., & Nguyen, D. C. (2023). *Intelligent Healthcare : Integration of Emerging Technologies*.

Diro, A. A., & Chilamkurti, N. (2018). Distributed attack detection scheme using deep learning approach for Internet of Things. *Future Generation Computer Systems*, *82*, 761–768. DOI: 10.1016/j.future.2017.08.043

El Houda, Z. A., Brik, B., & Senouci, S. M. (2022). A Novel IoT-Based Explainable Deep Learning Framework for Intrusion Detection Systems. *IEEE Internet of Things Magazine*, *5*(2), 20–23. DOI: 10.1109/IOTM.005.2200028

Elbir, A. M., Soner, B., Coleri, S., Gunduz, D., & Bennis, M. (2022). Federated Learning in Vehicular Networks. *2022 IEEE International Mediterranean Conference on Communications and Networking, MeditCom 2022*, 72–77. DOI: 10.1109/MeditCom55741.2022.9928621

Fadel, M. M., El-Ghamrawy, S. M., Ali-Eldin, A. M. T., Hassan, M. K., & El-Desoky, A. I. (2022). The proposed hybrid deep learning intrusion prediction IoT (HDLIP-IoT) framework. *PLoS ONE, 17*(7 July), 1–21. DOI: 10.1371/journal.pone.0271436

Gunupudi, R. K., Nimmala, M., Gugulothu, N., & Gali, S. R. (2017). CLAPP: A self constructing feature clustering approach for anomaly detection. *Future Generation Computer Systems*, *74*, 417–429. DOI: 10.1016/j.future.2016.12.040

Gupta, P., Yadav, L., & Tomar, D. S. (2022). Internet of Things: A Survey on Fused Machine Learning-Based Intrusion Detection Approaches. *Lecture Notes in Electrical Engineering*, *858*, 147–161. DOI: 10.1007/978-981-19-0840-8_11

Hasan, M. K., Akhtaruzzaman, M., Kabir, S. R., Gadekallu, T. R., Islam, S., Magalingam, P., Hassan, R., Alazab, M., & Alazab, M. A. (2022). Evolution of Industry and Blockchain Era: Monitoring Price Hike and Corruption Using BIoT for Smart Government and Industry 4.0. *IEEE Transactions on Industrial Informatics*, *18*(12), 9153–9161. DOI: 10.1109/TII.2022.3164066

Hizal, S., Cavusoglu, U., & Akgun, D. (2024). A novel deep learning-based intrusion detection system for IoT DDoS security. *Internet of Things : Engineering Cyber Physical Human Systems*, *28*, 101336. Advance online publication. DOI: 10.1016/j.iot.2024.101336

Husnain, M., Hayat, K., Cambiaso, E., Fayyaz, U. U., Mongelli, M., Akram, H., Ghazanfar Abbas, S., & Shah, G. A. (2022). Preventing MQTT Vulnerabilities Using IoT-Enabled Intrusion Detection System. *Sensors (Basel)*, *22*(2), 567. Advance online publication. DOI: 10.3390/s22020567

Karunarathne, S. M., Saxena, N., & Khan, M. K. (2021). Security and Privacy in IoT Smart Healthcare. *IEEE Internet Computing*, *25*(4), 37–48. DOI: 10.1109/MIC.2021.3051675

Kim, K., & Aminanto, M. E. (2017). Deep learning in intrusion detection perspective: Overview and further challenges. *Proceedings - WBIS 2017: 2017 International Workshop on Big Data and Information Security, 2018-Janua*, 5–10. DOI: 10.1109/IWBIS.2017.8275095

Liu, H., & Lang, B. (2019). Machine learning and deep learning methods for intrusion detection systems: A survey. *Applied Sciences (Basel, Switzerland)*, *9*(20), 4396. Advance online publication. DOI: 10.3390/app9204396

Lopez-Martin, M., Carro, B., Sanchez-Esguevillas, A., & Lloret, J. (2017). Conditional variational autoencoder for prediction and feature recovery applied to intrusion detection in iot. *Sensors (Basel)*, *17*(9), 1967. Advance online publication. DOI: 10.3390/s17091967

Malhotra, P., Singh, Y., Anand, P., Bangotra, D. K., Singh, P. K., & Hong, W. C. (2021). Internet of things: Evolution, concerns and security challenges. *Sensors (Basel)*, *21*(5), 1–35. DOI: 10.3390/s21051809

McDermott, C. D., Majdani, F., & Petrovski, A. V. (2018). Botnet Detection in the Internet of Things using Deep Learning Approaches. *Proceedings of the International Joint Conference on Neural Networks, 2018-July*. DOI: 10.1109/IJCNN.2018.8489489

Mehmood, T., & Rais, H. B. M. (2016). Machine learning algorithms in context of intrusion detection. *2016 3rd International Conference on Computer and Information Sciences, ICCOINS 2016 - Proceedings, April*, 369–373. DOI: 10.1109/ICCOINS.2016.7783243

Menon, I. U., Babu Kumaravelu, V., Kumar, V. C., Rammohan, A., Chinnadurai, S., Venkatesan, R., Hai, H., & Selvaprabhu, P. (2025). AI-Powered IoT: A Survey on Integrating Artificial Intelligence With IoT for Enhanced Security, Efficiency, and Smart Applications. *IEEE Access : Practical Innovations, Open Solutions*, *13*(February), 50296–50339. DOI: 10.1109/ACCESS.2025.3551750

Mishra, N., & Pandya, S. (2021). Internet of Things Applications, Security Challenges, Attacks, Intrusion Detection, and Future Visions: A Systematic Review. *IEEE Access : Practical Innovations, Open Solutions*, *9*, 59353–59377. DOI: 10.1109/ACCESS.2021.3073408

Mishra, P., Varadharajan, V., Tupakula, U., & Pilli, E. S. (2019). A detailed investigation and analysis of using machine learning techniques for intrusion detection. *IEEE Communications Surveys and Tutorials*, *21*(1), 686–728. DOI: 10.1109/COMST.2018.2847722

Oyelade, J., Isewon, I., Oladipupo, O., Emebo, O., Omogbadegun, Z., Aromolaran, O., Uwoghiren, E., Olaniyan, D., & Olawole, O. (2019). Data Clustering: Algorithms and Its Applications. *Proceedings - 2019 19th International Conference on Computational Science and Its Applications, ICCSA 2019, January 2020*, 71–81. DOI: 10.1109/ICCSA.2019.000-1

Pakrooh, R., Jabbari, A., & Fung, C. (2024). Deep Learning-Assisted Security and Privacy Provisioning in the Internet of Medical Things Systems: A Survey on Recent Advances. *IEEE Access : Practical Innovations, Open Solutions*, *12*(February), 40610–40621. DOI: 10.1109/ACCESS.2024.3377561

Patel, V. A., Bhattacharya, P., Tanwar, S., Gupta, R., Sharma, G., Bokoro, P. N., & Sharma, R. (2022). Adoption of Federated Learning for Healthcare Informatics: Emerging Applications and Future Directions. *IEEE Access : Practical Innovations, Open Solutions*, *10*(July), 90792–90826. DOI: 10.1109/ACCESS.2022.3201876

Qadri, Y. A., Ali, R., Musaddiq, A., Al-Turjman, F., Kim, D. W., & Kim, S. W. (2020). The limitations in the state-of-the-art counter-measures against the security threats in H-IoT. *Cluster Computing*, *23*(3), 2047–2065. DOI: 10.1007/s10586-019-03036-7

Qadri, Y. A., Nauman, A., Zikria, Y., Vasilakos, A. V., & Kim, S. W. (2020). The Future of Healthcare Internet of Things: A Survey of Emerging Technologies. *IEEE Communications Surveys and Tutorials*, *22*(2), 1121–1167. DOI: 10.1109/COMST.2020.2973314

Racherla, S., Sripathi, P., Faruqui, N., Alamgir Kabir, M., Whaiduzzaman, M., & Aziz Shah, S. (2024). Deep-IDS: A Real-Time Intrusion Detector for IoT Nodes Using Deep Learning. *IEEE Access : Practical Innovations, Open Solutions*, *12*(May), 63584–63597. DOI: 10.1109/ACCESS.2024.3396461

Ranjan, R., & Sahana, B. C. (2024). A Comprehensive Roadmap for Transforming Healthcare from Hospital-Centric to Patient-Centric through Healthcare Internet of Things (IoT). *Engineering and Science*, *30*, 1–16. DOI: 10.30919/es1175

Rashad, M., Hussein, D. L., Abdalkarim, H., & Azeez, R. (2022). Future IoT Software in Healthcare Also Exploring IoT Industry Application. *UHD Journal of Science and Technology*, *6*(1), 70–75. DOI: 10.21928/uhdjst.v6n1y2022.pp70-75

Rondon, L. P., Babun, L., Aris, A., Akkaya, K., & Uluagac, A. S. (2022). Survey on Enterprise Internet-of-Things systems (E-IoT): A security perspective. *Ad Hoc Networks*, *125*, 1–33. DOI: 10.1016/j.adhoc.2021.102728

Saranya, T., Sridevi, S., Deisy, C., Chung, T. D., & Khan, M. K. A. A. (2020). Performance Analysis of Machine Learning Algorithms in Intrusion Detection System: A Review. *Procedia Computer Science, 171*(2019), 1251–1260. DOI: 10.1016/j.procs.2020.04.133

Sarker, I. H., Abushark, Y. B., Alsolami, F., & Khan, A. I. (2020). IntruDTree: A machine learning based cyber security intrusion detection model. *Symmetry*, *12*(5), 1–15. DOI: 10.3390/sym12050754

Soldatos, J., Gusmeroli, S., Malo, P., & Di Orio, G. (2015). Internet of things applications in future manufacturing. *Digitising the Industry Internet of Things Connecting the Physical, Digital and Virtual Worlds*, 153–183. DOI: 10.1201/9781003337966-5

Sultana, N., Chilamkurti, N., Peng, W., & Alhadad, R. (2019). Survey on SDN based network intrusion detection system using machine learning approaches. *Peer-to-Peer Networking and Applications*, *12*(2), 493–501. DOI: 10.1007/s12083-017-0630-0

Ullah, F., Naeem, H., Jabbar, S., Khalid, S., Latif, M. A., Al-Turjman, F., & Mostarda, L. (2019). Cyber security threats detection in internet of things using deep learning approach. *IEEE Access : Practical Innovations, Open Solutions*, *7*, 124379–124389. DOI: 10.1109/ACCESS.2019.2937347

Williams, R., McMahon, E., Samtani, S., Patton, M., & Chen, H. (2017). Identifying vulnerabilities of consumer Internet of Things (IoT) devices: A scalable approach. *2017 IEEE International Conference on Intelligence and Security Informatics: Security and Big Data, ISI 2017, July*, 179–181. DOI: 10.1109/ISI.2017.8004904

Wyss, B. M. (2024). *CTC-SENTINEL-092024_cover-article-1*. 1–9.

Xiao, L., Wan, X., Lu, X., Zhang, Y., & Wu, D. (2018). *IoT Security Techniques Based on Machine Learning*. 1–20. https://arxiv.org/abs/1801.06275

Zheng, Y., Li, Z., Xu, X., & Zhao, Q. (2022). Dynamic defenses in cyber security: Techniques, methods and challenges. *Digital Communications and Networks*, *8*(4), 422–435. DOI: 10.1016/j.dcan.2021.07.006

# Chapter 3
# From Vulnerability to Resilience:
## Enhancing Security in Lightweight IoT Protocols

**Adelia Rizky Cantika**
*Esa Unggul University, Indonesia*

**Saelendra Farell Syahbana**
https://orcid.org/0009-0006-2249-6109
*Esa Unggul University, Indonesia*

**Binastya Anggara Sekti**
https://orcid.org/0000-0001-5489-4888
*Esa Unggul University, Indonesia*

## ABSTRACT

*The proliferation of Internet of Things (IoT) devices across critical sectors has intensified the adoption of lightweight security protocols designed to accommodate resource-constrained environments. However, the inherent trade-offs between computational efficiency and security robustness in these protocols have introduced significant vulnerabilities that threaten the integrity of IoT ecosystems. This chapter provides a comprehensive analysis of security weaknesses in prevalent lightweight IoT protocols, including MQTT, CoAP, LoRaWAN, and DTLS-based implementations. Through systematic vulnerability assessment and empirical security testing, this research identifies critical attack vectors, evaluates their potential impact on IoT infrastructures, and proposes a multi-layered mitigation framework.*

DOI: 10.4018/979-8-3373-7610-3.ch003

# INTRODUCTION TO LIGHTWEIGHT IOT SECURITY PROTOCOLS AND THREAT LANDSCAPE

## Introduction

The expansion of the Internet of Things (IoT) has introduced significant innovations across multiple industries, from healthcare to manufacturing. By connecting billions of devices and enabling real-time monitoring and control, IoT systems provide unmatched convenience, automation, and operational insight. This evolution is primarily supported by lightweight communication protocols, which have been engineered to operate under the strict power, memory, and bandwidth constraints of embedded and low-power devices. However, the same characteristics that make these protocols ideal for constrained environments also introduce vulnerabilities that malicious actors can exploit.

In this chapter, we provide an overview of lightweight communication protocols and assess their role in shaping the IoT security landscape. We examine the nature of current cyber threats targeting these protocols and present a foundational understanding of why security in resource-constrained environments remains a formidable challenge. By exploring the intersection of efficiency and exposure, we outline the necessity of evolving protocol-level defenses to ensure resilience in modern IoT deployments.

## Background: The Rise of Lightweight Protocols in IoT

Unlike traditional IT systems, many IoT devices operate under severe limitations. A battery-operated sensor node in a smart agriculture system, for instance, must conserve energy while transmitting critical environmental data. To enable efficient data exchange under such constraints, developers have adopted lightweight communication protocols such as MQTT (Message Queuing Telemetry Transport), CoAP (Constrained Application Protocol), and LoRaWAN (Long Range Wide Area Network)(Al-Na'amneh et al., 2025).

These protocols are designed to optimize resource use. MQTT, based on a publish-subscribe architecture, is popular for telemetry systems due to its minimal overhead and simplicity. CoAP offers REST-like messaging semantics over UDP, tailored for constrained environments with intermittent connectivity. LoRaWAN enables low-power, long-range communication, making it suitable for remote and wide-area applications.

While these protocols allow massive scaling and inter-device communication, their original design philosophy did not place security at the forefront. Instead, features such as authentication, integrity, and encryption are often treated as optional or implemented externally. This has resulted in diverse and inconsistent security postures across deployments.

## The Expanding IoT Threat Landscape

As IoT adoption continues to rise, the associated threat landscape has become more sophisticated. Attackers target not only high-value systems but also low-resource endpoints that may appear insignificant in isolation but are vital within the broader ecosystem. Lightweight protocols have become frequent entry points for exploitation due to their weak or misconfigured security controls.

Numerous IoT-specific malware strains have emerged in recent years. Botnets such as Mirai and Mozi exploit devices with open ports or weak credentials to perform distributed denial-of-service (DDoS) attacks. Once compromised, these devices can be coordinated to disable services, overwhelm networks, or serve as pivot points into secured environments. Many of these botnets leverage MQTT or similar lightweight protocols to communicate with command-and-control infrastructure.

Eavesdropping, message spoofing, and topic injection attacks are also prevalent. When lightweight protocols are used without proper encryption or authentication, attackers can intercept messages, impersonate devices, or disrupt application workflows. The lack of session validation, message integrity checks, and access control further aggravates the risk of unauthorized manipulation.

## Lightweight Protocols and Their Characteristics

To better understand their vulnerability profile, it is essential to examine the structural features of common lightweight IoT protocols.

MQTT operates on top of TCP and employs a broker-based model. Clients publish data to the broker, which then forwards it to subscribed clients. MQTT's strength lies in its simplicity and scalability. However, it lacks mandatory support for encryption or authentication, relying on implementations to enable Transport Layer Security (TLS) and access control lists.

CoAP, designed by the IETF, is an application-layer protocol that operates over UDP. It supports confirmable and non-confirmable messages and provides caching and resource discovery. While CoAP offers optional support for Datagram Transport Layer Security (DTLS), many implementations omit it due to resource limitations, leaving the protocol exposed to message replay and spoofing.

LoRaWAN, unlike MQTT and CoAP, is a physical and MAC layer protocol used for wide-area communications. It introduces some built-in security mechanisms, such as AES-128 encryption for payloads. However, mismanagement of keys and lack of secure device registration can lead to replay attacks, gateway spoofing, or unauthorized network access.(Jamwal et al., 2025)

Each of these protocols represents a trade-off between functionality and protection. While they are well-suited to their respective use cases, none can be considered secure by default. Security must be explicitly configured and regularly maintained, a task that is often neglected in real-world deployments.

## Challenges in Securing Lightweight Protocols

Securing communication in constrained environments presents a range of technical and operational challenges. Cryptographic algorithms require processing power and memory that are not always available on microcontroller-based IoT devices. As a result, system designers must strike a delicate balance between security and performance.

Several common challenges include:

1. Lack of standardized security profiles

Vendors often implement protocols inconsistently, leading to variations in how security features are applied. Some devices may support TLS or DTLS, while others may offer no encryption at all.

2. Infrequent firmware updates

Many IoT devices are deployed with no mechanism for over-the-air (OTA) updates. This makes it difficult to patch known vulnerabilities, leaving systems exposed for years.

3. Poor credential management

Default or hardcoded credentials remain one of the most frequently exploited weaknesses. In environments with hundreds or thousands of devices, managing unique and secure credentials becomes a logistical burden.

4. Physical exposure

IoT devices are often installed in unprotected environments such as public streets, remote agricultural sites, or factory floors. Physical access allows attackers to extract keys, clone firmware, or manipulate configuration settings.

5. Limited visibility and logging

Lightweight devices typically lack detailed logging capabilities. This hinders threat detection, forensic investigation, and anomaly analysis during or after an attack.

These issues highlight the need for a structured and layered approach to securing IoT protocols. Security must be embedded at every layer of the architecture, from hardware and firmware to communication and application logic.

## Comprehensive Vulnerability Analysis of MQTT Security Implementation

Message Queuing Telemetry Transport (MQTT) has become a foundational protocol in the Internet of Things (IoT) ecosystem. Designed for lightweight, low-bandwidth, and reliable message delivery, it plays a vital role in many IoT deployments such as industrial automation, smart homes, healthcare, and agriculture. Its publish-subscribe architecture enables asynchronous communication between devices while reducing network traffic and computational load. However, MQTT was not originally developed with security as a core consideration. In many real-world implementations, the protocol is deployed without adequate safeguards, leaving devices and systems vulnerable to various cyber threats.

This chapter provides a detailed analysis of vulnerabilities associated with MQTT protocol implementations. It investigates common misconfigurations, protocol design limitations, and real-world attack scenarios. The aim is to expose the security gaps that persist in MQTT deployments and to lay the groundwork for developing secure configurations and enhanced implementations discussed in subsequent chapters.

## Background: MQTT Protocol Architecture

MQTT is a client-server messaging protocol based on a brokered publish-subscribe model. Clients can either publish messages to specific topics or subscribe to topics to receive messages. The broker acts as an intermediary, routing published messages to the appropriate subscribers. This model decouples communication between endpoints and is especially well-suited for environments with intermittent connectivity or limited resources.

Key components of MQTT include the broker, publishers, subscribers, and topics. Topics are structured hierarchically and define the logical channels over which messages are exchanged. MQTT supports three Quality of Service (QoS) levels: 0 (at most once), 1 (at least once), and 2 (exactly once), allowing trade-offs between reliability and efficiency. (Almutairi & Sheldon, 2025)

While the protocol supports TLS for secure communication, it does not require its use. Similarly, authentication mechanisms such as username-password credentials or client certificates are optional and often omitted or misconfigured. These characteristics contribute to the protocol's operational flexibility but simultaneously introduce security weaknesses.

## Vulnerabilities Arising from Default Configurations

One of the primary sources of insecurity in MQTT deployments is the use of default or poorly configured broker settings. Many implementations prioritize ease of setup and operational simplicity over security, resulting in environments where:

- Authentication is disabled or weak
- Access control lists (ACLs) are nonexistent or permissive
- Transport Layer Security (TLS) is not enabled
- Wildcard subscriptions are allowed without restriction
- Message logging and audit trails are turned off

These practices create conditions where malicious actors can easily exploit MQTT-based systems. For instance, a broker that allows anonymous connections and has open topics effectively becomes a shared message board for anyone with network access. Attackers can publish fake telemetry data, subscribe to sensitive information, or disrupt communication flows.

In many cases, administrators are unaware of the exposure created by these configurations. Some brokers even ship with all security features disabled by default. This negligence not only endangers individual devices but also compromises entire IoT infrastructures connected to the broker.

## Protocol-Level Attack Vectors

The design of MQTT opens several avenues for attack. While not flaws in the protocol specification per se, these vectors emerge from how the protocol behaves under insecure conditions.

### Spoofing and Impersonation

Without strong authentication, an attacker can connect to the broker using any client ID. If a legitimate device disconnects and the attacker reconnects with the same ID, they may receive all messages intended for that device. This opens the door to eavesdropping, impersonation, and data manipulation.

### Topic Hijacking

In the absence of strict ACLs, an attacker can subscribe to sensitive topics or publish to control topics used for actuating devices. For example, in an industrial system, publishing to a topic used for motor control could start or stop machinery without authorization. (Elsisi & Bergies, 2025)

### Message Replay

MQTT lacks inherent protections against message replay. Attackers capturing messages on unsecured channels can replay them at a later time. If these messages trigger operations or commands, this could result in duplicated or unintended actions.

### Denial of Service

Brokers with minimal connection limits can be overwhelmed by repeated client connection attempts. Attackers can exploit this by exhausting broker resources using many dummy clients, causing legitimate devices to be denied access.

### Retention and Persistence Abuse

MQTT supports retained messages, where the last message on a topic is stored and sent to new subscribers. Attackers can exploit this by publishing malicious payloads with the retain flag set, causing all new subscribers to immediately receive compromised data. Similarly, persistent session exploitation can allow attackers to accumulate privileges or stale subscriptions over time

## Case Study: Vulnerable Smart Building Deployment

A real-world example illustrates the consequences of poor MQTT security. In a commercial smart building system, MQTT was used to coordinate lighting, HVAC, and security subsystems. The broker was hosted on a cloud virtual machine and allowed anonymous connections over port 1883. No TLS was enforced, and default credentials were used across all device clients.

Security researchers discovered the broker via internet scanning and were able to connect anonymously. They subscribed to various topics and immediately received data on occupancy, temperature, and security sensor status. Worse, they could publish to control topics and toggle HVAC systems remotely. This exposure remained undetected for months, highlighting the dangers of unsecured MQTT usage.

Although this deployment involved no malicious intent, it demonstrates how attackers could have easily gained control over critical infrastructure. The lack of encryption, authentication, and access control created a high-impact vulnerability surface that could have been prevented with basic security hygiene.

## Systemic Challenges in MQTT Security

The vulnerabilities in MQTT deployments are not limited to individual configuration errors. They reflect systemic issues in IoT development and operations. These include:

- Limited cybersecurity expertise among device integrators and operators
- Absence of security testing tools tailored to MQTT deployments
- Pressure to reduce costs and accelerate deployment timelines
- Use of outdated or unsupported MQTT broker implementations
- Lack of regulatory mandates for minimum IoT security standards

Compounding these issues is the difficulty of retrofitting security into legacy systems already in operation. In many cases, devices lack sufficient processing power to handle TLS, or firmware cannot be updated without physical access.

## Enhancing MQTT Security Posture

Securing MQTT requires a multi-layered approach that addresses both protocol-level defenses and operational practices. Recommendations include:

- Enabling TLS with mutual authentication between clients and brokers
- Implementing topic-based access control using granular ACLs
- Enforcing strong client identification and credential management
- Disabling anonymous access and wildcard subscriptions by default
- Using secure retain policies and managing persistent sessions carefully
- Logging all connection and publish/subscribe events for audit
- Segmenting MQTT traffic into dedicated virtual LANs or isolated VPNs
- Keeping broker software up to date and applying patches promptly

Emerging tools can aid in auditing and monitoring MQTT traffic for signs of abuse. Lightweight intrusion detection systems are being developed to recognize anomalous publishing rates, topic misuse, and client churn. The goal is to bring the same visibility and control to MQTT environments that exist in traditional IT networks.

## Toward Secure-by-Design Implementations

Long-term resilience requires MQTT to be deployed as part of a secure-by-design architecture. This involves designing devices and applications with built-in support for authentication, secure boot, encrypted storage, and update mechanisms. Security policies should be enforced from device provisioning through decommissioning.

Vendor guidelines and compliance frameworks are beginning to incorporate MQTT security benchmarks. However, widespread adoption will require collaboration across manufacturers, platform providers, and standardization bodies. By building secure MQTT implementations today, organizations can future-proof their IoT infrastructure against emerging threats and regulatory requirements.(M. Ali et al., 2025)

## CoAP Protocol Security Assessment and Attack Vector Analysis

The Constrained Application Protocol (CoAP) has gained recognition as a powerful lightweight protocol tailored for constrained devices and networks within the Internet of Things (IoT). Designed by the Internet Engineering Task Force (IETF), CoAP enables web-style communication using a compact binary format over the User Datagram Protocol (UDP). Its features are ideal for sensor-based networks where devices have limited processing capacity, energy reserves, and bandwidth. Despite its efficiency, CoAP presents a unique set of security challenges. The protocol's minimalism, while advantageous in performance terms, introduces several potential points of vulnerability when deployed without adequate controls.

This chapter provides an in-depth analysis of CoAP's architecture and identifies security gaps that emerge from its use in real-world applications. Through protocol examination, threat modeling, and review of known exploits, we develop a clear understanding of how CoAP may be attacked and how its security posture can be improved. The discussion sets the foundation for understanding protocol-level resilience and guides the development of secure-by-design CoAP deployments.

## Technical Overview of CoAP Protocol

CoAP is a web transfer protocol that replicates key HTTP functionalities such as GET, POST, PUT, and DELETE but in a form optimized for low-power devices and lossy networks. It supports a RESTful architecture, allowing devices to act as servers or clients. CoAP uses a compact binary message format and typically communicates over UDP to reduce overhead.

CoAP messages include a fixed-length header, optional token, and a variable-length payload. Message types include confirmable, non-confirmable, acknowledgment, and reset, enabling a flexible communication model that balances reliability with efficiency. The protocol is structured to support asynchronous interactions and observe resources, allowing clients to receive updates when sensor values change without repeated polling.

Security support in CoAP is provided through the Datagram Transport Layer Security (DTLS) protocol. DTLS enables encryption, message integrity, and authentication over UDP-based communication. However, the use of DTLS is optional and can be omitted to conserve resources. Furthermore, device manufacturers or system integrators may avoid implementing DTLS due to its perceived complexity, computational cost, or lack of embedded support. This leaves many CoAP-based deployments vulnerable to attacks that are otherwise preventable.(Alabdulatif, 2025)

## Vulnerabilities in CoAP-Based Systems

The vulnerabilities associated with CoAP deployments stem from both its core design and common implementation practices. Below are several security issues that arise when CoAP is deployed without proper protections.

### Lack of Transport Encryption

While CoAP is designed to be used with DTLS, many implementations skip encryption entirely to reduce latency or complexity. This results in messages being transmitted in plaintext, making them susceptible to interception, eavesdropping, and manipulation. In scenarios involving sensitive data transmission such as health metrics or environmental readings, this lack of confidentiality can lead to serious privacy violations.

### Message Spoofing and Forgery

Without authentication and message signing, CoAP messages can be forged by attackers. Devices may accept spoofed confirmable messages and respond to fake requests, leading to incorrect data handling or denial-of-service. Since CoAP is frequently used in critical control loops, a forged message could result in unintended actions such as actuating a valve or triggering an alarm.

### Resource Exhaustion

CoAP's design allows clients to initiate multiple concurrent requests, and devices are required to maintain transaction states during message exchanges. Attackers may exploit this feature by sending a flood of confirmable messages to force resource exhaustion on constrained devices. Since UDP is connectionless, these attacks are difficult to trace and mitigate at the network level.

### Amplification Attacks

CoAP responses are often larger than their corresponding requests. Malicious actors can exploit this asymmetry to carry out amplification attacks, where small requests sent with a spoofed source IP generate large replies directed at a victim. This characteristic has been exploited in distributed denial-of-service (DDoS) campaigns targeting CoAP servers. (Sharma & Shambharkar, 2025)

## Case Example: CoAP Misuse in Smart Metering Systems

An energy utility deployed a CoAP-based communication infrastructure to collect data from thousands of smart electricity meters in a regional grid. The implementation used UDP without DTLS, relying on a private network for security. However, network segmentation was weak, and some devices were reachable from the internet via exposed gateways.

Security researchers discovered that these endpoints were vulnerable to unauthorized access. By querying the resource discovery interface, they mapped meter IDs and resource URIs. They could then spoof POST requests to inject false consumption data. This attack not only corrupted utility records but could have impacted billing and energy load forecasting.

The incident underscored how reliance on network isolation is insufficient and that protocol-level security features must be implemented regardless of perceived perimeter protections.

## Security Gaps in Standard Implementations

Several open-source and commercial CoAP libraries demonstrate inconsistent support for security features. In some cases, DTLS implementations are incomplete or unstable. In others, configuration defaults disable authentication or allow unsafe cipher suites. Many libraries lack comprehensive documentation for enabling security, making it difficult for developers to apply best practices.

Firmware and application code built on these libraries often inherit these limitations. As a result, even when devices advertise support for secure CoAP, the underlying stack may be inadequate or broken. This inconsistency poses a systemic threat to the integrity of CoAP-based ecosystems.

## Mitigation Strategies

To reduce the attack surface and improve the resilience of CoAP deployments, a number of measures should be adopted. These include:

1. Enabling DTLS with strong cipher suites and mutual authentication between endpoints
2. Implementing nonce-based message authentication to prevent forgery and replay
3. Applying strict rate limiting and session tracking to mitigate flood and resource exhaustion attacks
4. Disabling resource discovery in production or restricting access through access control policies
5. Validating incoming payloads against schema and expected message types
6. Logging CoAP transaction metadata for anomaly detection and auditing
7. Using CoAP proxies or gateways that can enforce security policies and isolate constrained devices

Efforts are also underway to define lightweight object security mechanisms for CoAP. One such example is the Object Security for Constrained RESTful Environments (OSCORE) protocol, which provides end-to-end security at the application layer. OSCORE addresses many of the limitations of DTLS and is suitable for multicast, asynchronous, and group communication scenarios. Adoption of OSCORE or similar mechanisms may significantly improve CoAP security in future implementations.

As IoT ecosystems grow more complex and interdependent, isolated protocol vulnerabilities can cascade into system-wide failures. Treating CoAP security as optional or secondary is no longer sustainable. By recognizing and addressing its unique challenges, organizations can make informed decisions and build resilient infrastructure based on CoAP.

# LoRaWAN Security Evaluation and Long-Range Communication Threats

The Long Range Wide Area Network (LoRaWAN) protocol has emerged as one of the most widely adopted communication technologies for Internet of Things (IoT) deployments requiring low-power, long-range connectivity. Its energy efficiency and extended transmission capabilities have made it the protocol of choice for applications ranging from environmental monitoring and agriculture to smart cities and industrial automation. However, despite its suitability for constrained devices and wide-area communication, LoRaWAN presents several security challenges that stem from its design choices, physical layer characteristics, and operational assumptions.

This chapter presents a comprehensive evaluation of LoRaWAN's security model, explores its known weaknesses, and highlights attack vectors that exploit protocol features and deployment misconfigurations. Through technical analysis and real-world observations, the chapter reveals how LoRaWAN deployments are susceptible to both passive and active threats, particularly in environments lacking physical security and robust device authentication.

## Protocol Structure and Security Architecture

LoRaWAN operates on top of the LoRa physical layer, using spread spectrum modulation over unlicensed radio frequencies. The protocol defines communication between end devices and gateways, which relay messages to and from a centralized network server. LoRaWAN's architecture separates the physical network from the application logic, allowing scalable deployment of thousands of devices.

Key components of the architecture include:

- End Devices: Battery-powered sensors and actuators that transmit uplink messages or receive downlink messages.
- Gateways: Devices that forward messages between end devices and the network server over IP.
- Network Server: Centralized logic responsible for device authentication, message deduplication, and network-level routing.
- Application Server: The destination for decrypted messages and the source of control commands.

LoRaWAN incorporates two security layers: one for the network and another for the application. The Network Session Key (NwkSKey) is used to verify the integrity of messages between end devices and the network server, while the Application

Session Key (AppSKey) encrypts and decrypts payloads exchanged between devices and the application server.

Security is enforced through a join procedure. Devices either use Over-the-Air Activation (OTAA) or Activation By Personalization (ABP) to establish session keys. OTAA is considered more secure, as it involves a dynamic key exchange with the network server, while ABP stores keys locally and uses static identifiers that are vulnerable to cloning.

## Known Security Weaknesses

Despite the protocol's built-in cryptographic protections, LoRaWAN faces multiple security limitations in practice. Many of these issues originate from deployment errors, insufficient key management, and reliance on legacy activation methods.

### Static Keys in ABP

Devices activated through ABP use fixed keys and counters, making them vulnerable to replay attacks. If an attacker captures valid messages and reuses them, the receiving device or application may accept them as legitimate. In addition, ABP devices often fail to synchronize counters accurately during power cycles, leading to predictable values that can be exploited.

### Lack of Mutual Authentication

Although LoRaWAN authenticates devices via join requests in OTAA, gateways do not authenticate themselves to the end devices. This allows an adversary to introduce rogue gateways that capture uplink messages or inject malicious downlink responses. Since gateways operate in a non-exclusive mode and merely forward packets, the network lacks a mechanism to verify gateway trustworthiness.

### Payload Confidentiality Limitations

While the AppSKey protects application payloads, metadata such as device address, frame counters, and message types are transmitted in plaintext. This allows passive adversaries to analyze network behavior, infer device types, and map deployment topologies. In many smart city or agricultural deployments, such exposure could reveal sensitive operational details.

## Key Mismanagement

Key distribution and lifecycle management are often poorly implemented. In many deployments, session keys are manually assigned and stored insecurely. Developers sometimes reuse keys across multiple devices to simplify provisioning, which significantly weakens the security of the network. Once a key is compromised, all associated devices become exposed to data injection or interception.

## Physical Attacks and Device Cloning

LoRaWAN end devices are typically deployed in outdoor or unmonitored environments, making them susceptible to physical access. Attackers can extract firmware or keys using side-channel techniques or by exploiting insecure debug interfaces. Once credentials are retrieved, they can be used to clone devices and inject fake data or impersonate legitimate sensors.(Hernandez-Jaimes et al., 2025)

## Threat Landscape and Real-World Attack Scenarios

Several threat scenarios have been demonstrated by researchers and security practitioners that exploit LoRaWAN's weak points.

## Replay and Frame Counter Attacks

In one documented case, researchers captured uplink messages from a smart irrigation system using a software-defined radio. By replaying the messages using spoofed frame counters, they were able to repeatedly trigger irrigation without authorization. The system lacked proper counter synchronization and accepted duplicate messages, resulting in water waste and operational disruption.

## Jamming and Denial of Service

Because LoRaWAN operates over unlicensed bands, it is vulnerable to radio frequency interference. Attackers can disrupt communication by continuously transmitting noise on target channels. Due to its low data rate and long airtime, even short interference bursts can prevent message delivery. This technique can be used to isolate regions of a deployment or prevent specific devices from communicating with the network server.

## Rogue Gateway Injection

A notable attack involves the placement of unauthorized gateways that intercept uplink messages and modify or delay them before forwarding to the network server. If the attacker has control over the application server or can inject false downlink messages, they can manipulate device behavior or inject commands into actuators. The lack of gateway authentication in LoRaWAN permits this type of man-in-the-middle attack.

## Metadata Harvesting and Traffic Analysis

Researchers have shown that even without decrypting payloads, attackers can gather valuable insights by analyzing LoRaWAN metadata. By monitoring frame counters and timestamps, they can determine device uptime, usage patterns, and maintenance intervals. In critical infrastructure settings, this passive intelligence may be used to identify high-value targets or vulnerable periods.

## Mitigation and Hardening Strategies

Improving LoRaWAN security requires a combination of protocol compliance, secure deployment practices, and network monitoring. Recommended measures include:

## Adopt OTAA Exclusively

Deployments should avoid ABP whenever possible and rely exclusively on OTAA with dynamic session key derivation. This reduces exposure to static key exploitation and supports future updates to cryptographic algorithms.

## Enforce Frame Counter Validation

Devices and servers must validate that frame counters increment monotonically and discard duplicates. This protects against replay attacks and enforces message freshness. Devices should retain counter values across reboots or power loss events.

## Implement Gateway Whitelisting

Network servers should only accept traffic from registered gateways with known identifiers and IP addresses. Although this does not provide cryptographic authentication, it limits exposure to unauthorized infrastructure.

## Encrypt Metadata Where Possible

Advanced implementations should consider encrypting or obfuscating metadata such as DevAddr and message types. While LoRaWAN does not mandate such features, proprietary extensions or middleware layers can provide additional confidentiality.

## Enable Firmware Protection

Devices must be protected from physical tampering using secure boot mechanisms, tamper detection, and memory encryption. Debug interfaces should be disabled or password-protected. Devices should support secure firmware updates to allow patching of vulnerabilities post-deployment.(Almutairi & Sheldon, 2025)

## Monitor and Analyze Network Behavior

Operators should employ anomaly detection tools to identify unusual communication patterns, unexpected device activity, or traffic bursts. Combined with geolocation metadata, this allows rapid response to jamming or spoofing attempts.

## Toward a Secure LoRaWAN Ecosystem

LoRaWAN's promise of long-range, energy-efficient connectivity makes it a powerful enabler of large-scale IoT infrastructure. However, its security model requires careful implementation and constant vigilance. As attackers become more familiar with LoRaWAN deployments, reliance on default configurations and static keys will no longer suffice. Secure deployments must embrace best practices, audit their environments, and adapt their architectures to resist evolving threats.

# Emerging Threats and Protocol Vulnerabilities in Smart Environments

Smart environments represent a major evolution in how digital technologies are integrated into physical infrastructure. These environments encompass smart homes, smart cities, smart campuses, and industrial settings where interconnected devices continuously collect, process, and share data to optimize services and automate decision-making. The foundation of these systems lies in lightweight communication protocols that allow seamless interaction between constrained devices, centralized services, and user interfaces. However, the increasing complexity, heterogeneity, and scale of smart environments also introduce a host of emerging security threats.

This chapter explores the evolving threat landscape in smart environments by analyzing how protocol-level vulnerabilities are exploited by attackers. It identifies key systemic weaknesses in protocol deployment, contextualizes threats across use cases, and highlights the security gaps that must be addressed to ensure operational resilience.

## Protocol Exposure in Smart Infrastructure

In smart environments, a wide variety of devices including sensors, controllers, gateways, and cloud-based systems must communicate efficiently and reliably. Lightweight protocols such as MQTT, CoAP, and LoRaWAN are widely used due to their low power consumption, reduced bandwidth requirements, and architectural simplicity. These protocols enable real-time telemetry, remote control, and event-driven automation across distributed systems.

However, the same characteristics that support scalability and responsiveness also create exposure to adversaries. Lightweight protocols are often deployed without sufficient authentication, encryption, or access control. Devices may communicate over public networks, rely on weak keys, or use default credentials. In the absence of protocol-level security, the entire smart infrastructure can be compromised through relatively simple attacks.

## The Problem of Context-Agnostic Protocols

Most lightweight IoT protocols were not originally designed with application context in mind. For example, MQTT brokers handle all topics equally, regardless of whether the messages control lights or actuate emergency shutdown systems. Similarly, CoAP does not differentiate between low-priority environmental data and commands to industrial actuators. This lack of context awareness in protocol logic allows attackers to exploit uniform mechanisms for very different purposes.

A compromised client can misuse general-purpose protocols to inject commands, replay messages, or exfiltrate data. Since protocols do not validate the intent or criticality of transmitted messages, it becomes difficult to enforce policy or detect malicious behavior at the protocol layer alone. Smart environments that depend on autonomous responses may thus act on manipulated inputs without human oversight.

## Emerging Threat Vectors

As smart environments evolve, attackers adapt their methods to exploit new weaknesses. Below are several threat vectors that are increasingly prevalent in the modern landscape.

### Command Injection via Lightweight Protocols

Attackers have been able to manipulate MQTT and CoAP payloads to issue unauthorized commands to actuators in smart buildings, such as opening locks, disabling alarms, or switching off lighting in critical areas. In one example, malicious actors subscribed to public broker topics and waited for control commands. After learning the structure and sequence of legitimate messages, they injected forged messages to impersonate authorized devices.

### Credential Harvesting in Public Networks

Devices that communicate over unsecured networks using plaintext protocols can leak sensitive credentials, session tokens, or configuration data. In smart city deployments, street-level devices often connect through public Wi-Fi or cellular backhaul without encrypted channels. Sniffing tools can easily capture credentials that are reused across multiple devices, granting attackers access to entire segments of infrastructure.

### Multi-Protocol Exploitation

Smart environments frequently use multiple lightweight protocols within the same ecosystem. A gateway may support MQTT for data uplink and CoAP for control signals. Attackers can exploit inconsistencies between these protocols, such as injecting commands in one channel while spoofing device identity in another. The lack of unified identity and session management across protocols enables lateral movement within the network.

### Data Poisoning and Feedback Loop Manipulation

Autonomous systems that depend on real-time sensor inputs are vulnerable to data poisoning. By injecting fake or manipulated data into the protocol stream, attackers can disrupt feedback loops. For instance, a fake high-temperature reading could cause an HVAC system to overcool a building, resulting in energy waste or equipment strain. The simplicity of MQTT and CoAP payloads makes it easy to mimic legitimate data without raising immediate suspicion.

### Insecure Over-the-Air Updates

Smart environments often rely on remote firmware or configuration updates, delivered through lightweight protocols. Insecure update mechanisms can be hijacked to deploy malicious code. For example, an attacker who gains access to the MQTT topic used for updates can publish a forged update payload to multiple devices. Without signature validation or source authentication, devices may apply the malicious update automatically.

## Systemic Vulnerabilities Across Smart Environments

The threat vectors described above are compounded by systemic vulnerabilities in how smart environments are designed and managed. These vulnerabilities include:

### Inconsistent Security Policies

Smart environments often integrate devices from multiple vendors, each with its own implementation of protocols and security features. The result is a patchwork of inconsistent configurations, weak access control, and incompatible encryption schemes. Devices may support TLS, DTLS, or none at all, and network administrators may lack the tools to enforce security uniformly across the environment.

### Limited Device Visibility

As the number of devices scales into the thousands, maintaining visibility into each endpoint becomes difficult. Many lightweight devices do not support real-time monitoring or log generation. This makes it challenging to detect anomalous behavior or trace the origin of an attack. A compromised sensor may continue operating undetected while feeding malicious data into control systems.

### Lack of Device Identity Management

Most lightweight protocols do not include built-in device identity or provenance verification. Devices are identified by arbitrary IDs or network addresses, which can be spoofed. Without a strong identity management framework, it becomes impossible to verify the source of critical commands or telemetry. This undermines the trustworthiness of the system and enables impersonation attacks.

### Poor Patch Management

Devices in smart environments may lack support for secure remote updates or may be deployed in locations that are difficult to access physically. As a result, vulnerabilities in protocol stacks or firmware remain unpatched for years. Attackers can target known flaws in outdated software that remains in active use.

## Use Case: Smart Campus Building Automation System

A university deployed a smart building system that used MQTT to manage lighting, HVAC, and access control. Each floor was equipped with sensors and actuators connected through wireless gateways. While the system used TLS on external connections, internal traffic was unencrypted. An attacker connected to the campus network and used a packet sniffer to identify MQTT traffic.

By reverse-engineering topic names and message formats, the attacker subscribed to control topics and observed the sequence of commands used to unlock doors and adjust thermostats. They then injected their own commands, successfully bypassing access restrictions and adjusting climate settings in lecture halls. The breach went unnoticed for days due to the absence of device-level logging and access audits.

This scenario illustrates how lightweight protocol misuse can lead to unauthorized control of critical systems. It also demonstrates the importance of securing internal communication channels, monitoring traffic patterns, and implementing role-based access control.

## Toward Secure Protocol Integration in Smart Environments

To defend against these emerging threats, smart environments must adopt security as a core design principle rather than an afterthought. This involves standardizing secure configurations across protocols, enforcing encryption and authentication by default, and ensuring compatibility between systems.

Developers and integrators must design communication flows that validate identity, context, and intent. Devices should be provisioned with unique credentials, session keys, and digital signatures to prevent spoofing. Gateways and brokers must implement access control and anomaly detection to block unauthorized traffic and flag unusual behavior.

Security monitoring should extend across the full protocol stack, from message headers to payload semantics. Real-time traffic analysis and machine learning-based intrusion detection can help identify anomalies that indicate protocol abuse or coordinated attacks.

By adopting a proactive and layered approach to protocol security, smart environments can resist a broader spectrum of adversarial techniques. This ensures that the efficiency and convenience offered by lightweight communication technologies do not come at the expense of reliability and safety.

## Designing Resilient Architectures Using Secure Lightweight Protocols

The rapid deployment of Internet of Things (IoT) systems across industries has created a critical need for secure and resilient communication infrastructures. Lightweight protocols such as MQTT, CoAP, and LoRaWAN are commonly used in these systems due to their suitability for constrained environments. However, these protocols are often implemented without sufficient attention to secure architecture design, resulting in vulnerabilities that compromise system integrity, availability, and confidentiality.

This chapter presents principles and practical strategies for designing resilient architectures that incorporate lightweight protocols securely. It explores layered defense mechanisms, architectural patterns, and real-world practices that strengthen protocol usage across device, network, and application layers. By embedding security into every layer of system architecture, developers can mitigate common attack vectors and ensure that IoT deployments remain robust under operational and adversarial conditions.

## Design Principles for Resilience in Constrained Networks

Designing a secure and resilient system begins with a set of core principles that guide the structure and interaction of system components. These principles serve as the foundation for building layered security mechanisms that compensate for limitations in individual protocol capabilities.

### Defense in Depth

The defense-in-depth approach layers multiple protective measures across the architecture to ensure that the failure of one control does not compromise the entire system. For lightweight protocols, this involves implementing encryption, access control, monitoring, and physical safeguards at different levels of the communication stack.

### Least Privilege

Every device, user, and application should operate with the minimum set of permissions necessary for its function. For instance, a sensor node that only sends temperature data should not have the ability to execute remote control commands. Using access control lists (ACLs) in MQTT brokers or role-based permissions in CoAP gateways enforces this principle.

### Segmentation and Isolation

Logical and physical separation of communication channels reduces the blast radius of security breaches. Network segmentation using VLANs, firewalls, or protocol gateways prevents unauthorized traffic from propagating laterally. Isolating critical devices from public-facing services limits their exposure to external threats.

### Redundancy and Failover

To maintain availability during attacks or outages, resilient architectures incorporate redundancy in communication paths, brokers, and edge nodes. Protocol implementations should support automatic reconnection, message retries, and state persistence to recover gracefully from disruptions.

### Monitoring and Observability

Resilience depends not only on prevention but also on detection and response. Architectures should include logging, telemetry, and alerting mechanisms that track protocol usage, message anomalies, and device behavior. These observability features are critical for identifying active threats and recovering from incidents.

## Secure Device Bootstrapping and Provisioning

A critical phase in any IoT deployment is the onboarding of new devices. Secure bootstrapping ensures that devices are authenticated and configured correctly from the outset. For lightweight protocol environments, this involves generating and distributing keys securely, verifying device identity, and limiting the use of static credentials.

Protocols such as LoRaWAN with Over-the-Air Activation (OTAA) offer better security than Activation by Personalization (ABP) due to their dynamic session key generation. In MQTT, pre-shared keys or client certificates can be used during Transport Layer Security (TLS) handshake for mutual authentication. Provisioning platforms must include mechanisms for secure credential injection, revocation, and rotation to accommodate the device life cycle.

## Gateway-Centric Security Enforcement

Given the resource constraints of end devices, security responsibilities are often delegated to gateways. These intermediary devices can act as enforcement points for protocol security, handling authentication, message filtering, encryption, and traffic shaping.

Gateways should terminate and re-encrypt insecure protocol traffic, validate payload formats, and enforce topic-level or URI-level access policies. They can also serve as telemetry aggregators, forwarding metadata and usage statistics to security information and event management (SIEM) platforms for analysis.

By positioning gateways as control points, architectures benefit from a balance between scalability and protection without overburdening constrained endpoints.

## Protocol Proxying and Edge Intelligence

To enhance resilience further, architectures may incorporate proxying and edge computing techniques. In this model, lightweight protocol traffic is terminated at an edge proxy or edge analytics node, where additional logic is applied. This includes anomaly detection, message validation, normalization, and caching.

For instance, MQTT messages arriving at an edge proxy can be sanitized and inspected for rate anomalies before being forwarded upstream. CoAP requests can be proxied with replay protection, and LoRaWAN gateways can apply geolocation validation to verify device movement patterns.

Edge intelligence not only increases resilience by offloading processing from cloud services but also reduces latency and improves detection response times for localized threats.

## Secure Communication Patterns

Architectures should enforce secure communication patterns by default. This includes:

- Encrypted Transport: Use TLS or DTLS for all MQTT and CoAP traffic, even within local networks.
- Payload Signing: In cases where end-to-end encryption is not feasible, digitally signing payloads ensures integrity and non-repudiation.

- Session Control: Limit session duration and rotate session keys periodically to reduce exposure.
- Message Authentication Codes (MACs): Apply MACs to prevent message tampering or spoofing.
- Anti-Replay Mechanisms: Use counters, timestamps, or nonces to prevent replay attacks on critical control commands.

## Architectural Pattern: Secure Smart Agriculture Network

Consider a smart agriculture deployment that uses LoRaWAN for field sensor communication, MQTT for gateway-to-cloud uplink, and CoAP for irrigation control. A resilient architecture integrates security across each segment as follows:

1. LoRaWAN sensors use OTAA to securely join the network. Device keys are stored in tamper-resistant hardware and rotated periodically.
2. Gateways validate device identity and detect frame counter anomalies. They report unusual message timing or geolocation mismatches to the central dashboard.
3. MQTT brokers enforce TLS with client certificates. Each device has a unique certificate and publishes to a restricted set of topics based on its function.
4. CoAP-based actuators use DTLS with mutual authentication. All commands are validated using payload signatures before execution.
5. Gateways proxy CoAP and MQTT traffic through edge analytics nodes that normalize data, apply business rules, and detect out-of-policy behavior.
6. A centralized SIEM system collects logs from gateways, brokers, and proxies. It uses machine learning to detect anomalies such as sudden message floods, new topic usage, or off-hour activity.
7. An update management platform ensures firmware for all devices is signed, validated, and delivered securely.

This architecture demonstrates how layering secure protocol usage within an integrated framework protects against both internal and external threats.

## Secure Configuration and Maintenance

Resilient architectures must also support ongoing maintenance, updates, and audits. Configuration management systems should maintain inventory of all deployed devices, protocol versions, cryptographic keys, and policy settings. Configuration drift and undocumented changes pose risks that compromise security integrity.

Patch management systems should support over-the-air (OTA) updates that are cryptographically signed and version-verified. Automated update policies can ensure that security patches are applied across fleets without requiring manual intervention. Logging and version tracking help maintain compliance with organizational and regulatory standards.

Security testing and verification should be integrated into development and deployment pipelines. Protocol simulators, fuzzers, and penetration testing frameworks can be used to identify weaknesses before they reach production environments.

### Future-Proofing with Modular Design

Resilient architectures should also be modular to accommodate protocol upgrades and evolving threat models. By abstracting protocol interfaces behind service APIs or middleware components, organizations can replace or upgrade communication stacks without affecting business logic.

For example, a CoAP-based communication module can be replaced with a secure gRPC implementation or upgraded to support OSCORE without rewriting application logic. This abstraction decouples protocol choice from functionality and allows systems to adapt to advances in protocol security over time.

## EVALUATION METRICS AND PERFORMANCE IMPACT OF SECURITY ENHANCEMENTS

### Introduction

The integration of security mechanisms in lightweight IoT protocols is essential for protecting data confidentiality, ensuring message integrity, and enforcing access control. However, these enhancements often introduce computational and communication overhead that can impact system performance, especially in constrained environments. Evaluating this trade-off is a critical step in designing secure and efficient IoT systems.

This chapter presents a comprehensive framework for evaluating the performance impact of security enhancements applied to lightweight communication protocols. It discusses key performance indicators, experimental methodologies, and benchmarking tools. Through comparative analysis, the chapter also highlights how various security configurations affect latency, memory usage, energy consumption, and throughput. Understanding these trade-offs allows practitioners to make informed decisions when selecting security measures for real-world deployments.

## Framework for Security Evaluation

To assess the impact of security features, a structured evaluation framework is necessary. This framework should include:

- Definition of baseline performance using unsecured protocol implementations
- Identification of security configurations under test (e.g., TLS, DTLS, MAC, encryption, authentication)
- Measurement of protocol-level and system-level performance indicators
- Analysis of variance across device classes, network conditions, and message types

The evaluation must be conducted in conditions that reflect real-world operating environments. Tests should include both synthetic loads (e.g., simulated message floods) and operational traffic patterns typical of smart homes, cities, or industrial automation. Devices used in testing should represent a range of computational capabilities, from microcontrollers to gateway-class hardware.

## Key Performance Metrics

Several metrics are critical for evaluating the performance of lightweight protocols with and without security features. These metrics can be grouped into communication overhead, computational cost, energy usage, and latency.

### Latency

Latency refers to the time required for a message to be transmitted from sender to receiver and acknowledged, if applicable. Security features such as encryption, key negotiation, and message signing increase this time due to processing and handshake overhead. For time-sensitive applications such as remote actuation or real-time monitoring, added latency may be unacceptable.(Elsisi & Bergies, 2025)

### Troughput

Throughput measures the number of successful message transactions per unit of time. Cryptographic processing and increased message size due to added headers can reduce throughput. Protocols like CoAP, which operate over UDP, may be more sensitive to processing delays than MQTT, which runs over TCP.

## CPU Utilization

Lightweight devices have limited processing power. The use of public-key cryptography, mutual authentication, or digital signing can increase CPU load significantly. Evaluation should measure peak and average CPU usage during different protocol operations to identify potential bottlenecks.

## Memory Footprint

Security libraries and protocol stacks consume RAM and flash storage. The size of encryption buffers, key storage, and session state tables must be quantified, especially on microcontrollers with 64 KB or less RAM. Excessive memory usage may lead to device instability or crash under load.

## Energy Consumption

Battery-powered devices must optimize energy usage. Each cryptographic operation, message retransmission, or handshake affects battery life. Evaluations should include current consumption measurements during idle, transmission, and secure handshake phases.

## **Packet Size and Bandwidth**

An evaluation testbed typically consists of three layers: endpoint devices (e.g., sensors or actuators), edge gateways, and a central server. The testbed is instrumented with software tools to collect and analyze performance data.(Rawat et al., 2025)

Tools such as Wireshark can be used to capture and analyze packet-level metrics. Embedded OS instrumentation (e.g., FreeRTOS trace hooks) can monitor CPU and memory usage. Power measurement tools such as Monsoon Power Monitor or Joulescope capture real-time current draw for energy profiling.

Test scenarios should include:

- Unsecured communication (baseline)
- Basic authentication (e.g., username-password or pre-shared keys)
- Encrypted channels (TLS/DTLS)
- Payload signing with symmetric or asymmetric cryptography
- Full-stack protection with encryption, authentication, and replay prevention

## Experimental Results: Protocol Comparisons

To illustrate trade-offs, consider a comparison of CoAP and MQTT implementations using DTLS and TLS respectively on a 32-bit ARM Cortex-M4 device with 128 KB RAM. Messages were transmitted at 10-second intervals over Wi-Fi to a local broker or server.

### Scenario A: MQTT with TLS (Client Authentication Disabled)

- CPU utilization increased from 8% (baseline) to 18%
- RAM usage grew by 14 KB due to TLS stack
- Average latency rose by 120 ms
- Packet size increased from 220 to 390 bytes
- Energy consumption increased by 23% per message
- Throughput decreased by 12% compared to baseline

### Scenario B: CoAP with DTLS and Mutual Authentication

- CPU utilization increased from 6% to 22%
- RAM usage grew by 22 KB
- Latency increased by 180 ms
- Payload success rate dropped under 80% when signal strength decreased
- Battery life estimate reduced by 28% under constant message load

### Scenario C: CoAP with OSCORE (Object Security)

- Lower RAM footprint than DTLS by 30%
- Latency increased only by 60 ms
- Energy impact minimal due to efficient symmetric encryption
- Security persisted across proxy routing and multicast
- Most suitable for constrained group communication

## Trade-Off Analysis

The results indicate that while TLS and DTLS offer strong protection, they introduce significant latency and resource overhead. Devices operating on low-frequency networks or using small batteries may not tolerate these impacts. OSCORE and similar lightweight application-layer security models offer better efficiency, particularly when end-to-end security is needed without always-on session management. (Sharma & Shambharkar, 2025)

Symmetric cryptography (e.g., AES-CMAC, HMAC) is more energy-efficient than asymmetric schemes (e.g., RSA, ECDSA) and should be preferred for constrained endpoints. However, asymmetric methods remain necessary during key exchange or firmware verification.

Security feature selection should depend on:

- Device class and resource availability
- Network reliability and bandwidth constraints
- Required security guarantees (e.g., confidentiality vs. integrity only)
- Regulatory compliance and auditability
- Expected lifespan and update capability of the system

## Adaptive Security Strategies

One emerging approach is to implement adaptive security mechanisms that scale based on device state or operating conditions. For example:

- Devices may start with full authentication during bootstrapping but fall back to lightweight MAC verification during routine data transmission
- Protocol stacks may adjust cipher suite strength based on power availability or signal strength
- Gateways may proxy and offload heavy cryptographic operations on behalf of constrained clients

These strategies allow systems to balance protection and performance dynamically, improving resilience without exhausting device resources.

## Guidance for Protocol Developers

Protocol designers and library developers should support modular security stacks that allow selective enabling of features. Developers should:

- Provide lightweight cipher suites optimized for embedded use
- Implement pre-shared key (PSK) profiles that avoid certificate chains
- Expose API hooks for application-layer security customization
- Ensure interoperability testing with major gateway and cloud platforms

Documentation should include clear benchmarks and configuration guidance for developers targeting various device classes

## Toward a Unified Security Framework for Lightweight IoT Protocols

The increasing ubiquity of lightweight communication protocols in IoT systems has led to a profound transformation in how devices interact, exchange data, and make autonomous decisions. Protocols such as MQTT, CoAP, and LoRaWAN have empowered innovation in areas including smart homes, industrial automation, healthcare, and environmental monitoring. Yet, the growing dependence on these protocols exposes organizations to evolving cybersecurity risks. Security in lightweight IoT communication has historically been addressed in a fragmented and ad hoc manner, with inconsistent implementations, varying cryptographic policies, and limited interoperability.

This chapter proposes a unified security framework that provides a cohesive, standards-aligned, and modular approach to securing lightweight protocols. It integrates the lessons, analyses, and evaluations presented in earlier chapters to form a practical model for enhancing the resilience of protocol deployments across heterogeneous environments. The chapter also offers policy recommendations, architectural alignment strategies, and final reflections on the role of protocol security in sustainable IoT growth.

## Rationale for a Unified Framework

The fragmentation of security practices across IoT protocols presents significant challenges:

- Devices from different vendors implement the same protocol differently, leading to unpredictable behavior
- Security measures such as encryption or authentication are applied inconsistently across the stack
- Developers and system integrators lack clear guidance on selecting and combining security features
- Protocols lack a common interface for interoperable security configuration and policy enforcement

A unified framework addresses these gaps by establishing a structured security architecture that can be applied across protocol types, device classes, and use cases.

It provides a foundation for standardization, automation, and certification while preserving the lightweight nature of underlying protocols.

## Core Components of the Framework

The proposed framework consists of six integrated layers that work in concert:

1. Identity and Provisioning Layer

This layer establishes device identity through digital certificates, pre-shared keys, or secure element integration. It supports secure bootstrapping, device onboarding, and credential management. The layer ensures that each endpoint is uniquely identifiable and traceable.

2. Transport Security Layer

Protocols operating over IP or radio links are secured using appropriate transport mechanisms such as TLS, DTLS, or OSCORE. The framework enforces mandatory encryption and authentication for all bidirectional communication unless constrained by strict hardware limits. Cipher suite negotiation and key exchange mechanisms are modular.

3. Application Layer Security

To ensure end-to-end integrity and confidentiality, application payloads are signed and optionally encrypted. This allows messages to traverse untrusted intermediaries such as proxies or brokers without loss of trust. Standardized payload encryption formats are encouraged for cross-vendor interoperability.

4. Access Control and Policy Management

Access is governed by role-based access control (RBAC) or attribute-based access control (ABAC). Each device or service is associated with a set of permissions based on function, context, and sensitivity. Policies can be enforced at the gateway, broker, or cloud interface levels.

5. Threat Detection and Monitoring

A distributed security monitoring subsystem collects protocol metadata, device logs, and network telemetry for real-time analysis. Anomaly detection algorithms identify behavioral deviations, while dashboards provide visibility into attack surfaces, system health, and compliance.

6. Update and Recovery Layer

This layer supports secure firmware and configuration updates via digitally signed packages. It also defines rollback procedures, patch verification, and lifecycle management protocols to maintain long-term system security.

## Integration Strategy for Heterogeneous Protocols

The framework promotes protocol-agnostic integration by abstracting security responsibilities from the protocol logic. Each layer can be implemented as a service module that interfaces with the underlying protocol stack. For example:

- MQTT brokers integrate access control, TLS support, and logging extensions via plug-ins
- CoAP stacks support DTLS or OSCORE with key storage modules
- LoRaWAN gateways apply frame counter validation and forward logs to monitoring services
- Proxy servers enforce application-layer validation for all inbound and outbound traffic

This modular architecture allows developers to implement consistent security behavior across different communication channels without rewriting protocol-specific code.

## Standardization and Compliance Alignment

To support broad adoption, the unified framework should align with existing industry standards and regulatory requirements. These include:

- ISO/IEC 30141: Reference Architecture for IoT
- IETF RFCs for CoAP (RFC 7252), MQTT (ISO/IEC 20922), and LoRaWAN (LoRa Alliance specifications)
- ETSI TS 103 645: Cybersecurity for Consumer IoT
- NIST SP 800-213 and SP 800-82 for securing industrial control systems and IoT devices

By mapping framework components to standard controls, organizations can simplify audits, streamline certification processes, and demonstrate conformance with data protection laws such as GDPR and HIPAA.

## Policy Guidelines and Best Practices

To operationalize the framework, organizations should implement a set of core policies:

- All device communications must be encrypted and authenticated unless explicitly exempted
- Device credentials must be unique, securely stored, and periodically rotated
- Security configurations should be automated during provisioning, with templates based on device type and risk profile
- All protocol activity must be logged and retained for forensic analysis
- All devices must support secure updates, and patches should be deployed within defined service-level agreements
- Anomaly detection thresholds and alert channels must be defined and tested periodically

These guidelines should be adapted based on system scale, criticality, and environmental constraints.

## Future Directions

As IoT ecosystems continue to expand, the need for autonomous and self-adapting security architectures will grow. The proposed framework lays the foundation for emerging directions, including:

- AI-driven adaptive security that adjusts controls based on behavior and context
- Blockchain-based credential verification and device identity management
- Quantum-resistant cryptographic primitives for long-term confidentiality
- Zero-trust architectures where trust is continuously evaluated based on telemetry and policy

Incorporating these trends into the unified framework will enable next-generation IoT systems to remain secure under evolving threat landscapes.

## General Conclusion

The progression from vulnerability to resilience in lightweight IoT protocols is not simply a technical journey but also an architectural and organizational one. Throughout this book, we examined the structure and security properties of protocols such as CoAP, MQTT, and LoRaWAN. We explored their vulnerabilities, assessed the impact of integrating security features, and proposed robust architectural patterns to mitigate threats.

The lessons drawn across eight chapters highlight the complexity of securing distributed, resource-constrained systems. Protocols that prioritize efficiency must be complemented with security frameworks that are equally lightweight yet comprehensive. The proposed unified security framework brings together identity management, transport protection, policy enforcement, and observability in a modular and scalable structure.(M. Ali et al., 2025)

Security in IoT must no longer be an afterthought or optional feature. As smart environments grow increasingly critical to economic, environmental, and societal functions, the resilience of communication protocols becomes paramount. By adopting standardized, layered, and integrated security strategies, we can ensure that the potential of lightweight IoT protocols is realized without compromising safety or trust.

## REFERENCES


Al-Na'amneh, Q., Hazaymih, R., Al-Harasis, T., Almaiah, M., Aljawarneh, M., Qadoumi, B., & Shah, S. M. (2025). Enhancing IoT security RPL attack detection using sine cosine algorithm with XGBoost. In *Cryptography* (pp. 1–28). Biometrics, and Anonymity in Cybersecurity Management., DOI: 10.4018/979-8-3693-8014-7.ch001

Alabdulatif, A. (2025). A Novel Ensemble of Deep Learning Approach for Cybersecurity Intrusion Detection with Explainable Artificial Intelligence. *Applied Sciences (Basel, Switzerland)*, *15*(14), 7984. Advance online publication. DOI: 10.3390/app15147984

Ali, M., Saleem, Y., Hina, S., & Shah, G. A. (2025). DDoSViT: IoT DDoS attack detection for fortifying firmware Over-The-Air (OTA) updates using vision transformer. *Internet of Things : Engineering Cyber Physical Human Systems*, *30*, 101527. Advance online publication. DOI: 10.1016/j.iot.2025.101527

Almutairi, M., & Sheldon, F. T. (2025). IoT–Cloud Integration Security: A Survey of Challenges, Solutions, and Directions. *Electronics (Basel)*, *14*(7), 1394. Advance online publication. DOI: 10.3390/electronics14071394

Alzahrani, A. I. A. (2025). Exploring AI and quantum computing synergies in holographic counterpart frameworks for IoT security and privacy. *The Journal of Supercomputing*, *81*(11), 1194. Advance online publication. DOI: 10.1007/s11227-025-07682-0

Elsisi, M., & Bergies, S. (2025). A robust IoT architecture for smart inverters in microgrids using hybrid deep learning and signal processing against adversarial attacks. *Internet of Things : Engineering Cyber Physical Human Systems*, *31*, 101576. Advance online publication. DOI: 10.1016/j.iot.2025.101576

Hernandez-Jaimes, M. L., Martinez-Cruz, A., Ramírez-Gutiérrez, K. A., & Morales-Reyes, A. (2025). Network traffic inspection to enhance anomaly detection in the Internet of Things using attention-driven Deep Learning. *Integration (Amsterdam)*, *103*, 102398. Advance online publication. DOI: 10.1016/j.vlsi.2025.102398

Jamwal, Y., Kumari, P., Mishra, A., Goel, N., & Goswami, M. (2025). Security challenges and solutions in IoT: Analyzing threats, architectures, and policies. In *Hardware Security* (pp. 215–238). Challenges and Solutions., DOI: 10.1007/978-3-031-81213-2_10

Rawat, R. S., Diwakar, M., Garg, U., & Srivastava, P. (2025). Developing an Intelligent System for Efficient Botnet Detection in IoT Environment. *International Journal of Mathematical. Engineering and Management Sciences*, *10*(2), 537–553. DOI: 10.33889/IJMEMS.2025.10.2.027

Sharma, N., & Shambharkar, P. G. (2025). Transforming security in internet of medical things with advanced deep learning-based intrusion detection frameworks. *Applied Soft Computing*, *180*, 113420. Advance online publication. DOI: 10.1016/j.asoc.2025.113420

# Chapter 4
# Zero Trust Architecture in Healthcare IoT

**Arnika Jain**
https://orcid.org/0000-0001-9527-2209
*Manav Rachna University, Faridabad, India*

**Pramod Kumar Sagar**
https://orcid.org/0009-0009-7979-2939
*Raj Kumar Goel Institute of Technology, Ghaziabad, India*

**Anu Chaudhary**
*Ajay Kumar Garg Engineering College, Ghaziabad, India*

**Pawan Kumar Goel**
https://orcid.org/0000-0003-3601-102X
*Raj Kumar Goel Institute of Science and Technology, Ghaziabad, India*

## ABSTRACT

*The exponential growth of Healthcare Internet of Things (H-IoT) technologies has introduced unprecedented opportunities for patient monitoring, diagnostics, and operational efficiency. However, these advancements have also magnified the cybersecurity risks inherent in distributed, device-rich environments. Traditional perimeter-based security models have proven inadequate in addressing the evolving threat landscape, necessitating the implementation of Zero Trust Architecture (ZTA), which adheres to the principle of "never trust, always verify." In this chapter the applicability of ZTA in H-IoT settings has been critically analyzed, with focus placed on its core principles—least privilege access, micro-segmentation, continuous monitoring, and context-aware policy enforcement. Implementation strategies such as dynamic access control, software-defined segmentation, and machine learning-based anomaly detection have been discussed to offer a comprehensive security posture.*

DOI: 10.4018/979-8-3373-7610-3.ch004

## 1. INTRODUCTION

The evolution of the Internet of Things (IoT) has revolutionized healthcare by enabling continuous monitoring, remote diagnostics, and intelligent data-driven decision-making. Healthcare IoT (H-IoT) encompasses interconnected medical devices, wearables, sensors, and cloud-based analytics platforms, all working together to enhance patient outcomes and operational efficiency. However, the proliferation of these interconnected systems introduces significant security challenges. Traditional perimeter-based security models are insufficient in addressing the dynamic, distributed, and heterogeneous nature of H-IoT systems. This necessitates the adoption of a more robust, identity-centric security framework — the Zero Trust Architecture (ZTA) (Chen et al, 2020).

Zero Trust is a cybersecurity paradigm centered on the principle of "never trust, always verify." It assumes that threats can originate from inside or outside the network and therefore mandates strict access controls and continuous verification of every device, user, and network flow. This chapter explores the application of Zero Trust Architecture in Healthcare IoT, examining the motivations, architectural models, implementation strategies, and future directions.

## 2. NEED FOR ZERO TRUST IN HEALTHCARE IoT

### 2.1 Rising Threat Landscape

The healthcare sector is increasingly targeted by cybercriminals due to the high value of medical data, the sensitivity of patient records, and the critical nature of healthcare operations. Patient health records, insurance details, genomic data, and clinical trial information hold immense monetary and strategic value on the black market, making healthcare organizations prime targets for cybercrime. Furthermore, the increasing adoption of connected devices such as wearable monitors, infusion pumps, and smart diagnostic tools introduces an ever-expanding digital footprint that is often undersecured. Many of these Healthcare IoT (H-IoT) devices are designed with minimal security features to prioritize usability and cost-efficiency, making them highly vulnerable to exploitation.

High-profile ransomware attacks have paralyzed hospital operations, delayed surgeries, and jeopardized patient safety. Attackers exploit vulnerabilities in unpatched software, unsecured network protocols, and poorly segmented systems. Unauthorized access to patient monitoring devices can enable malicious actors to manipulate vital signs or intercept real-time data streams, leading to severe clinical and legal consequences. As these devices operate in critical care settings, even a momentary disruption can pose life-threatening risks (Maji et al., 2025).

Traditional network security approaches, which rely on a hardened perimeter and implicit trust within the internal network, are no longer sufficient to deal with the scale and sophistication of modern threats. These outdated models assume that actors inside the network are trustworthy, ignoring the fact that many attacks now originate from compromised internal systems or malicious insiders. Moreover, with the increased integration of third-party vendors, cloud services, and remote access tools, the concept of a fixed security boundary has effectively dissolved. Therefore, healthcare institutions must transition to a more resilient and adaptive security posture that emphasizes continual verification, strict access controls, and contextual risk assessment at every interaction point — the foundational principles of Zero Trust Architecture.

## 2.2 Challenges of Traditional Security Models

Perimeter-based models assume that everything inside the network can be trusted. This assumption fundamentally breaks down in a distributed environment like Healthcare IoT (H-IoT), where medical devices, wearables, sensors, and gateways are spread across various physical and logical boundaries — such as hospital departments, remote clinics, patient homes, and mobile health units (Kumar et al., 2023). This geographical and functional dispersion greatly increases the complexity of enforcing centralized security policies and creates numerous blind spots where attackers can infiltrate undetected.

Additionally, many H-IoT devices operate on lightweight operating systems and have limited computational power, memory, and battery life. These constraints make it impractical to deploy conventional endpoint security tools like antivirus software, intrusion detection systems, or full-disk encryption. Compounding the issue is the presence of legacy systems that were not designed with modern security standards in mind, making them susceptible to vulnerabilities and difficult to update or patch (Ali et al., 2025).

The increasing reliance on remote patient monitoring, cloud-based EHR systems, and mobile applications further expands the attack surface. Data now flows through diverse channels, from edge devices to centralized analytics platforms, making it imperative to monitor and control access at every point in the communication chain. These limitations highlight the need for a paradigm shift — moving away from static trust boundaries and toward a dynamic model that continuously verifies the legitimacy of every access request, regardless of its origin or location (Adil et al., 2024). Zero Trust Architecture offers this exact capability by enforcing a security-first approach that evaluates user identity, device posture, access context, and behavior before allowing any interaction with sensitive systems or data.

## 3. PRINCIPLES OF ZERO TRUST ARCHITECTURE

Zero Trust Architecture (ZTA) is founded upon a fundamental rethinking of traditional network security practices (Edo et al., 2024). It challenges the long-standing assumption that everything inside a network perimeter can be trusted. Instead, ZTA operates on the premise that trust must be continuously earned and never automatically granted. This security model is especially relevant in dynamic and heterogeneous environments like Healthcare IoT (H-IoT), where users, devices, and applications frequently interact across organizational boundaries. The shift to Zero Trust ensures that no user or device—regardless of whether it resides inside or outside the organization's physical network—has access to resources without explicit, context-aware authorization (Sultana et al., 2020).

As shown in figure 1, a core principle of ZTA is Least Privilege Access, which stipulates that users and devices should be granted the minimum level of access required to perform their duties. By minimizing the number of permissions, organizations reduce the risk of misuse or exploitation of elevated privileges. In a hospital setting, this could mean that a nurse has access to patient monitoring dashboards but not to administrative system configurations (Sammartino & Baiardi, 2024). Least privilege enforcement reduces the attack surface and limits the damage that could result from a compromised account or device.

Another critical tenet is Micro-Segmentation (Sukumar & Aline, 2013), which divides the network into smaller, isolated zones to contain potential breaches and prevent lateral movement by attackers. In a micro-segmented H-IoT environment, each group of devices—such as infusion pumps, diagnostic equipment, or patient wearables—is treated as a separate security domain with its own access policies. If one device or zone is compromised, the intrusion is contained and cannot easily propagate to others, significantly improving overall network resilience.

Continuous Monitoring and Validation (Abideen et al., 2017) further reinforces Zero Trust by ensuring that all interactions within the network are constantly scrutinized for signs of abnormal or unauthorized behavior. This involves real-time inspection of user actions, device communications, and data flows to detect anomalies. For example, if a medical device suddenly begins transmitting large volumes of data at odd hours, this behavior can be flagged and investigated, potentially preventing a data breach or denial-of-service attack.

*Figure 1. Zero Trust Architecture*

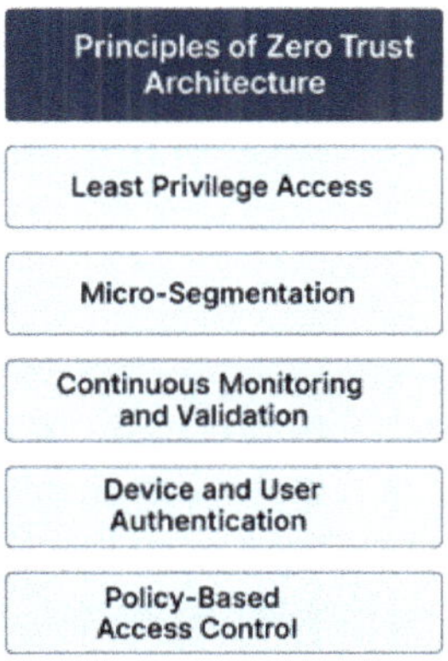


Device and User Authentication is also indispensable to ZTA (Dhillon & Kalra, 2018). Strong authentication mechanisms such as multi-factor authentication (MFA), biometric verification, and digital certificates are employed to validate the identity of every actor before granting access. This reduces reliance on easily compromised credentials like passwords and ensures that only verified entities can access sensitive data or systems. In the healthcare context, this could mean requiring biometric login for access to electronic health records or using device attestation to verify the integrity of a connected insulin pump.

Lastly, Policy-Based Access Control ensures that access decisions are not static but instead dynamically adapt to contextual factors such as the user's role, the device's security posture, geolocation, time of access, and even current threat intelligence (Khan & Sakamura, 2020). Policies can be updated in real-time to reflect evolving security requirements or respond to detected threats. For example, access to patient data might be restricted if a device is found to be operating with outdated firmware or if a user logs in from an unfamiliar location.

Together, these principles create a holistic security framework that is both preventive and adaptive, offering robust protection for the complex, data-intensive, and life-critical domain of Healthcare IoT. By continuously validating trust and limiting access based on strict policies, Zero Trust minimizes the likelihood of breaches and ensures that when attacks do occur, they are swiftly contained and neutralized.

## 4. ZERO TRUST FOR H-IOT: ARCHITECTURAL INTEGRATION

Implementing Zero Trust Architecture (ZTA) in Healthcare IoT (H-IoT) environments is a multifaceted process that necessitates careful consideration across various architectural layers (Pandey et al., 2024). Given the diversity of devices, communication protocols, and data processing workflows involved in modern healthcare, each layer—ranging from the physical endpoint to the cloud—requires a tailored approach to integrate ZTA principles effectively.

## 4.1 Device Layer Security

At the foundational level, H-IoT devices must be fortified against compromise. This involves embedding secure boot processes to ensure devices boot only with authenticated software, alongside employing firmware integrity checks to detect tampering. Additionally, incorporating device identity and attestation mechanisms allows each device to present verifiable credentials when connecting to a network or application (Mrabet et al., 2020). By establishing a root of trust, these measures prevent rogue or counterfeit devices from infiltrating the system.

In an expanded approach, device telemetry should also be continuously analyzed to assess the operational health and behavioral patterns of devices. Any deviation from baseline activity could signal compromise, triggering automated responses such as quarantine or privilege reduction.

## 4.2 Network Layer Security

The network layer serves as the connective tissue for all H-IoT components and thus is a critical domain for Zero Trust integration as shown in figure 2. Implementing Software-Defined Networking (SDN) allows administrators to dynamically segment the network, creating secure zones based on context and need. Dynamic segmentation ensures that even if one device or user is compromised, their ability to move laterally across the network is severely limited (Swamy et al., 2017).

Moreover, encrypted communication protocols such as TLS and VPN tunneling should be enforced across all device-to-device and device-to-server interactions. Isolation policies should be adaptive and enforced through centralized control planes, allowing for real-time changes based on the threat landscape. This approach enhances resilience against eavesdropping, man-in-the-middle attacks, and unauthorized surveillance.

## 4.3 Application Layer Security

The application layer is where most data transactions occur, and it demands rigorous security scrutiny. Integration of access tokens, JSON Web Tokens (JWT), and API gateways ensures that only authorized applications and users can access specific services and datasets (Nebbione & Calzarossa, 2020). These tools offer granular access control and help in monitoring API traffic for signs of misuse or abuse.

In addition to static controls, runtime application self-protection (RASP) and behavioral analysis should be considered to dynamically monitor application behavior. Suspicious requests, unexpected input patterns, or anomalous usage trends should trigger alerts or automated mitigations.

*Figure 2. H-IoT Architecture*

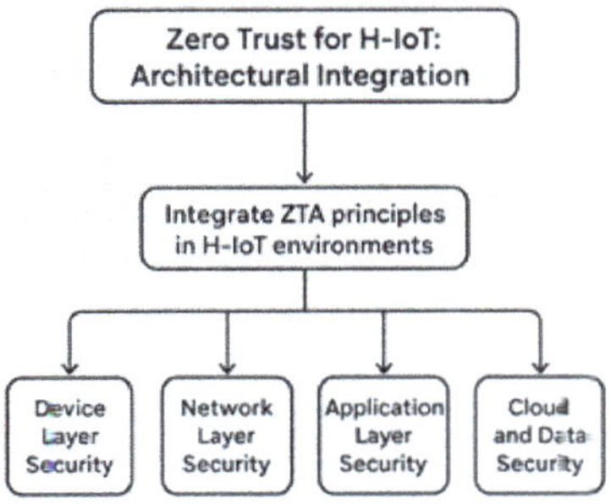


## 4.4 Cloud and Data Security

The cloud is often the backbone of data aggregation, analysis, and long-term storage in H-IoT systems (Khadidos et al., 2022). To align with Zero Trust principles, data must be encrypted both in transit and at rest using modern encryption standards such as AES-256 and end-to-end encryption methodologies. Data access should be governed by attribute-based access controls (ABAC) that evaluate real-time parameters before granting access.

Activity monitoring tools should be deployed to capture access logs, user actions, and system events (Manogaran et al., 2017). These logs must be continuously analyzed to detect policy violations or unusual behavior patterns. Additionally, cloud security posture management (CSPM) tools can help identify misconfigurations that may lead to vulnerabilities.

By integrating Zero Trust principles across these layers, healthcare organizations can create a resilient and adaptable security architecture that evolves in tandem with emerging threats and technological advancements.

## 5. IMPLEMENTATION STRATEGIES

Implementing Zero Trust Architecture in Healthcare IoT environments requires a systematic and well-coordinated approach. Each strategy must be aligned with the overarching goal of eliminating implicit trust and promoting continuous validation. Below are essential implementation strategies, each of which must be tailored to the specific needs and constraints of the healthcare ecosystem. In addition to implementing technical controls, it is crucial to foster a culture of security awareness among staff and establish governance frameworks to guide secure decision-making (Kodali et al., 2015).

### 5.1 Risk Assessment and Asset Inventory

Begin by identifying and categorizing all IoT assets within the healthcare infrastructure. This includes patient monitoring devices, diagnostic tools, smart wearables, medical imaging systems, gateways, and associated cloud services (Salih et al., 2019). Each asset must be documented with attributes such as device type, firmware version, network location, and communication behavior. Evaluate their risk profiles based on factors like criticality to patient care, exposure to external networks, and existing security controls. This foundational knowledge enables the creation of context-aware access policies and highlights areas requiring immediate security enhancement. Furthermore, this inventory process should be continuous and automated where possible, as the dynamic nature of H-IoT environments often leads to frequent additions, removals, and changes in asset configurations.

### 5.2 Identity and Access Management (IAM)

Strong IAM is the backbone of Zero Trust. Implementing robust identity governance ensures that only authenticated and authorized entities interact with system resources. Use role-based access control (RBAC) to limit access according to user roles, and supplement it with attribute-based access control (ABAC) for more granular enforcement. Ensure that all users—clinicians, technicians, administrators, and vendors—are authenticated using multi-factor authentication (MFA). Device identity provisioning should incorporate digital certificates and cryptographic tokens to verify authenticity and integrity before a device is allowed to connect to the network or exchange data (Alamri et al., 2022). Periodic access reviews and identity audits should also be enforced to detect dormant or misused accounts.

## 5.3 Network Micro-Segmentation

Segment the H-IoT environment into smaller, logically defined zones that isolate devices, departments, and workflows. Each segment should have strict access control policies and traffic filtering mechanisms. For instance, patient monitoring devices in the ICU should not have network access to administrative systems or unrelated clinical departments. Use virtual LANs, firewalls, and SDN to enforce these boundaries dynamically. Micro-segmentation also simplifies breach containment by limiting the lateral movement of attackers, thereby reducing the blast radius of any potential compromise. Additionally, organizations can define segmentation policies based on device function, operational schedule, or behavior patterns, further tightening the scope of access (Bellamkonda et al.).

## 5.4 Monitoring and Analytics

Deploy centralized monitoring platforms, such as Security Information and Event Management (SIEM) systems, to collect and correlate logs from across the H-IoT environment as shown in figure 3. Supplement these platforms with machine learning-based anomaly detection systems that establish behavioral baselines for devices and users, enabling the identification of deviations that may indicate security incidents. Proactive alerting mechanisms should be integrated with automated response workflows to ensure rapid containment and remediation (Tan & Abdul Halim, 2019). Visualization dashboards and key performance indicators (KPIs) should be utilized to support security operations teams in assessing the effectiveness of implemented controls and guiding strategic improvements.

*Figure 3. Implementation strategies for zero trust architecture in H-IoT*

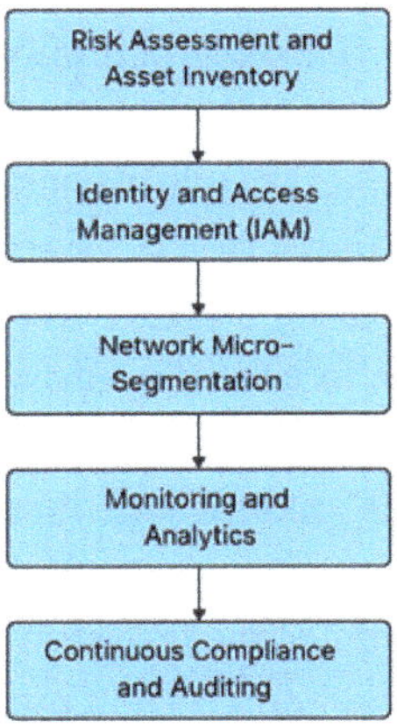

## 5.5 Continuous Compliance and Auditing

Ensure regular audits, compliance with healthcare regulations (like HIPAA, GDPR), and continuous policy updates. Regulatory compliance is not a one-time event but an ongoing process that must evolve in response to technological changes and threat intelligence. Automated compliance validation tools should be integrated into the CI/CD pipeline and runtime environment to detect deviations from required standards in real-time. Additionally, audit trails should be preserved and regularly reviewed to demonstrate due diligence during inspections and to support forensic investigations in the event of a breach (Boda & Allam, 2021).

A successful implementation strategy for ZTA in Healthcare IoT must be both comprehensive and iterative, evolving in tandem with the organization's technological landscape and threat profile. Through careful planning, execution, and monitoring, healthcare organizations can build a more secure and resilient infrastructure centered on Zero Trust principles.

# 6. CASE STUDY: IMPLEMENTING ZTA IN A SMART HOSPITAL

A large hospital system undertook a comprehensive Zero Trust Architecture (ZTA) deployment to protect its rapidly growing Healthcare IoT (H-IoT) infrastructure. The implementation began with a detailed asset inventory and classification of all connected devices, including infusion pumps, telemetry monitors, diagnostic imaging tools, and patient wearables. Each device was assigned a unique digital identity, enabling granular access control and contextual verification based on location, function, and usage patterns.

Software-Defined Networking (SDN) was leveraged to segment network traffic by department and function. For example, laboratory devices were logically isolated from administrative systems, and surgical suite systems were further segmented from outpatient diagnostic tools. This segmentation significantly reduced the blast radius of any potential compromise and helped enforce device-specific policies.

To secure user interactions, the hospital mandated multi-factor authentication (MFA) for all personnel accessing critical systems, including electronic health records (EHRs), clinical dashboards, and IoT device management consoles. This was supplemented with identity federation, allowing integration with third-party services while maintaining control over access privileges. The hospital also implemented AI-driven behavioral analytics to monitor real-time communications between devices, detect abnormal patterns, and respond to anomalies proactively. For instance, a sudden surge in data transmission from a bedside monitor outside typical operation hours would trigger alerts and prompt investigation. Coupled with automated incident response workflows, this significantly improved the mean time to detect and respond (MTTD/MTTR).

Encryption protocols, including TLS and AES-256, were enforced for both data in transit and at rest. Continuous monitoring systems were deployed to ensure HIPAA compliance, and audit logs were reviewed weekly to maintain visibility into access events and policy enforcement. The integration of ZTA led to a marked decline in security incidents, including unauthorized access attempts and internal misconfigurations. Furthermore, staff reported increased confidence in the security of systems, and the IT team observed a measurable improvement in threat detection and mitigation timelines. This case study demonstrates the feasibility and impact of Zero Trust in a complex, multi-layered healthcare environment.

## 7. CHALLENGES AND FUTURE DIRECTIONS

Despite its many advantages, implementing Zero Trust Architecture (ZTA) in Healthcare IoT (H-IoT) environments introduces several significant challenges that must be carefully navigated to realize its full potential as shown in figure 4:

- **Scalability:** Managing identities, policies, and access controls for tens of thousands of heterogeneous IoT devices presents a formidable scalability issue. Each device must be authenticated, monitored, and governed by dynamic access policies, which can become computationally intensive and administratively overwhelming without automation and efficient orchestration tools. Additionally, as more medical devices become connected, the complexity of maintaining secure interoperability grows exponentially.
- **Legacy Systems:** A substantial portion of healthcare infrastructure still relies on outdated devices and systems that lack the necessary computational capabilities or firmware support to integrate with ZTA frameworks. These legacy systems may not support secure communication protocols, multi-factor authentication, or device attestation, creating potential blind spots in a Zero Trust ecosystem. Retrofitting these devices with modern security layers or isolating them through strict segmentation and proxying mechanisms can be difficult and costly.
- **Performance Overhead:** Implementing comprehensive security controls—such as encryption, continuous monitoring, and dynamic policy evaluation—can introduce latency and performance degradation in latency-sensitive clinical environments. Real-time monitoring of patient vitals or automated drug delivery systems may be impacted by even slight delays, making it impera-

tive to optimize ZTA solutions for minimal performance overhead. Balancing strong security with clinical efficiency remains a key challenge.

- **Interoperability and Standardization:** The diversity of vendors, protocols, and platforms in H-IoT can hinder the seamless integration of ZTA. Lack of standardized frameworks and interoperability guidelines often leads to fragmented security implementations, reducing overall effectiveness. Establishing industry-wide protocols and certification schemes is essential to ensure consistent adoption.

*Figure 4. Implementation of Zero Trust Architecture in H-IoT*

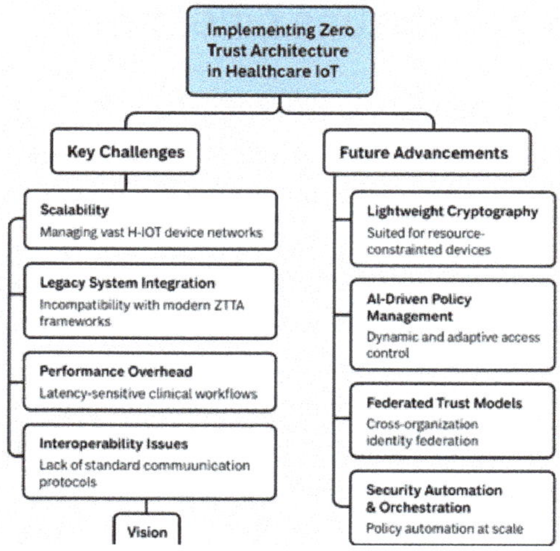


Future directions in ZTA research and development will likely emphasize:

- **Lightweight Cryptographic Techniques:** To accommodate the resource constraints of IoT devices, lightweight encryption algorithms and authentication methods are being explored that maintain strong security without overloading system resources.
- **AI-Powered Policy Management:** Artificial Intelligence and Machine Learning can assist in dynamically adapting access policies based on contextual data such as device behavior, threat intelligence feeds, and user activity. This helps reduce manual policy maintenance while increasing responsiveness to new threats.

- **Federated Trust Models:** As healthcare ecosystems grow to include external stakeholders such as labs, pharmacies, insurers, and telehealth providers, federated identity and trust models will be crucial for secure cross-domain collaboration. These models can facilitate secure, interoperable access to shared resources without compromising Zero Trust principles.
- **Automation and Orchestration:** Greater reliance on automation for provisioning, monitoring, incident response, and compliance tracking will be essential for scaling ZTA in complex H-IoT environments. Automated tools can help enforce policies consistently, respond to threats in real time, and reduce administrative burden.

By addressing these challenges and focusing on the emerging technologies that support scalable, efficient, and interoperable Zero Trust models, the healthcare industry can move toward a more secure and resilient future.

## 8. CONCLUSION

Zero Trust Architecture represents a transformative approach to securing Healthcare IoT systems. By shifting from implicit trust to continuous verification, ZTA addresses the fundamental security challenges posed by distributed, heterogeneous, and often insecure IoT devices. While implementation requires significant planning and investment, the long-term benefits in terms of patient safety, data protection, and regulatory compliance make it a vital strategy for the future of healthcare cybersecurity. By ensuring that no component of the system is implicitly trusted, ZTA offers a proactive defense against insider threats and advanced persistent threats that often go undetected by traditional security models. Moreover, as healthcare organizations increasingly adopt telemedicine, wearable health devices, and cloud-based patient data systems, the attack surface continues to expand. Zero Trust provides the necessary framework to manage this complexity by unifying access control, monitoring, and threat response mechanisms across diverse environments. In doing so, it enhances the resiliency and trustworthiness of healthcare systems. Looking ahead, the integration of artificial intelligence and machine learning into ZTA promises to bring adaptive, context-aware security policies that respond in real-time to emerging risks, ultimately creating a safer and more reliable digital healthcare ecosystem.

## REFERENCES


Abideen, Z. U., & Shah, M. A. (2017). "An IoT based robust healthcare model for continuous health monitoring." *2017 23rd international conference on automation and computing (ICAC)*. IEEE, DOI: 10.23919/IConAC.2017.8082012

Adil, M., Khan, M. K., Kumar, N., Attique, M., Farouk, A., Guizani, M., & Jin, Z. (2024). Healthcare Internet of Things: Security threats, challenges, and future research directions. *IEEE Internet of Things Journal*, *11*(11), 19046–19069. DOI: 10.1109/JIOT.2024.3360289

Alamri, B., Crowley, K., & Richardson, I. (2022). "Blockchain-based identity management systems in health IoT: A systematic review." Bellamkonda, Srikanth. "Network Segmentation and Micro-Segmentation: Reducing Attack Surfaces in Modern Enterprise Security."

Ali, T. E., et al. (2025). "Trends, prospects, challenges, and security in the healthcare internet of things." *Computing* 107.1-28.

Boda, V. V. R., & Allam, H. (2021). Automating Compliance in Healthcare: Tools and Techniques You Need. *International Journal of Emerging Trends in Computer Science and Information Technology*, *2*(3), 38–48. DOI: 10.63282/3050-9246.IJETCSIT-V2I3P105

Chen, B., Qiao, S., Zhao, J., Liu, D., Shi, X., Lyu, M., Chen, H., Lu, H., & Zhai, Y. (2020). A security awareness and protection system for 5G smart healthcare based on zero-trust architecture. *IEEE Internet of Things Journal*, *8*(13), 10248–10263. DOI: 10.1109/JIOT.2020.3041042 PMID: 35783535

Dhillon, P. K., & Kalra, S. (2018). Multi-factor user authentication scheme for IoT-based healthcare services. *Journal of Reliable Intelligent Environments*, *4*(3), 141–160. DOI: 10.1007/s40860-018-0062-5

Edo, O. C., Ang, D., Billakota, P., & Ho, J. C. (2024). A zero trust architecture for health information systems. *Health and Technology*, *14*(1), 189–199. DOI: 10.1007/s12553-023-00809-4

Khadidos, A.O., et al. (2022). "Healthcare data security using IoT sensors based on random hashing mechanism." *Journal of Sensors* 2022.1 8457116.

Khan, M. F. F., & Sakamura, K. (2020, December). A context-policy-based approach to access control for healthcare data protection. In *2020 International Computer Symposium (ICS)* (pp. 420-425). IEEE.

Kodali, R. K., Swamy, G., & Lakshmi, B. (2015). *"An implementation of IoT for healthcare." 2015 IEEE Recent Advances in Intelligent Computational Systems (RAICS)*. IEEE.

Kumar, M., et al. (2023). "Healthcare Internet of Things (H-IoT): Current trends, future prospects, applications, challenges, and security issues." *Electronics* 12.9 2050.

Maji, R., Gayen, B., & Saha, S. (2025). *A Robust IoT-Based Approach to Enhance Cybersecurity and Patient Trust in the Smart Health Care System: Zero-Trust Model*. Design and Forecasting Models for Disease Management. DOI: 10.1002/9781394234073.ch12

Manogaran, G., et al. (2017). "Big data security intelligence for healthcare industry 4.0." Cybersecurity for Industry 4.0: Analysis for Design and Manufacturing. Cham: Springer international publishing, 103-126.

Mrabet, H., et al. (2020). "A survey of IoT security based on a layered architecture of sensing and data analysis." *Sensors*20.13 3625.

Nebbione, G., & Calzarossa, M. C. (2020). Security of IoT application layer protocols: Challenges and findings. *Future Internet*, *12*(3), 55.

Pandey, S., Bhushan, B., & Hameed, A. A. (2024). Securing Healthcare 5.0: Zero-Knowledge Proof (ZKP) and Post Quantum Cryptography (PQC) Solutions for Medical Data Security. In *Soft Computing in Industry 5.0 for Sustainability* (pp. 339–355). Springer Nature Switzerland. DOI: 10.1007/978-3-031-69336-6_15

Salih, F. I., Abu Bakar, N. A., Hassan, N. H., Yahya, F., Kama, N., & Shah, J. (2019). IOT security risk management model for healthcare industry. *Malaysian Journal of Computer Science*, •••, 131–144. DOI: 10.22452/mjcs.sp2019no3.9

Sammartino, V., & Baiardi, F. (2024). Database Decomposition to satisfy the Least Privilege Principle in Healthcare. *ARIS2 : Advanced Research on Information Systems Security*, *4*(1), 47–69. DOI: 10.56394/aris2.v4i1.43

Sukumar, S. R., & Aline, F. (2013). "Application of micro-segmentation algorithms to the healthcare market: A case study." *2013 Biomedical Sciences and Engineering Conference (BSEC)*. IEEE, DOI: 10.1109/BSEC.2013.6618489

Sultana, M., et al. (2020). "Towards developing a secure medical image sharing system based on zero trust principles and blockchain technology." *BMC Medical Informatics and Decision Making* 20.1 256.

Swamy, S. N., Jadhav, D., & Kulkarni, N. (2017). "Security threats in the application layer in IOT applications." *2017 International conference on i-SMAC (iot in social, mobile, analytics and cloud)(i-SMAC)*. IEEE, DOI: 10.1109/I-SMAC.2017.8058395

Tan, E. T., & Abdul Halim, Z. (2019). Health care monitoring system and analytics based on internet of things framework. *Journal of the Institution of Electronics and Telecommunication Engineers, 65*(5), 653–660. DOI: 10.1080/03772063.2018.1447402

# Chapter 5
# Building Trustworthy AI for Healthcare Privacy:
## First Approaches With Federated Learning and IoMT

**Abhinav Upadhyay**
https://orcid.org/0009-0003-7951-6447
*Manipal University Jaipur, India*

**Ayush Raj**
*Manipal University Jaipur, India*

**Mridul Maheshwari**
https://orcid.org/0009-0008-5415-5231
*Manipal University Jaipur, India*

**Swayam Bansal**
*Manipal University Jaipur, India*

## ABSTRACT

*Healthcare data contains highly sensitive information, making privacy a top priority in AI-based medical systems. Traditional centralized machine learning aggregates data from multiple sources, raising concerns about privacy breaches, data ownership, and regulatory compliance. Federated Learning (FL) offers a solution by allowing AI models to be trained across decentralized data sources without moving patient data. Only model updates are shared, preserving privacy. FL uses tools like differential privacy and secure multi-party computation to enhance security. Algorithms such as FedAvg and FedProx enable collaborative training without exposing individual data. FL also supports IoMT devices, allowing them to contribute to model training while*

DOI: 10.4018/979-8-3373-7610-3.ch005

*keeping data local. This not only safeguards patient privacy but also addresses the challenge of limited, diverse medical data across institutions. Federated Learning helps build secure, compliant, and flexible AI systems in healthcare, ensuring both innovation and protection of sensitive patient information.*

## INTRODUCTION

The movement to digitize healthcare systems has increased significantly because of the introduction of Artificial Intelligence (AI), Machine Learning (ML), and the Internet of Medical Things (IoMT). All three, along with IoMT devices (wearables, implantables, and monitoring devices), can provide exciting possibilities for real-time diagnosis, individualized treatment, and smart healthcare delivery. IoMT devices produce abundant medical data, which, in real-time, can be processed by AI, further guiding clinical judgment in order to optimize patient outcomes (Nguyen, 2021).

However, the traditional centralized AI structure dictates that the collection and aggregation of sensitive health and medical data, be it sourced from healthcare providers' information systems or organizations, must be stored in a central server or the cloud. This leads to serious challenges in privacy, security, and data ownership. First, that risks breaches in the data constitutes a violation of patient confidentiality, and it usually doesn't comply with health regulations like the Health Insurance Portability and Accountability Act (HIPAA) and the General Data Protection Regulation (GDPR) (Ali et al., 2022; Mosaiyebzadeh et al., 2023). Second, such an architecture doesn't scale across diverse and distributed medical institutions at a time when health data itself is becoming decentralized and heterogeneous.

With these limitations in mind, Federated Learning (FL) is a privacy-preserving distributed machine learning framework that leverages the collaborative abilities of clients—such as hospitals, clinics, and IoMT devices—to train one global model without sharing raw data. Federated Learning relies on the clients producing model updates (e.g., gradients, weights) as their contributions instead of sharing any raw data (Nguyen, 2021; Ali et al., 2022). Since only model updates are shared, the client's data is never sent or shared and maintained at its source, similar to naive malicious data (i.e., default data hiding). FL can improve the sharing of non-domain data while gaining roughly comparable privacy benefits to other approaches. The benefits of FL include decreased communication latency and concerns about data governance across jurisdictions.

FL is particularly synergistic with systems based on IoMT/sensors, where massive amounts of data are being generated across different healthcare contexts like home monitoring, hospital devices, and mHealth/telemedicine apps (Mosaiyebzadeh et al., 2023). These contexts necessitate low-latency, secure, and trustworthy learning mechanisms that consider the privacy of individual users. FL provides a built-in contractual assumption of privacy, but for further privacy guarantees of sensitive records being generated by individual users, we can embed PETs such as Differential Privacy, Homomorphic Encryption, or Secure Multi-party Computation (SMPC) alongside our FL protocols (Mosaiyebzadeh et al., 2023).

Creating trustworthy AI in healthcare is more than applying technical security. It must also include fairness, transparency, explainability, and ethical use in model conduct. Trust is a requirement for acceptance of AI by clinicians and patients alike when patient welfare (and sometimes life) is at stake. Numerous recent studies cite the combination of FL and PETs as a foundational approach to creating AI systems that are high performing, but also ethically attuned and compliant with the law (Ali et al., 2022; Kumari et al., 2025).

This chapter seeks to address privacy-first AI frameworks for healthcare, specifically regarding the anatomy of Federated Learning and the Internet of Medical Things. We give a technical background on FL, survey privacy-preserving methods, and discuss prominent application domains of remote health monitoring, electronic health records (EHR), medical imaging, and cybersecurity for IoMT. Furthermore, we detail some of the open challenges and research avenues for creating secure, scalable, and trusted AI systems.

## BACKGROUND

### The Evolution of AI in Healthcare

AI has shown strong potential across multiple facets of healthcare -- disease diagnosis, medical imaging, drug discovery, and remote patient monitoring, for example. Approaches like deep learning have proven effective in modeling the intrinsic high dimensionality of complex biomedical data, while maintaining an improved accuracy of diagnostic decision-making and clinical diagnostic decision support systems (in figure 1) (Nguyen, 2021; Ali et al., 2022) However, these successes have often depended on centralized data storage and training architectures, raising serious concerns related to the privacy and security of medical data.

There will always be more health devices relying on the connectivity of the internet, and the amount and sensitivity of data being produced will only grow with it. For example, “Internet of Medical Things” (IoMT) devices including wearable monitor devices (e.g., Fitbit), smart pumps for insulin delivery, implantable glucose sensors, and other medical devices continuously collect data about an individual's physiology (e.g., heart rate, glucose levels, oxygen content) (Mosaiyebzadeh et al., 2023; Kumari et al., 2025). These data streams have tremendous value for real-time assessment of health status but can also be subject to cyber-attacks, unauthorized access, and privacy violations.

*Figure 1. A timeline of key advancements in healthcare AI, from rule-based systems to Federated Learning and IoMT.*

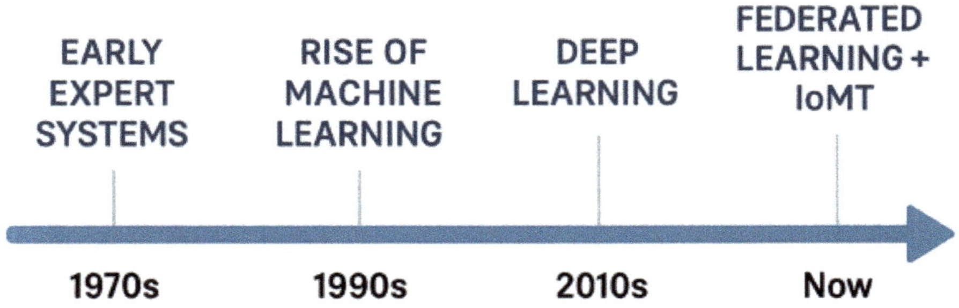


Source: Synthesized from Nguyen (2021), Ali (2022)

## Limitations of Centralized Learning in Healthcare

In a conventional centralized machine learning framework, a healthcare organization must put all patient data at a single location (e.g., cloud or data center) to train a machine-learning model. This creates three main challenges:

- Risks to privacy: Centralized storage poses greater risk to data breaches and compliance lapses, especially transmitting sensitive data across different networks.
- Data silos: Institutions are not willing to share their data, due in part to legal, ethical, or competitive issues, creating a set of data silos, and limiting collaborative development of AI.
- Scalability: As the amount of medical data continues to grow, transmitting a large data set and also carrying a high volume of data for the storage is impractical and inefficient.

## Federated Learning: A Paradigm Shift

In order to address these issues, Federated Learning (FL) has emerged as a collaborative-based, decentralized learning approach that allows for collaborative training without the sharing of raw data. Because in FL, each participating entity (e.g., hospital, clinic, IoMT device) trains a local model using its private dataset, and only sends encrypted model updates to a central server, which then aggregates the local updates to form a global model (Nguyen, 2021).

Advantages of this paradigm include:

- Data stays local and therefore has lower privacy risks.
- Regulatory compliance is more achievable.
- Various data sources (e.g., rural clinics, urban hospitals) can contribute to model trainings without exposing private information.
- Data transfer overheads and costs are minimized which improves training efficiencies.

FL is ideal for healthcare applications in which patients' data is varied, private, and distributed across a variety of edge and institutional sources.

## Role of IoMT in Smart Healthcare

The IoMT space comprises a diversity of smart medical devices which capture real-time patient data outside the clinical environment. These smart medical devices are the foundation of these continuous health monitoring systems, enabling proactive delivery of care. However, their use also incurs unique privacy and cybersecurity risks:

- Man-in-the-middle attacks, replay attacks, and data tampering are a growing threat in IoMT settings (Kumari et al., 2025).
- The myriad device manufacturers and communication protocols make security standardization even more challenging.

FL together with privacy-preserving technologies such as Differential Privacy, Homomorphic Encryption, and Blockchain provide a solid foundation to secure learning on IoMT networks while sustaining patient privacy.

## Fundamentals of Federated Learning and IoMT

The merging of Federated Learning (FL) and the Internet of Medical Things (IoMT) is revolutionizing healthcare by facilitating intelligent, privacy-preserving, and decentralized health data analytics. In this section, we provide an overview of the fundamental concepts of FL, the IoMT, its various types, architectures, and their applications in healthcare.

## Federated Learning: Concept and Working Principle

Federated Learning is a distributed machine learning framework that allows multiple clients (including hospitals, wearable devices, or clinics) to develop a shared global model while ensuring that raw data is never shared. Rather than sending data to a central server where it can be unelaborated data shared, each client trains the model locally and only sends the updates of the model (weights/gradients) to a server to combine/disseminate (see figure 2) (Nguyen, 2021).

The essential steps of the standard FL workflow include:

- Client Selection: The server determines which clients it will include, based on their availability or, in some cases, capability.
- Local Model Training: Each client takes its local dataset and trains the model.
- Sending model updates: Clients send encrypted updates of the model to the server.
- Model Aggregation: The central server will aggregate the updates.
- Broadcasting: Once the updates are aggregated and the new global model has been created, the server shares the improved model back to clients who will then have access on their next round.

The clients/servers will continue in this manner, potentially uninterrupted, until the global model converges.

*Figure 2. Illustration of how hospitals and IoMT devices train local models and share only updates with a central server for aggregation.*

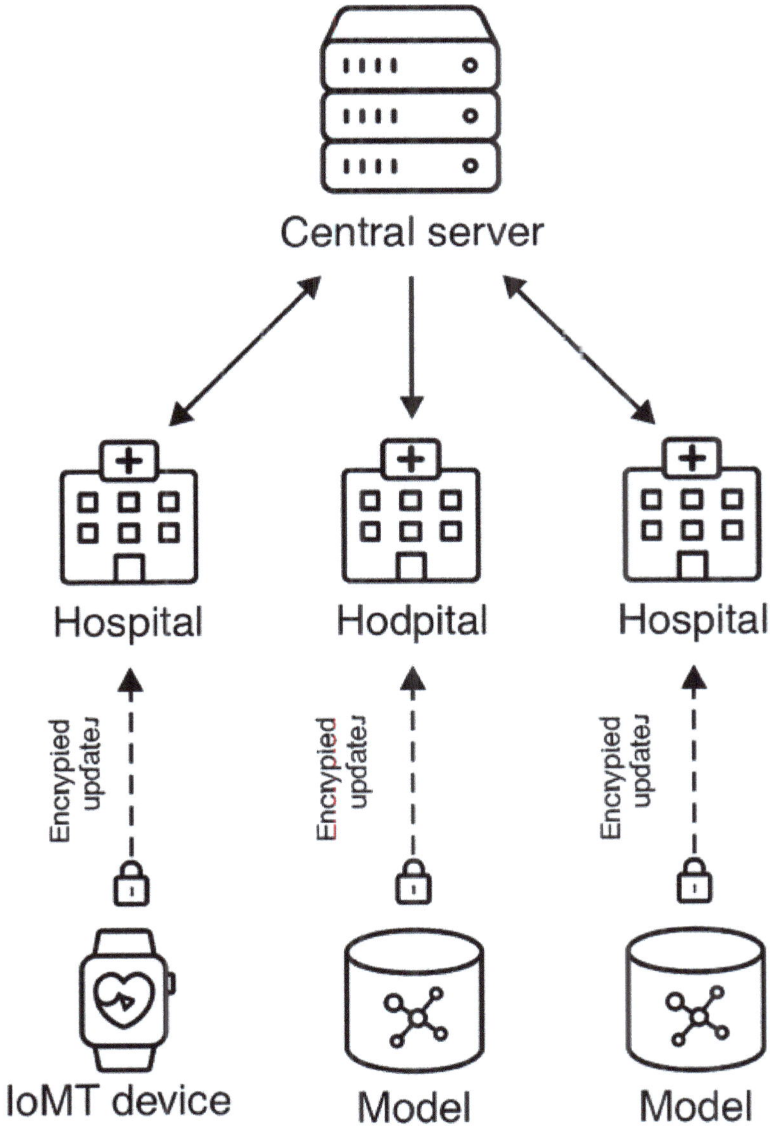

## Types of Federated Learning in Healthcare

FL can be subdivided into different categories based on how data is distributed among clients:

- Horizontal Federated Learning (HFL):
    - Each client shares the same feature space but different samples of data.
    - *Example*: Multiple hospitals train a model of patient vitals with the same feature space (e.g., heart rate, BP) but with different populations of patients.
- Vertical Federated Learning (VFL):
    - Each client has the same samples of data, but they have different features.
    - *Example*: A hospital and insurance company collaborating on patient data—information that one has from clinical history, whereas the other has information from billing.
- Federated Transfer Learning (FTL):
    - Some clients have different features and samples, but they can collaborate through transfer learning.
    - Transfer learning is useful when dataset sizes/heterogeneity are somewhat aligned.

## Core Algorithms in Federated Learning

Many algorithms have been proposed specifically for FL in healthcare settings:

- FedAvg (Federated Averaging) – An algorithm that performs model parameter-averaging over clients depending on the size of the dataset used.
- FedProx – Regularization is used to reduce client drift—heterogeneity is taken into account.
- FedMA (Federated Matched Averaging) – Matches and averages layers of heterogeneous model architectures.
- MOON, Scaffold, and FedDyn – Balance improvements regarding data that are not IID (non-independent and identically distributed) with respect to personalized scenarios (Nguyen, 2021).

These algorithms are particularly important in the healthcare setting because of such data which are typically not IID at each institution.

## IoMT: Architecture and Data Flow

The Internet of Medical Things (IoMT) is defined as connected health care devices, systems, and applications that use internet-based technologies to collect, process, and analyze patient data (Ali et al., 2022; Kumari et al., 2025).

A typical architecture of IoMT has the following levels:

- Sensing Layer: Wearable and implantable devices that collect physiological data (e.g., glucose monitors, smart ECGs, etc.).
- Network Layer: Transfers data over secure protocols (e.g., Wi-Fi, 5G, BLE).
- Processing Layer: Edge devices or servers that filter data, provide feature extraction, and use real-time analytics.
- Application Layer: Health-care applications that provide insights, alerts, and remote monitoring dashboards (Bashir et al., 2023).
- The IoMT provides for continuous, real-time monitoring and collection of data that could be used for federated AI model training in Pi (see in figure 3) (Bashir et al., 2023).

*Figure 3. A layered structure of IoMT showing sensing, network, processing, and application layers for real-time healthcare data flow.*

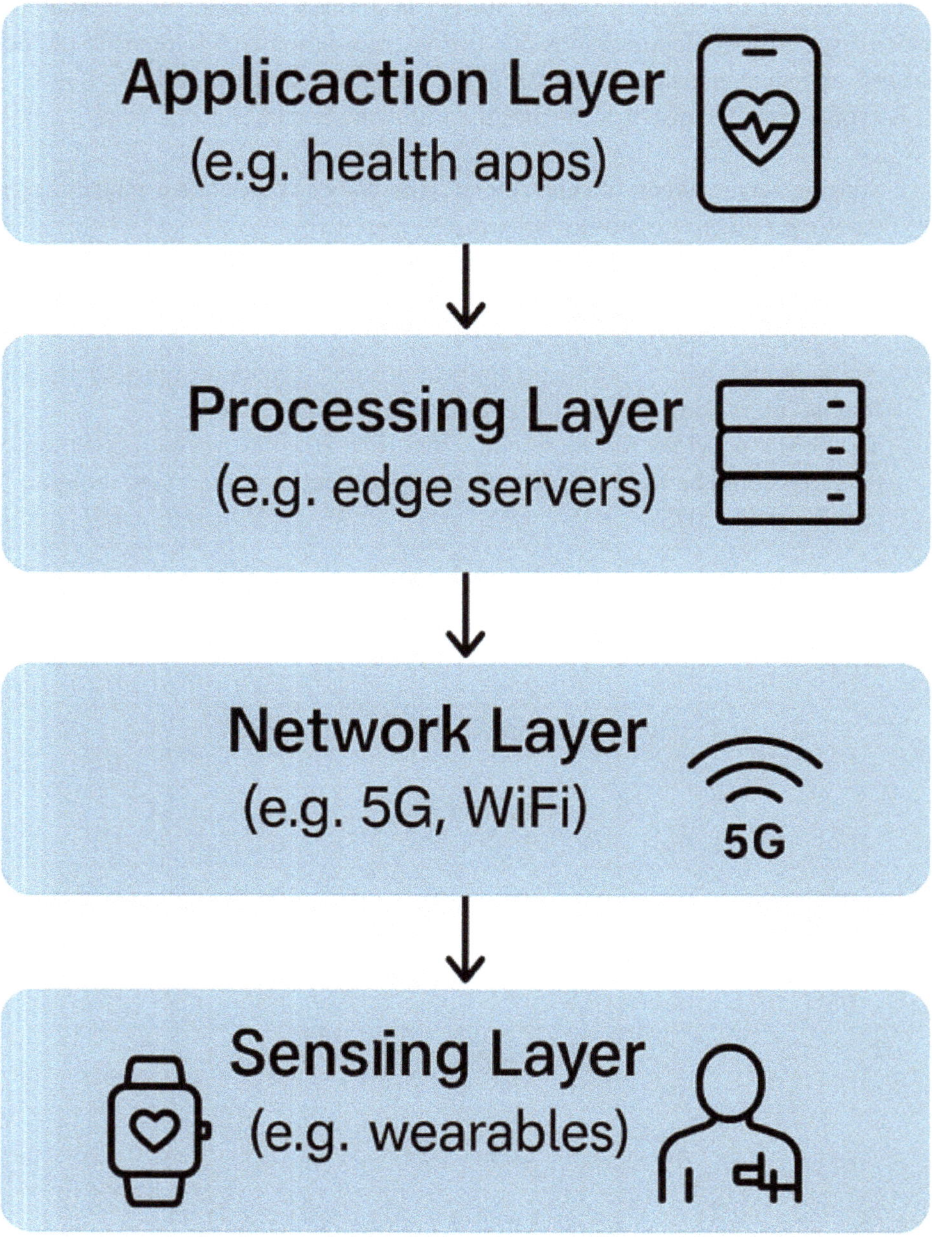

## Integration of FL and IoMT in Healthcare

The incorporation of FL into IoMT creates a privacy-first approach for use cases for real-time AI applications in health care.

- On-device Learning: Since IoMT devices perform local training with FL algorithms already embedded in the devices, they are capable of using on-device learning.
- Privacy-by-Design: Patient data lives only on the device, which significantly mitigates privacy risks.
- Low Latency: IoMT inherently provides edge computing, and this is critical for immediate response when monitoring health outcomes (e.g., anomaly detection, arrhythmia).
- Personalized Models: FL allows local personalisation of models based on patients' ongoing behaviour or healthcare conditions.

This combination, the symbiotic relationship of IoMT and FL, can create a framework that enables intelligent diagnosis, management of chronic disease, and early warning systems, all while maintaining patient confidentiality (Mosaiyebzadeh et al., 2023).

## Security Challenges in FL-IoMT Systems

Despite helping increase privacy, FL is prone to similar types of risks as a centralized model. Here are some of the frequently cited threats:

- Poisoning Attacks: Malicious clients may inject poisoned or corrupted updates to inject bias into the model.
- Inference Attacks: Clients may reconstruct sensitive information from the model updates and gradients shared.
- Communication Overhead: The frequent exchange of models with clients consumes bandwidth that is often already limited for IoMT networks.

A combination of privacy-enhancing technologies like Differential Privacy, Secure Multi-party Computation (SMPC), and Blockchain with FL will also have increasing importance.

## Privacy-Enhancing Technologies in Federated Learning

Federated Learning (FL) is a promising way to implement decentralized, privacy-preserving AI in healthcare, but it is not immune to privacy attacks. Sharing model updates could leak sensitive health-related information through inference, reconstruction, or poisoning attacks even without shared raw data. Therefore, it will be important to implement Privacy-enhancing Technologies (PETs) and other privacy protections to strengthen FL-based systems, e.g., in sensitive environments, such as the Internet of Medical Things (IoMT).

In this section, we will provide an overview of the key PETS that can be used in conjunction with FL to increase privacy, particularly the risks of data leakage, as well as provide secure collaborative learning in healthcare.

## Differential Privacy (DP)

Differential Privacy is a mathematical framework that says adjusting a single data point will not dramatically change the value of a computation. It provides formal privacy guarantees in theoretical terms by adding noise to the learning/training process as well as the model parameters, through the definition of "epsilon".

- Use Cases in Federated Learning:
  - The aggregator adds noise to the model updates (i.e., gradients, weights) before they send them to the aggregation server.
  - The most common use of differential privacy is known as "epsilon-differential privacy," where a smaller epsilon value results in greater privacy protection
- Advantages:
  - Reduces the threat of membership inference and/or model inversion attacks.
  - Obtain compliance with regulations such as GDPR and HIPAA.
- Disadvantages:
  - Reducing the accuracy of the model from adding noise can be problematic in small datasets (Mosaiyebzadeh et al., 2023; Ali et al., 2022).

## Secure Multi-party Computation (SMPC)

SMPC allows multiple parties to jointly compute a function on their inputs, while neither of the parties will learn any information about the inputs except for the output of the computation. In the context of FL, SMPC will allow for secure aggregation of model updates so that no party (including the servers) can see the individual updates.

- Application in FL:
  - o Each client will encrypt their model updates into shares and send the shares to multiple servers.
  - o The servers will then collaboratively perform the aggregation without ever seeing the raw updates.
- Benefits:
  - o Prevents honest-but-curious servers from ever gaining access to the individual updates from clients.
  - o Provides strong protection against the risks of centralized aggregation.
- Limitations:
  - o High computational and communication overhead, which is problematic for low-power IoMT devices (Mosaiyebzadeh et al., 2023).

## Homomorphic Encryption (HE)

Homomorphic Encryption permits computations to occur while the data remains encrypted, yielding encrypted outputs that can be decrypted and yield the correct result.

- Application in FL:
  - o Clients encrypt their model updates before sending them to the server.
  - o Server can perform a meaningful aggregation over the encrypted data.
- Benefits:
  - o Data is encrypted end-to-end - this is a very strong confidentiality guarantee.
  - o There is no intermediate exposure of sensitive model updates
- Limitations:
  - o Very high computational overhead, and not good enough support yet for more complex operations, such as deep learning.

## Blockchain for Federated Learning

Blockchain is a decentralized, tamper-proof ledger that has the potential to improve trust, auditability, and data provenance in Federated Learning (FL)

- Application in FL:
  - o Log all model update transactions to create transparency and traceability of models.
  - o Utilize smart contracts for the governance of rules and incentive mechanisms in FL.

- Benefits:
    - o Builds trust among the many non-collaborative actors in healthcare.
    - o Allow auditable and verifiable FL workflows across multiple institutions (Mosaiyebzadeh et al., 2023; Bashir et al., 2023).
- Limitations:
    - o Scalability issues and additional latency.
    - o Energy inefficiency of some consensus protocols (e.g., Proof-of-Work).

## Trusted Execution Environments (TEEs)

Trusted execution environments (TEEs), like Intel SGX, provide secure, insulated environments within the processing power of devices for performing sensitive computations.

- Application in FL:
    - o Server-side aggregation of model updates can be done safely within a TEE so that the host OS or attackers cannot access the raw model updates.
- Benefits:
    - o Low-latency, lightweight protection, with no noise or cryptographic overhead.
    - o Very appropriate for real-time IoMT use cases.
- Limitations:
    - o Specific hardware requirements (and vulnerability to side-channel attacks).

## Multi-PET Integration for Healthcare AI

Hybrid approaches often appear due to trade-offs. For example:

- Combining DP + SMPC so that model aggregation occurs in secure and private environments.
- Using Blockchain + DP to certify and create an audit log that is privacy-compliant.
- Encoding TEEs + DP into IoMT edge devices to secure real-time training of the model.

This rationale in layered approaches enables balance between the privacy-accuracy-efficiency triangle, which is vitally important in practical and medical environments.

## Comparison and Selection of PETs in Healthcare FL

*Table 1. Comparison of PETs in Federated Learning for Healthcare Settings*

| Privacy-Enhancing Technology (PET) | Privacy Level | Computation Cost | Communication Cost | Use Case Suitability |
|---|---|---|---|---|
| Differential Privacy | High (with noise) | Low to Moderate | Low | EHRs, mobile devices |
| Secure Multi-party Computation (SMPC) | Very High | High | High | Inter-hospital FL |
| Homomorphic Encryption | Very High | Very High | High | Encrypted model updates |
| Blockchain | Medium (Audit) | Moderate | Moderate to High | Model audit trails |
| Trusted Execution Environments (TEE) | High (Hardware-based) | Low to Moderate | Low | Edge/IoMT computation |

*Figure 4. A visual comparison of PETs used in Federated Learning based on privacy level, computation cost, communication cost, and use case suitability.*

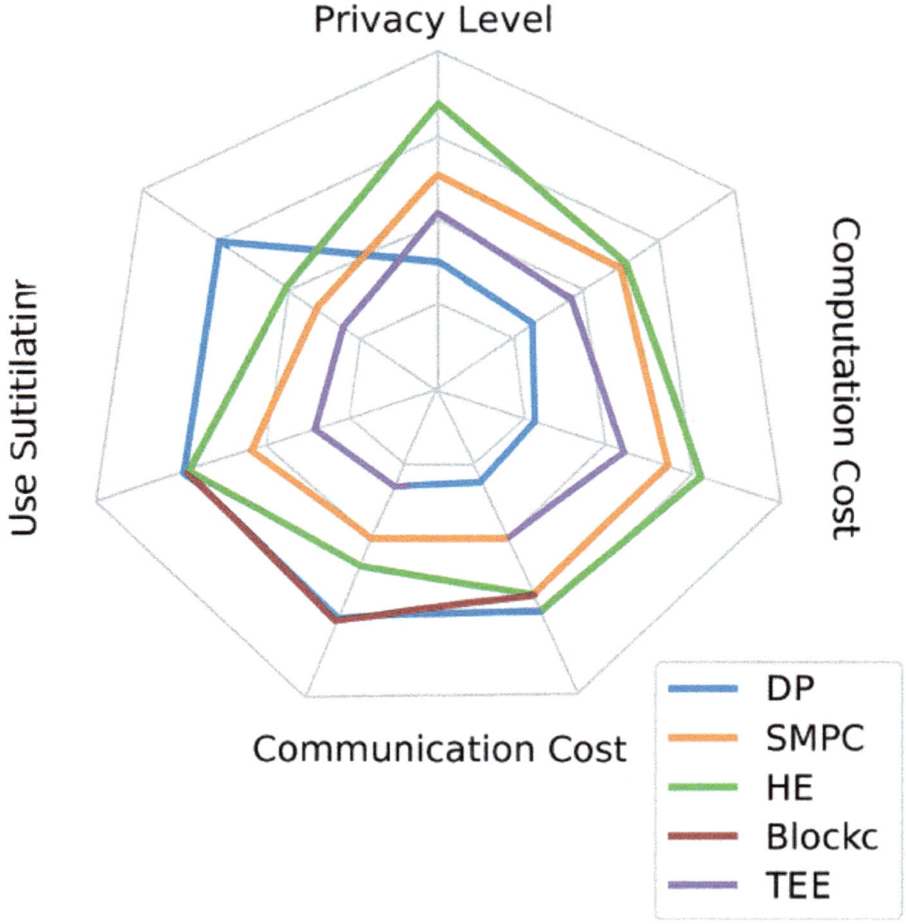


## Use Cases and Applications

The combination of Federated Learning (FL) and the Internet of Medical Things (IoMT) is changing how healthcare systems manage, analyze, and secure medical data. FL is well-suited to a variety of healthcare applications because of its privacy-preserving features, especially in scenarios where sensitive patient data is gathered from multiple types of sources, including hospitals to clinics, and sensors to wearables.

This section discusses important applications in which FL is being utilized or has the potential to be implemented in the real world when combined with IoMT. (see in figure 5)

*Figure 5. Overview of key FL applications in healthcare, including EHR sharing, remote monitoring, medical imaging, disease surveillance, and mental health support.*

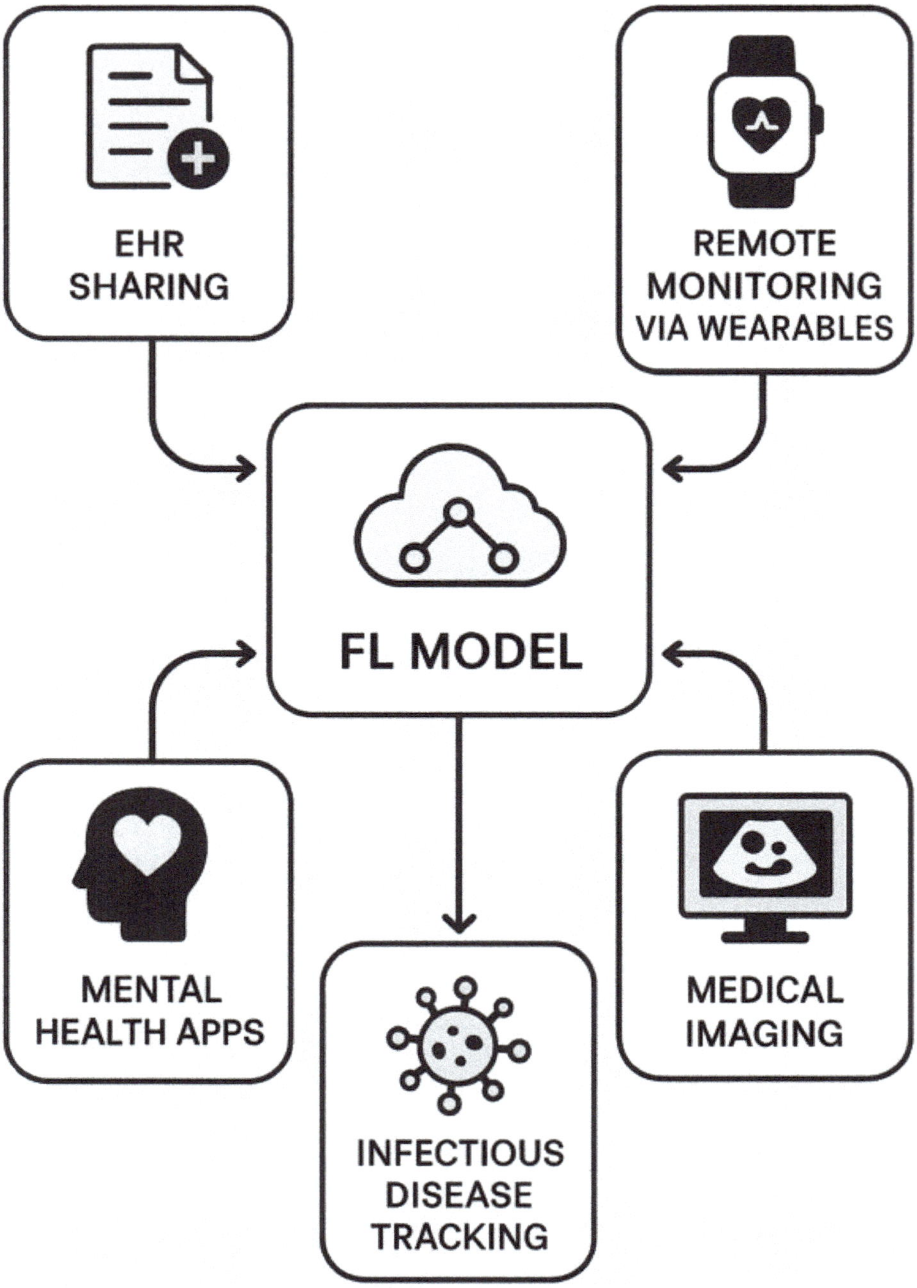

## Federated Electronic Health Record (EHR) Management

Electronic Health Records (EHRs) are institutionally stored and accessed digital records relating to patients' medical information. The data is usually siloed due to privacy protections and institutional silos.

- How FL would work:
  - o Hospitals can partner to create a global model predicting disease, forecasting readmissions, or identifying drug-drug interactions without the need to share patients' records.
  - o With FL, hospitals can share knowledge across institutions from the locally held data while preserving private attributes like diagnosis, prescriptions, and patient identifiers, within their organizational structure (Nguyen, 2021).

For example, FL was used in a collaborative study among hospitals to develop a model to predict mortality from COVID-19 using non-shared records of electronic health records. The results indicated that the model produced comparable accuracy to centralized models while preserving patient privacy (Ali et al., 2022).

## Remote Health Monitoring via IoMT

IoMT devices like wearables (e.g., smart watches, ECGs, glucose monitors, blood pressure cuffs) are widely used to remotely monitor a variety of chronic conditions, including diabetes, hypertension, and heart disease.

- Application of FL:
  - o Models can be trained on a device, using edge FL, to detect anomalies like heart arrhythmia, glucose variations, or respiratory problems.
  - o On-device training updates the model locally, improving personalization for the individual and responsiveness, without exposing the raw physiological data (Mosaiyebzadeh et al., 2023).

For example, a federated architecture was developed where wearables trained local models to identify sleep apnea; the aggregated cloud models provided equivalent performance without losing data privacy.

## Federated Medical Imaging

Medical imaging (CT scans, MRIs, X-rays, etc.) is essential in diagnostic medicine and often contains sensitive information within a given hospital's PACS (Picture Archiving and Communication Systems) data sets. The data sets very rarely leave their repository because of legal and ethical concerns.

- Application of FL:
  - Multiple institutions, respectively, could train their own deep learning model, either for tumor detection, lung segmentation, or fracture classification, without requiring access or centralized storage of their imaging data.
  - FL models have proven to achieve high accuracy and generalizability from multiple imaging sources (Nguyen, 2021).

For example, the NVIDIA Clara platform has demonstrated that universities and institutions can leverage FL across institutions for MRI scans of brain tumor segmentation and achieve high dice scores while remaining HIPAA compliant.

## Federated Learning for Infectious Disease Surveillance (COVID-19 and Beyond)

To realize timely detection and monitoring for infectious diseases, public health organizations need to coordinate with hospitals, which is often limited by data-sharing agreements or limitations.

- Application of FL:
  - FL could be applied to monitor disease progression, identify areas (hotspots) affected by outbreaks, and forecast patterns of outbreaks by sharing real-time case data in a federated manner.
  - Governments and international health organizations can work together with regionally and nationally distributed patient data securely and privately, again without revealing sensitive information about individual patients (Ali et al., 2022).

For example, FL frameworks during the COVID-19 pandemic were used to compile and share a variety of patient data, including vital signs, lab test results, and CT images, collected from a diverse array of hospitals throughout the world in a decentralized manner to build models to forecast the severity of the disease.

## Cybersecurity and Intrusion Detection in IoMT

Healthcare decreases security with the proliferation of connected devices, increasing attack surfaces. Threats such as man-in-the-middle attacks, data spoofing, and unauthorized access are common in IoMT networks, mobile health devices, and wearables (Kumari et al., 2025).

- Application of FL:
  - FL-based Intrusion Detection Systems (IDS) can be deployed to learn on distributed devices in the IoMT, which can detect irregular activities and/or malicious activity.
  - FL prevents the need to send security logs and telemetry data to a centralized cloud, thus reducing the exposure.

For example, one example is the secure FL framework that used Variational Autoencoders (VAEs) and deep learning, which was deployed on individual edge IoMT nodes to detect network intrusions with better than 91% accuracy without having to expose raw traffic data (Kumari et al., 2025).

## Personalized Federated Learning for Mental Health and Rehabilitation

Mental health applications such as mood management applications, cognitive-behavioral apps, and virtual reality (VR) rehabilitation all rely on user-specific behaviors and sensitive mental health records.

- Application of FL:
  - With personalized FL, adaptive models can be created based on the interaction and behavioral data of each user, while mental health records are only kept private on the device itself.
  - Systems like these can provide better therapeutic outcomes while protecting user anonymity.

FL has been successfully used to train on the use of smartphones to understand the patterns of depression in a user or the levels of stress in a user. None of the data is ever transmitted, and there is no personal data collected on the central server (see in figure 6) (Bashir et al., 2023).

*Figure 6. Depiction of how personalized FL enables adaptive local models on user devices, supporting privacy-preserving mental health and rehabilitation applications.*

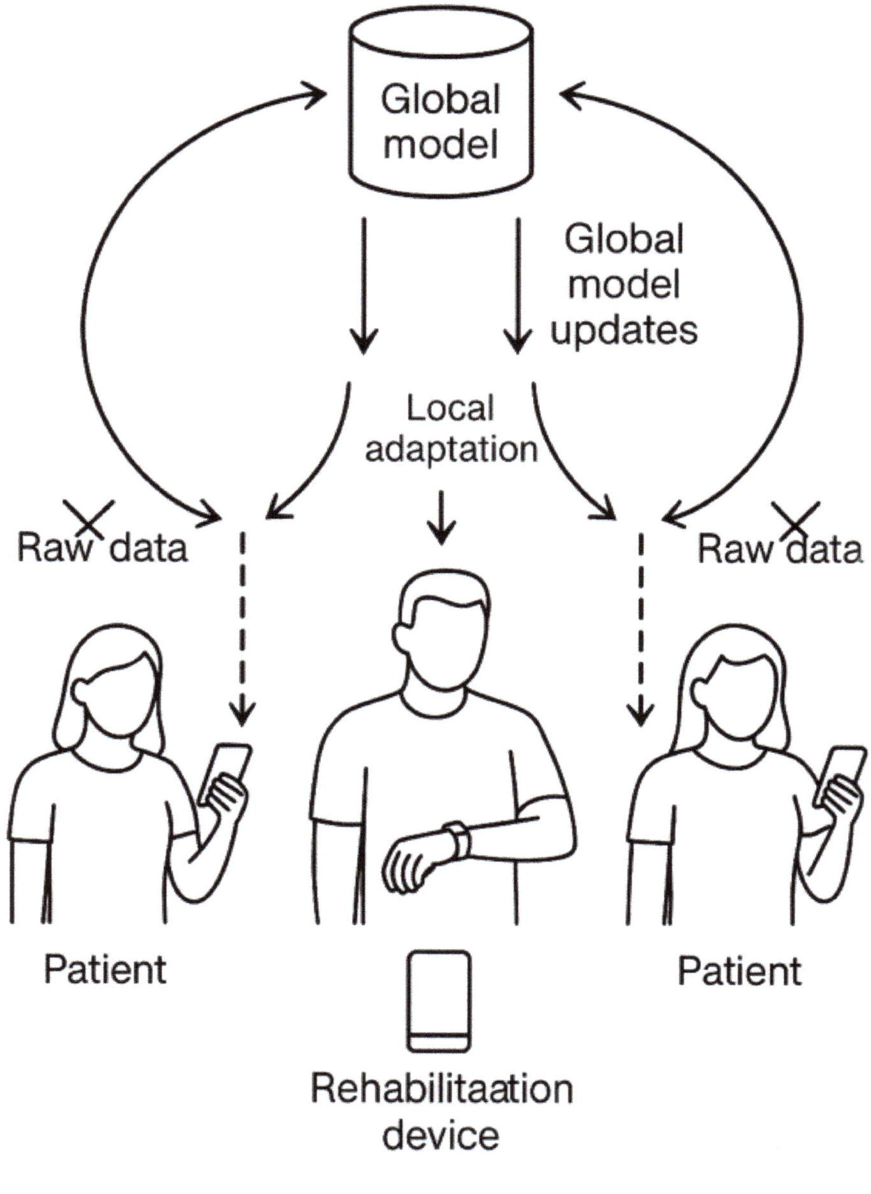

## Drug Discovery and Clinical Trial Optimization

Drug discovery and clinical trials generate a large quantity of data, often from genomics, pharmacology, and patients' responses, and distributed across institutions.

- Application of FL:
  - o Many pharmaceutical companies may collaborate on a project and commission research with limited proprietary sharing or access, allowing team members to exchange and share "code" while reducing time and expenses related to sharing, while preserving the long-term integrity of data.
  - o FL allows for integration of real-world evidence (RWE) and electronic health data in a model to create a drug efficacy model across populations of patients.

Use of FL in a collaboration between research hospitals and pharmaceutical companies to predict side effects of drugs from patient level and optimize recruiting so patients would be the "right" patient for the drug, and consider machine learning to optimize recommendations to prescribe personalized drugs for personal use.

## Trust and Reliability in Federated Healthcare AI

The integration of AI into healthcare and other domains is about more than performance—it is about trust! When the lives and safety of patients are at stake, users (including patients, physicians, policymakers, etc.) must be assured that AI models are safe, reliable, correct, trustworthy, fair, and accountable. In the context of Federated Learning (FL), the question of trust becomes exponentially harder due to the distributed nature of data and collaborative model training.

This section will examine the characteristics of trust and reliability in Federated AI in healthcare, the associated essential characteristics, and how these characteristics work collaboratively to mitigate risks in real-world situations.

## Dimensions of Trust in Healthcare AI

In healthcare AI, trust is multidimensional, including:

- Privacy & Security: Users should rely on healthcare AI that technically protects privacy and protects against misuse and breaches.
- Model Accuracy & Robustness: Reliability of AI systems should be demonstrated concerning performance with diverse and unseen patient populations.

- Fairness & Reduction of Bias: AI outputs should not be substantively discriminatorily disbalanced in respect to analysis of any demographic or clinical subpopulation.
- Transparency & Explainability: Clients and patients should be fully understanding in respect to high-confidence modelling.
- Compliance and Accountability: Systems should adhere to useable standards concerning HIPAA, GDPR, and ethical AI goals.

FL enables improvement of these aspects: privacy and decentralised data to improve privacy features, but poses challenges with respect to viewability of models, standards of uniformity, and verifiability that could potentially deter trust from stakeholders (Ali et al., 2022; Mosaiyebzadeh et al., 2023).

## Privacy Assurance in Federated Environments

Trust in FL depends on how FL can safeguard sensitive health data. While raw data never leaves the client device, it is still possible to expose the information relating to the health data in the context of adversarial data users. The methods suggested for decreasing risks, such as Differential Privacy (DP), Secure Multi-party Computation (SMPC), and Homomorphic Encryption (HE), discussed in Section 4, would apply here.

Although PETs may improve the privacy assurances of a model, models may not perform as well with the increased complexity, depending on the hardware and data availability in small clients or devices. As a result, managing a privacy versus utility trade-off will be critical. Aggressive implementation of privacy can result in a less accurate model and reduce trust in model predictions.

To strengthen privacy assurances:

- Clients receive clear guarantees on what data is collected, what data is used, and how it is safeguarded.
- Aggregators provide cryptographic or hardware-backed assurances that compromise states will not infer through various attack types.
- Policies facilitate auditing and access inspection logs to identify the behavior of models across time.

## Fairness and Bias in Federated Healthcare AI

Bias in healthcare AI may lead to unequal treatment or inequalities in health outcomes across various groups of patients. In FL systems, this is exacerbated by the non-IID (non-identically distributed) nature of data across the clients (e.g., a rural clinic may exclusively serve older patients with chronic comorbidities, whereas an urban hospital may serve younger patients with a mix of chronic and community-dominating backgrounds). If the global model learns predominantly from only a small subset of clients, it will likely perform poorly on the other client populations.

When attempting to build equitable and inclusive FL systems:

- We should apply weighted averaging algorithms (e.g., one method is FedAvg with client-aware tuning) to ensure equal representation from individual client populations.
- We must design our client sampling strategies to mitigate overfitting to the dominant institutions.
- We can include fairness constraints in our loss function if we wish to penalize our model for discriminatory predictions.

Recent work has also discussed applying personalized federated learning, whereby a model is locally fine-tuned for each user, to deal with variability between users while preserving privacy as an avenue to reduce bias (Nguyen, 2021; Kumari et al., 2025).

## Explainability and Interpretability

Trust is highly dependent on how interpretable a model is, particularly in high-stakes situations such as diagnostics or prognosis. It's unlikely that a healthcare professional will trust a model that behaves like a "black box".

In FL, achieving explainability is more difficult because of:

- Distributed model updates are less conducive to global interpretability.
- Availability of client-specific data for post-hoc analysis is limited.

Some options include:

- Using interpretable models (e.g., logistic regression, decision trees) instead of fine-tuning a complex deep network when it isn't necessary.
- Using federated explainability frameworks, such as FL-shared SHAP or LIME processes, which apply local computation of feature attributions.
- Visual dashboards for a healthcare professional to review the rationale for predictions across federated institutions.

Explainability is particularly important in applications such as radiology, oncology, or the prediction of cardiac events, where the model outcome frequently influences clinical judgment.

## Robustness and Security Against Adversarial Attacks

In terms of reliability, an equally important consideration is robustness to random noise and deliberate attacks. FL systems are vulnerable to:

- **Poisoning attacks**, such as malicious clients making invalid updates to the overall model.
- **Back door attacks**, which include small changes in the model being made to yield malicious results when properly requested.
- **Inference attacks**, which try to reconstruct private data from a gradient update or weight release.

Ways to ensure robustness include:

- An anomaly detection system to filter out abnormal client updates before aggregation.
- Robust aggregation algorithms (e.g., Krum, Trimmed Mean) that should handle adversarial inputs adequately.
- Adversarial training approaches that build robustness against maliciously manipulated input data.

Healthcare systems should have a continuous monitoring and rollback process in case harmful behavior is detected in an ML model. Being only able to rollback one version can interrupt service (Kumari et al., 2025).

## Accountability, Auditing, and Compliance

Trustworthy AI systems must be auditable and accountable, particularly given the high levels of regulation in fields like healthcare. FL allows organizations to gather relevant patient data while mitigating privacy risks compared to traditional machine learning approaches; however, the distributed model and reliance on cooperating participants can create challenges for accountability.

Some measures to improve auditability are:

- Enablements to blockchain so that there is an immutable record of auditable information, including: model updates, identities of the participants, and the path of decisions.
- Smart contracts to ensure compliance and the mechanisms for incentive arrangements between healthcare institutions.
- Model cards created for federated models, including model training procedures, data provenance, and known restrictions.

AI models used in healthcare are often also subject to international regulatory frameworks like:

- HIPAA (USA): required safeguards protecting Health Information (PHI).
- GDPR (EU): several requirements related to minimization of data, transparency of data, and data generally under user control.
- ISO/IEC 27701: a privacy information management standard relating to AI.

Integrating technical safeguards with ethical and regulatory compliance will allow FL systems to achieve compliance-by-design with established and accepted privacy frameworks and maintain trust.

## Challenges and Open Research Problems

The integration of Federated Learning (FL) with the Internet of Medical Things (IoMT) promises a privacy-preserving, distributed paradigm for artificial intelligence (AI) in healthcare. However, the practical realization of this vision faces numerous technical and systemic challenges. This section explores some of the most pressing and open research problems impeding the deployment of scalable, trustworthy AI in healthcare, specifically focusing on scalability and interoperability, communication and energy constraints, and data and label heterogeneity. Understanding and addressing these challenges is critical to building resilient, ethical, and privacy-first healthcare systems powered by FL and IoMT.

## Scalability and Interoperability in Healthcare Systems

Modern healthcare systems are heterogeneous and fragmented, with institutions operating on disparate digital infrastructures and storing patient data in incompatible formats. As healthcare becomes increasingly digitized and interconnected, scalability and interoperability emerge as foundational challenges for deploying FL and IoMT at scale (in figure 7) (Govardanan, 2023).

*Figure 7. Illustration of challenges in scaling Federated Learning with IoMT, including client management, device heterogeneity, and communication overhead.*

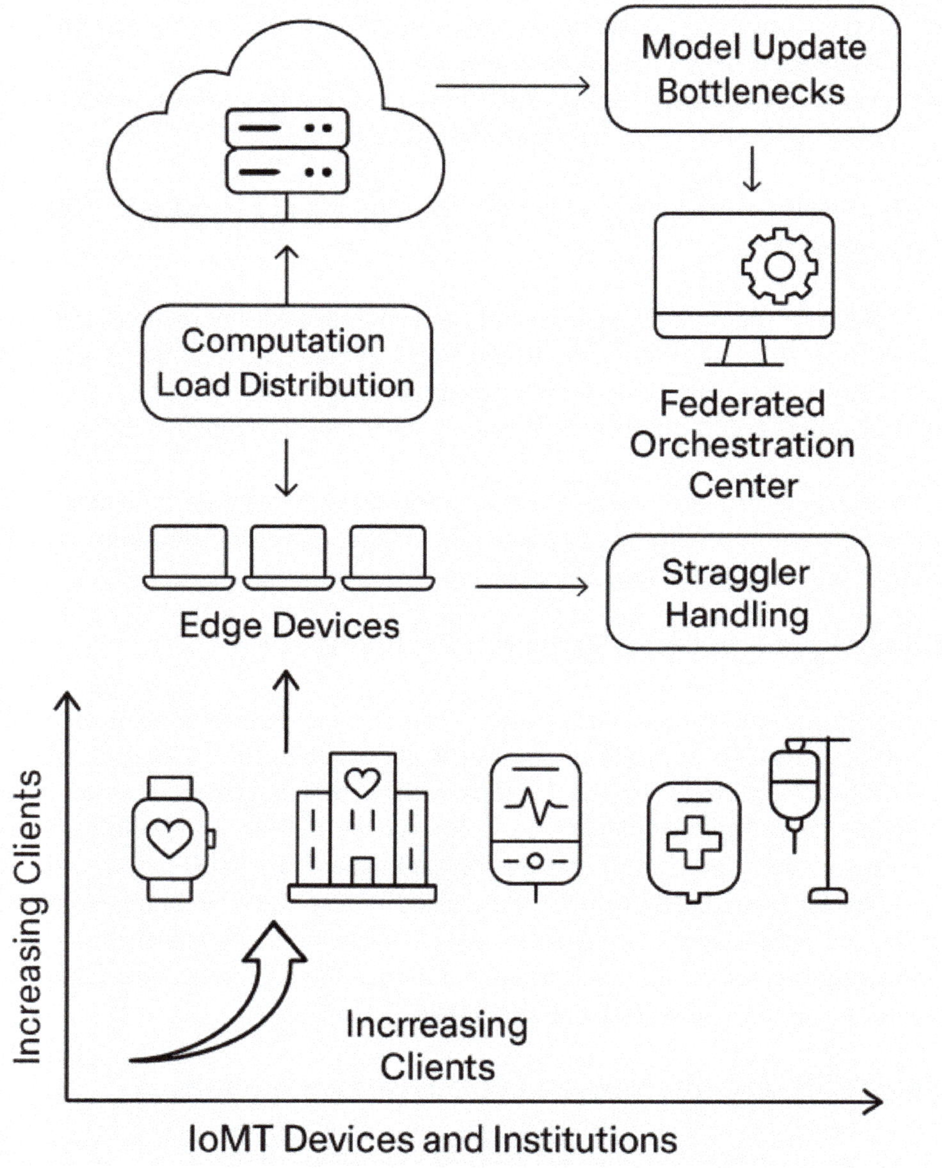

## Scalability Challenges

Scalability in this context refers to the ability of an FL-based healthcare system to effectively include a growing number of data sources, institutions, and IoMT devices without degrading performance or accuracy. Real-world healthcare environments can involve thousands of hospitals, clinics, and wearable devices, each with its unique latency, bandwidth, hardware capabilities, and privacy requirements (Mosaiyebzadeh et al., 2023; Annappa et al., 2024).

- Client Management: Managing thousands of edge clients in federated settings can overwhelm central servers. FL systems must be able to dynamically select participants and handle stragglers—clients with slower updates—without compromising global model performance (Singh et al., 2023; Vivian, n.d.).
- Computation Load Balancing: Not all clients are equal; some devices may be resource-constrained while others are more capable. FL must adaptively distribute training tasks to optimize computation and maintain fairness across clients.
- Model Size and Update Frequency: Large deep learning models and frequent updates can burden networks and edge devices. Scalable compression and quantization techniques are needed to reduce model size while preserving accuracy.

## Interoperability Challenges

Interoperability ensures that healthcare systems and IoMT devices can communicate seamlessly, exchange data accurately, and integrate AI insights meaningfully (Juan, n.d.; SH, n.d.).

- Data Standards and Protocols: Healthcare data is stored in various formats (e.g., HL7, FHIR, DICOM) and across different platforms (EHRs, mobile apps, cloud services). Harmonizing these standards to enable cross-platform federated learning remains a key challenge.
- Semantic Interoperability: Beyond technical format conversion, semantic interoperability—ensuring consistent meaning of data across systems—is harder to achieve. Variations in how diagnoses, procedures, or symptoms are coded (e.g., ICD-10, SNOMED CT) can impact the quality and interpretability of AI models.
- Device Heterogeneity: IoMT devices vary in manufacturers, operating systems, sensor precision, and communication protocols. Enabling these devices

to participate in a federated learning network requires standardized APIs and middleware layers.

Addressing scalability and interoperability is not merely a technical challenge—it requires policy-level coordination, regulatory compliance, and industry-wide co-operation. Open-source platforms and common data models could play a pivotal role in standardizing how FL is deployed in heterogeneous healthcare environments (Bashir et al., 2023; Govardanan, 2023).

## Communication and Energy Constraints in IoMT

IoMT devices, ranging from wearable fitness trackers to implantable medical sensors, are often deployed in energy- and bandwidth-constrained environments. When federated learning is introduced into this equation, the limitations of IoMT infrastructure become a bottleneck (Zheng et al., 2021; Ahmed R., n.d.).

### Communication Constraints

Federated learning relies on frequent communication between edge clients and the central server for model updates. However, continuous data exchange is infeasible for IoMT devices due to:

- Limited Bandwidth: Many IoMT devices rely on low-power wide-area networks (LPWANs) such as LoRaWAN, NB-IoT, or Bluetooth Low Energy (BLE), which are not designed for high-throughput data exchange (Zheng et al., 2021).
- Intermittent Connectivity: In remote or mobile environments, consistent internet access may not be available. This causes delays in model updates, introduces stale gradients, and potentially biases the global model (Zheng et al., 2021).
- Latency Sensitivity: Medical applications such as real-time monitoring or emergency alerts are latency-sensitive. Prioritizing these over model training is necessary, making FL less feasible during critical operations (Ahmed R., n.d.).

Communication-efficient FL algorithms such as SparseFL, FedAvg with compression, or adaptive aggregation can help reduce the volume of data exchanged. Local update steps and fewer synchronization rounds can also minimize communication overhead, though they risk slowing convergence or reducing model accuracy.

### Energy Constraints

Battery life is a primary concern in wearable and implantable IoMT devices. The additional computational burden of training deep learning models locally can significantly reduce device lifetime.

- Local Training Overhead: Performing gradient updates requires both memory and compute cycles. For energy-constrained devices, this can lead to overheating or premature battery drainage (Tran et al., 2020).
- Model Complexity: Complex neural architectures with millions of parameters are impractical for edge devices. There is a trade-off between model expressiveness and feasibility (Mohammad et al., 2020).
- Scheduling and Duty Cycling: Energy-aware scheduling algorithms are needed to determine when a device should participate in training versus sleep modes (Mohammad et al., 2020).

Hardware-aware model design, including TinyML and pruned neural networks, can help minimize energy consumption. Research into FL-aware chipsets and edge accelerators (e.g., Google Coral, NVIDIA Jetson) is also a promising direction.

## Data and Label Heterogeneity

Healthcare data is inherently non-uniform, varying across institutions, populations, and devices. This heterogeneity poses one of the most profound challenges to FL and IoMT.

### Statistical Heterogeneity

- Non-IID Data: In federated settings, each client may hold data from a unique population subset (e.g., pediatric vs. geriatric patients, urban vs. rural clinics), leading to significant distributional shifts. This violates the IID (independent and identically distributed) assumption common in centralized ML (Usevalad, n.d.).
- Label Imbalance: Some rare diseases or conditions may be overrepresented in certain hospitals and absent in others. This can lead to model bias and poor generalization (Zhang et al., 2022).
- Concept Drift: Over time, patient demographics, disease prevalence, and clinical practices change. FL models must be robust to such dynamic data environments (Usevalad, n.d.).

### Annotation and Label Quality

- Inconsistent Annotations: Labels in healthcare are often derived from clinician inputs, which may vary in accuracy and consistency. This inter-rater variability reduces the signal-to-noise ratio in training data (Zhang et al., 2022).
- Missing Labels: Electronic health records often contain incomplete labels or rely on weak supervision (e.g., ICD codes rather than detailed clinical annotations), which can affect training quality.
- Multi-modal and Multi-task Learning: IoMT devices capture data across modalities (e.g., ECG, accelerometry, glucose levels). Aligning these data types with consistent labels for multi-task FL is an ongoing challenge.

Solutions such as personalized federated learning, clustered FL, and meta-learning approaches are being explored to mitigate heterogeneity. However, designing algorithms that can generalize while respecting local data peculiarities remains a major open research problem (Zhang et al., 2022; Usevalad, n.d.).

## FUTURE DIRECTIONS

This section outlines four promising future directions: the integration of digital twins and the metaverse, the advancement of explainable AI (XAI), the formation of global FL collaborations, and insights from real-world deployments and case studies.

### Integration of Digital Twins and the Metaverse in FL-Enabled Healthcare Digital Twins

A digital twin is a dynamic, virtual representation of a physical entity or system. In healthcare, digital twins can simulate a patient's anatomy, physiology, disease progression, and treatment response in real-time. These personalized models could revolutionize preventive care, precision medicine, and remote monitoring.

Federated Learning enables the safe development of digital twins by allowing institutions to collaboratively train predictive models without exposing sensitive patient data. For example, multiple hospitals could contribute to a model that simulates cardiac function or cancer progression, using local datasets to refine a universally applicable digital twin framework.

Key future applications include:

- Chronic disease management: Continuously updating digital twins can simulate treatment outcomes for diabetes, hypertension, or heart failure, enabling real-time adjustments.
- Surgical planning and training: Virtual replicas of patient anatomy can assist surgeons and trainees in simulated environments, with data-driven updates through FL.

However, significant research is needed to address:

- High-fidelity modeling across diverse patient populations
- Privacy-preserving real-time synchronization between digital twins and FL models
- Integration of multi-modal data from wearables, imaging, and EHRs

## Metaverse and Immersive Healthcare Environments

The metaverse, an immersive virtual environment powered by extended reality (XR), can complement healthcare by enabling virtual consultations, collaborative diagnostics, and remote patient engagement. Within the FL context, the metaverse can serve as:

- A simulated training environment for AI systems using synthetic patient interactions
- A collaborative clinical space where healthcare professionals and AI agents co-exist and test models safely before real-world deployment

FL will be vital in enabling distributed learning for these virtual environments while safeguarding user privacy. Coupled with digital twins, the metaverse could support highly personalized, interactive models for patient care and clinical decision-making.

## Explainable AI for Healthcare Decision-Making

As AI becomes embedded in diagnostic tools, treatment planning, and risk prediction, transparency and interpretability are essential for clinical trust and adoption. Explainable AI (XAI) addresses this by providing insights into model decisions.

## Importance in Federated Settings

In federated healthcare AI, clinicians and patients are one step further removed from the training process, increasing the need for interpretable outputs. Unlike centralized models, federated models are trained on unseen and often non-IID data. Without interpretability:

- Clinicians may mistrust AI recommendations
- Errors may be difficult to debug
- It becomes harder to ensure fairness and accountability

## XAI Techniques for Federated Healthcare

Several XAI techniques are being adapted to FL frameworks:

- **SHAP** (SHapley Additive exPlanations): Quantifies feature contributions to individual predictions
- **LIME** (Local Interpretable Model-agnostic Explanations): Approximates local decision boundaries for black-box models
- **Attention mechanisms and saliency maps**: Provide visual cues in imaging or time-series data, useful in radiology, pathology, or ECG interpretation

Future research must address:

- Efficient deployment of XAI methods in edge environments (e.g., wearables, remote clinics)
- Federated training of inherently interpretable models
- Clinician-centered design of explanations that match domain reasoning

Explainability also plays a critical role in ethical AI, enabling transparency in decision pathways and supporting informed consent by patients and practitioners.

## Global FL Healthcare Collaborations

Federated learning uniquely positions itself as a vehicle for global collaboration in healthcare AI, especially valuable for improving equity, accelerating medical discovery, and addressing rare diseases.

## Cross-Border Health AI Development

Countries and institutions with diverse populations, disease burdens, and medical technologies can collaboratively develop AI models without compromising patient data privacy. For instance:

- Pandemic surveillance models (e.g., COVID-19, influenza) can be trained across national health systems in real-time
- Rare disease diagnosis can benefit from pooled data, where each institution contributes cases too infrequent to train standalone models

FL enables cross-border model training without cross-border data movement, mitigating regulatory hurdles such as GDPR and HIPAA.

## Challenges to Global Federated Collaborations

Despite its promise, global FL in healthcare faces several challenges:

- Legal interoperability: Aligning diverse data protection laws, ethics guidelines, and institutional review protocols
- Infrastructure disparities: Ensuring equitable participation by under-resourced regions with limited connectivity or computing
- Language and coding standards: Harmonizing clinical terminologies and EHR systems across countries

International initiatives and open-source FL platforms (e.g., OpenFL, Flower) are emerging to tackle these challenges and promote inclusive, global FL ecosystems.

## Real-World Deployments and Case Studies

Several real-world deployments and pilot studies are now showcasing the feasibility of FL in healthcare.

## Federated Tumor Segmentation (FeTS)

The Federated Tumor Segmentation (FeTS) initiative, led by the University of Pennsylvania and other global partners, is a landmark FL project in neuroimaging. It involves over 30 institutions collaborating on brain tumor segmentation using MRI scans. No raw data is shared; instead, local models are trained and aggregated securely.

## Outcomes:

- Comparable performance to centralized models
- Preservation of patient privacy
- Standardization of clinical workflows for multi-institutional AI

## Federated Learning in Diabetes Prediction

Wearable glucose monitors and smartphones enable the collection of rich behavioral and physiological data. Several studies have used FL to build personalized diabetes risk prediction models without transmitting user data to central servers. These models adapt locally while benefiting from global learning, improving prediction accuracy in resource-constrained and privacy-sensitive environments.

## Industry and Health System Adoption

- Owkin has deployed FL to study cancer treatment response across hospitals in Europe.
- Mayo Clinic and NVIDIA's Clara FL platform have explored federated learning for pathology and radiology AI.
- Healthchain and IBM **Federated Learning** offer enterprise-grade frameworks for secure AI collaborations.

These examples highlight how FL can move from concept to clinical reality, provided trust, governance, and performance criteria are met.

In conclusion, the future of trustworthy, privacy-preserving AI in healthcare is being shaped by the convergence of federated learning, IoMT, digital twins, the metaverse, and global partnerships. Each frontier—whether it's personalized virtual patient models, explainable AI tools for decision support, or real-world collaborations—contributes to a robust ecosystem where innovation doesn't compromise privacy or equity.

To unlock the full potential of FL in healthcare, several imperatives must be addressed:

- Build governance models for international and multi-institutional cooperation
- Embed explainability and accountability into every stage of the AI lifecycle
- Invest in infrastructure to support real-time, energy-efficient federated systems
- Foster inclusive innovation, ensuring that AI benefits are globally distributed

By aligning technological advances with ethical, clinical, and regulatory frameworks, federated learning can transform not just how healthcare AI is built, but who it serves and how safely it does so.

## CONCLUSION

As healthcare increasingly turns to data-driven intelligence, the demand for privacy-first, secure, and ethically aligned AI systems has never been more urgent. Federated Learning (FL), combined with the Internet of Medical Things (IoMT), offers a compelling solution by enabling collaborative model training without transferring sensitive patient data. This chapter has explored the foundations, challenges, and future directions of Privacy-Preserving Federated Learning (PPFL) in healthcare, emphasizing that building trustworthy AI requires a comprehensive approach that integrates technology, ethics, governance, and real-world constraints.

We've examined how PPFL addresses critical privacy concerns by keeping data decentralized, using cryptographic safeguards like differential privacy and secure aggregation. At the same time, we have highlighted real challenges that must be overcome: scalability and interoperability across healthcare systems, communication and energy limitations in IoMT devices, and data heterogeneity across populations and institutions. These technical barriers underscore the need for intelligent system design and adaptive FL algorithms capable of functioning under real-world constraints.

Equally vital is ensuring trust and reliability in federated healthcare AI. We explored the necessity of governance frameworks, institutional accountability, and robust defenses against adversarial attacks. Addressing bias and fairness emerged as both a technical and ethical imperative, especially given healthcare's direct impact on human well-being. Solutions like personalized FL, fairness-aware optimization, and participatory design were proposed as ways to ensure equitable outcomes.

Looking ahead, the future of PPFL in healthcare is being shaped by emerging technologies and paradigms. Digital twins and the metaverse offer immersive, personalized environments for modeling health states and treatments, while Explainable AI (XAI) ensures clinicians can interpret and trust model decisions. Global federated collaborations promise to democratize access to medical AI innovations across borders, fostering inclusivity while respecting regulatory diversity. These developments are no longer theoretical, real-world deployments such as FeTS for brain tumor segmentation, Mayo Clinic's work in radiology, and wearable-based diabetes prediction platforms are demonstrating the tangible potential of FL in clinical practice.

In conclusion, building trustworthy, privacy-preserving AI in healthcare is not a destination but a journey. It requires the seamless fusion of technology, trust, transparency, and thoughtful design. By embracing federated learning and IoMT, and addressing the challenges outlined in this chapter, we move closer to a healthcare future where AI is not just intelligent, but also secure, ethical, and worthy of trust, for every patient, everywhere.

## REFERENCES


Ali, M., Naeem, F., Tariq, M., & Kaddoum, G. (2022). Federated Learning for Privacy Preservation in Smart Healthcare Systems: A Comprehensive Survey. *arXiv preprint*. https://arxiv.org/abs/2203.09702

Annappa, B., Hegde, S., Abhijit, C. S., & Ambesange, S. (2024). Fedcure: A heterogeneity-aware personalized federated learning framework for intelligent healthcare applications in iomt environments. *IEEE Access*. https://ieeexplore.ieee.org/abstract/document/10412046/

Bashir, A. K., Victor, N., Bhattacharya, S., Huynh-The, T., Chengoden, R., Yenduri, G., Praveen, K. R. M., Pham, Q.-V., Gadekallu, T. R., & Liyanage, M. (2023). A Survey on Federated Learning for the Healthcare Metaverse: Concepts, Applications, Challenges, and Future Directions. *arXiv preprint*. https://arxiv.org/abs/2304.00524

Govardanan, C. S., Murugan, R., Yenduri, G., Gurrammagari, D. R., Bhulakshmi, D., Kandati, D. R., ... & Jhaveri, R. H. (2024). The amalgamation of federated learning and explainable artificial intelligence for the internet of medical things: a review. Recent Advances in Computer Science and Communications (Formerly: Recent Patents on Computer Science), 17(4), 1-19.

Tran, H. V., Kaddoum, G., Elgala, H., Abou-Rjeily, C., & Kaushal, H. (2020). Lightwave power transfer for federated learning-based wireless networks. *IEEE Communications Letters*, *24*(7), 1472–1476.

Kumari, M., Gaikwad, M., & Chavan, S. A. (2025). A secure IoT-edge architecture with data-driven AI techniques for early detection of cyber threats in healthcare. *Discover Internet of Things*, *5*(1), 54.

Mohammad, U., Sorour, S. M., & Hefeida (2020). Task Allocation for Mobile Federated and Offloaded Learning with Energy and Delay Constraints. *2020 IEEE International Conference on Communications Workshops (ICC Workshops)*. https://ieeexplore.ieee.org/document/9145450/

Mosaiyebzadeh, F., Pouriyeh, S., Parizi, R. M., Sheng, Q. Z., Han, M., Zhao, L., & Batista, D. M. (2023). Privacy-enhancing technologies in federated learning for the internet of healthcare things: A survey. *Electronics (Basel)*, *12*(12), 2703.

Nguyen, D. C., Pham, Q. V., Pathirana, P. N., Ding, M., Seneviratne, A., Lin, Z., & Hwang, W. J. (2022). Federated learning for smart healthcare: A survey. *ACM Computing Surveys*, *55*(3), 1–37.

Singh, C., Mishra, R., Gupta, H. P., & Banga, G. (2023). A Federated Learning-Based Patient Monitoring System in Internet of Medical Things. *IEEE Transactions on Computational Social Systems*. https://ieeexplore.ieee.org/document/9994660/

Zhang, M., Qu, L., & Singh, P. (2022). Splitavg: A heterogeneity-aware federated deep learning method for medical imaging. https://ieeexplore.ieee.org/abstract/document/9806163/

Zheng, X., Shah, S. B. H., Ren, X., & Li, F. (2021). Mobile edge computing enabled efficient communication based on federated learning in internet of medical things. https://onlinelibrary.wiley.com/doi/abs/10.1155/2021/4410894

# Chapter 6
# Anomaly-Resilient Digital Health Integrating AI, IoT, and Privacy Frameworks for Secure Patient Monitoring

**Abhinav Upadhyay**
https://orcid.org/0009-0003-7951-6447
*Manipal University Jaipur, India*

**Ridhi Kulshreshtha**
https://orcid.org/0009-0000-7989-5019
*Manipal University Jaipur, India*

**Ram Mohan Bhola**
https://orcid.org/0009-0000-2281-2411
*Manipal University Jaipur, India*

**Saurabh Mishra**
*Indian Institute of Information Technology, Allahabad, India*

## ABSTRACT

*The advent of digitalized patient monitoring systems marks a major breakthrough in healthcare. IoT, cloud computing, and AI generate behavior-driven big data but this integration also raises concerns about anomalies and cybersecurity threats. This chapter explores two types of anomalies: patient-centered irregular medical activity and system- centered network threats. Traditional methods are often inade-*

DOI: 10.4018/979-8-3373-7610-3 ch006

*quate compared to machine learning approaches like SVM, unsupervised learning, LSTM, and autoencoders for real-time detection. We examine how cloud-enabled IoT systems manage patient data amid potential breaches, supported by compliance frameworks like HIPAA and GDPR. Federated Learning enhances data privacy in monitoring devices. Two case studies are presented: one using wearable ECG devices for patient anomaly detection, and another using the NbaIoT dataset for identifying security breaches. This chapter outlines a path toward a trust-centric, secure, AI-enabled healthcare monitoring framework.*

# 1 INTRODUCTION

## 1.1 Rise of IoT and Cloud in wearable Healthcare devices

Healthcare systems, especially patient monitoring, saw revolution with the amalgamation of Internet of things (IoT) and Cloud systems that support Artificial Intelligence (AI) integration. Wearable technologies are ubiquitous, not to mention in home-based healthcare, ranging from smartwatches to biosensor-enabled tracking of heart rate, $SpO_2$, ECG, blood glucose, etc. To enhance performance and resource utilization, cloud platforms with real-time data integrity, centralised storage and analytics paves way for an intelligent and patient-focused care system.

Internet of Medical Things (IoMT) promotes personalized remote care in real-time by connecting patients to healthcare assistance via easy to operate devices. These devices are non-invasive compared to traditionally uncomfortable or intrusive ones. The data collected by these devices is transmitted to cloud-based servers following communication protocols (see Figure 1). This exchange of data demands a robust platform that not just stores data but also helps analyse it. Thus, cloud computing offers scalable infrastructure that handles streams of big data, behavioral in nature captured via utilization patterns. After this, when AI tools perform analysis on this stored data that the system alerts patient as well as health care practitioners about any anomaly, be it in the system or patient condition related. These practices lead to effective outcomes, efficiency and service delivery by medical practitioners towards patient care.

While we get continuous, real-time monitoring instead of appointments which aids in early diagnosis, applications in healthcare field come with challenges such as privacy and cybersecurity with the integration of AI.

*Figure 1. IoT-Based Patient Monitoring Device Architecture*

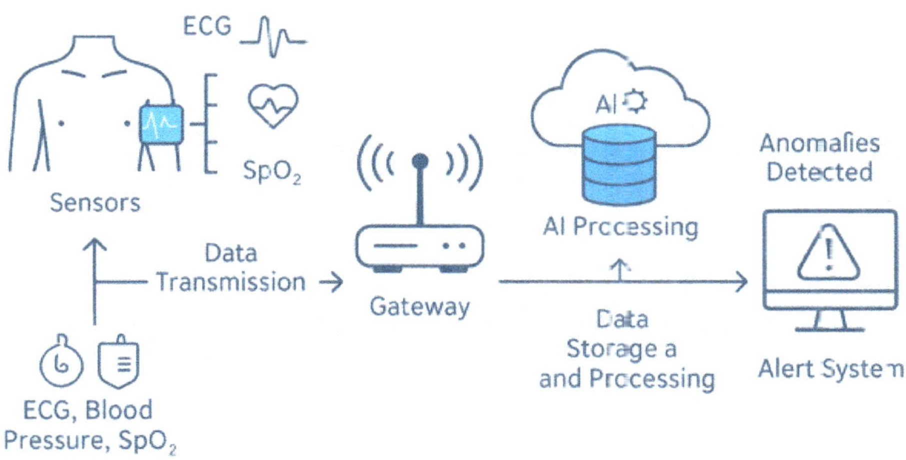


## 1.2 Defining the Central Problem: What Constitutes a Behavioral Anomaly?

Challenges in medical patient monitoring devices are rising due to behavioral anomalies. These anomalies rise from aberrations – either in user's established routine or in the system itself (See Figure 2). These values may fall out outside expected and later help us flag potential risk. Hence anomalies, in this book chapter, refers to two broad categories.

First are anomalies reported by AI monitoring devices to aware users about arrhythmia, drop in SpO$_2$, etc in the form of smartwatches, trackers, or even smart clothing. They help flag irregularity in activity metrics and may even provide communication with healthcare professionals. The second anomaly category apprises us about network and system level one that arise as a result of technologies like IoT infrastructure in activities like data transfer interruption, abnormal traffic or even unauthorized access as cybersecurity issues.

*Figure 2. Dual Nature of Behavioral Anomalies: Patient or System-Centric*

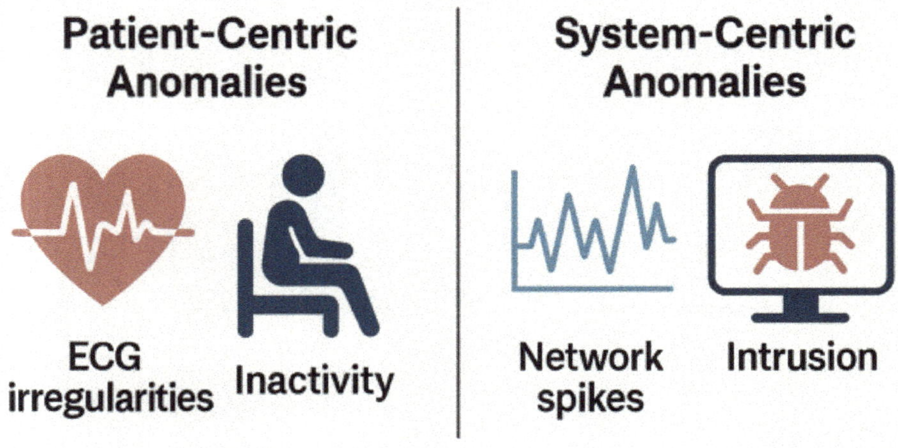


A major challenge to tackle is the real-time detection of these deviations from routine changes cause by temporary misalignment of sensors or a simple lifestyle change. Traditional models for anomaly detection struggle due to unforeseen circumstances and the complex nature of data. Hence come into the picture, AI-based solutions that adapts by learning patterns from data.

The problem being addressed by this book chapter is the dual nature of behavioral anomalies in recognizing the medical irregularities as well as network cybersecurity threats concerning wearable monitoring devices in the field of healthcare.

## 1.3 The Importance of Behavioral Monitoring

The tracking of physiological parameters can prove to be prognosis for chronic diseases, health assessment and even recovery. These monitoring devices provide feedback and tailored care transforming healthcare. Over 80% consumers across globe are enthusiastic to adopt wearable devices for health tracking. (Soto et al.,2024) In terms of patient care, it helps us collect volumes of data that patients might forget otherwise and covers long-term evaluation giving data for anomaly assessment. (Vijayan et al.,2021) An example can be ECG devices that can help flag arrhythmias which may not be noticed in check-ups. Even tracking sleep may help uncover neurological issues.

A point to note is that this behavioral data also helps flag any misuse or malfunction in these devices. Some cybersecurity activities include unusual patterns in data transfer, unexpected device behavior or any tampering involved. This behavioral data due to its volume and velocity is considered big data which helps with training ML models and predicting or flagging by finding patterns. However, this continuous use of data can risk patients' privacy. The sensitivity of the scenario, while following compliance regulations, calls for a framework that ensures trust while flagging anomalous behavior.

The aim of this book chapter is to explore how IoT devices integrated with cloud infrastructure, along with AI methodologies can face the dual challenge of physiological and system aberrations. The main objectives covered during the course of this chapter are:

1. To explore the role of cloud infrastructure, IoT devices and AI in the field of patient monitoring devices
2. To analyse the dual nature of behavioral anomalies in healthcare monitoring systems: patient and system centric
3. To introduce concept of federated learning as privacy preserving solution to comply with Health Insurance Portability and Accountability Act (HIPAA) and the General Data Protection Regulation (GDPR)
4. To demonstrate how machine learning and deep learning models enable real time adaptive detection
5. To validate the effectiveness of AI driven frameworks with the help of two case studies – one focused on patient anomaly using wearable ECG device and another on cybersecurity threat using NbaIoT dataset

# 2 BEHAVIORAL ANOMALIES IN HEALTHCARE: SCOPE AND SIGNIFICANCE

## 2.1 Patient-Centric Anomalies: Medical Behavioral Deviations

In an individual's physiological data, irregularities deviating from their expected health patterns are known as patient-centric anomalies, for example, erratic heart rates and inactivity. Erratic heart rates signal conditions like arrhythmia, which is among adults with congenital heart disease, a major cause of mortality (Menachem et al., 2017). A unique pattern linked to behavioral and emotional disturbances can be seen when monitoring heart rate changes which suggests that physiology and mental states are intertwined (Freeman et al., 1999).

Another critical patient-centric anomaly, contributing to major public health problems; prolonged physical inactivity has been recognized as a cardiovascular risk associated with placing an enormous burden on healthcare services and costs

(Prasad & Das, 2009). Healthcare industry has seen a rise of IoT devices, such as sensors that monitor vitals like heart rate and blood pressure, increasing the risk of irregular patterns or outliers in patient data highlighting the need for robust anomaly detection mechanisms so that early signs of deterioration can be identified (Kadir et al., 2024).

## 2.2 Device / Network-Centric Anomalies

Another kind of anomalies involving cyber and usage irregularities affecting the security of healthcare systems and operational integrity is the Device/network-centric anomalies. A key example being unexpected spikes in network traffic. Given the fact that the data transferred on healthcare networks involves sensitive information, secure network operations become very crucial as network faults can take place due to anomalous traffic (Lee et al., 2015).

Usage anomalies such as loosely attached leads, compromising signal quality can be seen in Body Sensor Networks (BSNs) such as those monitoring Electrocardiogram (ECG) can directly impact diagnosis (Chen & Bate., 2016). From a network-centric perspective, AI and Machine Learning method are now being integrated to detect abnormalities like unusual device behaviour in real-time improving the operational integrity (Fan et al., 2023). As the use of Healthcare IoT increases, the threats across security layers also increases making intrusion detection and secure data transmission more important than ever.

## 2.3 Interconnectivity Between Patient-Centric and Device/Network-Centric Anomalies

The above mentioned two types of anomalies are often connected. For instance, to detect anomalies, data flow characteristics alongside patient biometrics are being used in modern healthcare monitoring systems mirroring real-life applications in clinical environments (Hady et al., 2020).

The interconnectivity is seen in hospital settings where IoT sensors are used to monitor patient vitals such as heart rate and blood pressure. These patient-centric data streams generate vast amounts of data directly linking to the security of the network and robust decision mechanisms, avoiding the risk of distorted clinical insight or delays of any kind (Kadir et al., 2024). Additionally, in the case of body sensors, such as the ones used to detect anomalous ECG signals, there is always a possibility that abnormality may arise due to issues like incorrect device usage (Chen & Bate., 2016).

Furthermore, to detect anomalies that suggests both health issues and device-related irregularities, there are real-time monitoring systems that compare expected user behavior with actual events using physiological sensing devices to identify irregularities relating to medical problems, device misuse, or security breaches

(Parvin, 2018). This interplay shows the importance of designing anomaly detection frameworks in patient monitoring systems.

## 2.4 Importance of Real-Time Detection

To ensure safety of the patient and operational efficiency, real-time detection is of utmost importance in responding to behavioral anomalies. Early detection, especially for elderly people, can prevent severe injuries and save lives (Moore & Lu., 2020). Healthcare industry must move beyond analysing health history to managing future health which makes real-time analytics, particularly in applications like arrhythmia detection using electrocardiogram (ECG) monitoring, increasingly essential (Agneeswaran et al., 2013).

Recent frameworks can identify anomalies with high precision in the data collected from sensors in wearables and medical devices demonstrating the importance of Real-time anomaly detection to protect patient data and device integrity in Healthcare IoT environments.

## 2.5 Limitations of Rule-Based Systems

Due to their intrinsic intricacy and strict constraints, rule-based systems suffer from limitations when it comes to detecting behavioral anomalies in healthcare, often leading to false alerts and not being able to detect all potential errors in areas such as medication prescription. Furthermore, healthcare systems are complex and more often than not these systems are inadequate in enhancing anomaly detection due to their static nature limiting their ability to adapt to real-time variations in patient behavior (Raghavan., 2025). Although it has been used in some contexts, applicability of rule-based systems in pervasive healthcare has been limited especially for nuanced anomalies and abnormal patient behaviours (Mitchell & Chen., 2014).

To overcome these limitations, hybrid approaches are gaining traction that combine the rule-based reasoning with the adaptability and flexibility of Machine Learning (ML) Techniques to provide more efficient and accurate anomaly detection (S Kierner, J Kucharski, & Z Kierner, 2023). One such instance of this hybrid approach demonstrated strong performance by achieving 76% interception rate for high-risk prescriptions and a precision-rate of 75% showcasing the superior performance of the ML-enhanced Medical Decision Support System over the traditional rule-based systems (Rahman, F. 2024). In fields like Cybersecurity and healthcare, where precision and real-time responsiveness are critical, these findings signal the need for more advanced anomaly detection systems to surpass the constraints of traditional rule-based systems.

# 3 IoT-ENABLED PATIENT MONITORING DEVICES: A SOURCE OF BEHAVIORAL DATA

## 3.1 IoT powered Monitoring Devices

The required data for behavioral analysis comes from IoT-enabled patient monitoring devices. These devices help in continuously collecting this stream of data, utilising plethora of sensors or modern-day technologies. There are various types of devices for measuring different parameters (see Figure 3). This captured data is then used for early detection in medical care. Before we understand the data, we need to understand the source of it. Table 1 below explains the various types of such wellbeing devices used in medical field along with their implementation. It shows how different devices look out for different parameters and with the help of these try to collect data. Even the technology used for measuring different physiological parameters is varying with use case.

*Figure 3. Types of IoT-Enabled Monitoring Devices for Various Physiological Parameters*

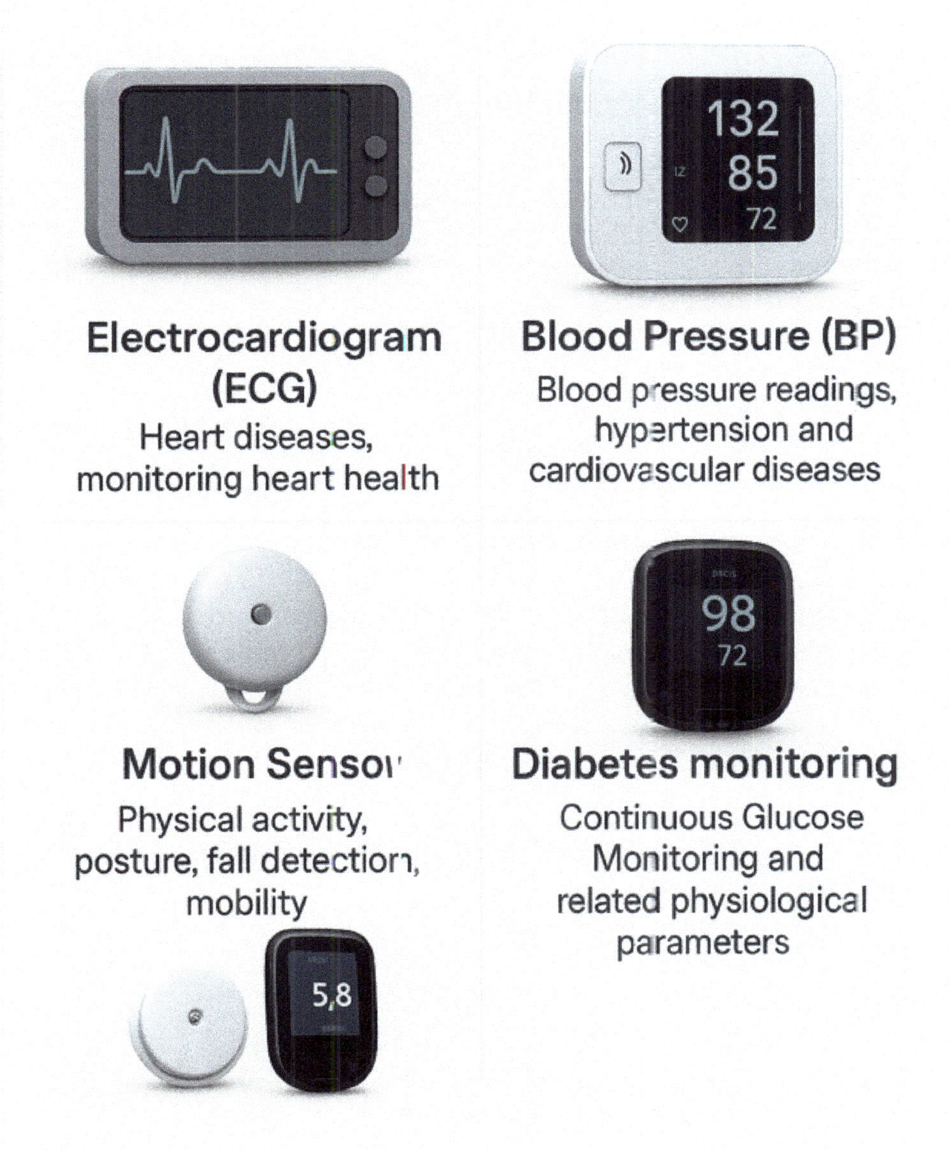


The above-mentioned systems can also combine multiple systems in order to predict a combination of physiological parameters together. For example, ECG monitoring can be combined with $SpO_2$ for comprehensive assessment (Fanucci et al 2012). As mentioned by Murugan et al., 2024, systems may use Galvanic Skin

Response (GSR) sensors and even use cameras to note the activity levels. They also recognize retinopathy images to assess diabetic conditions in patients.

*Table 1. Types of IoT-Enabled Monitoring Devices and Their Behavioral Parameters*

| Device Type | Monitored Parameters | Technology used |
|---|---|---|
| Electrocardiogram (ECG) | Heart diseases, monitoring heart health | Three-lead and five-led ECG sensors |
| Blood Pressure (BP) | Blood pressure readings, hypertension and cardiovascular diseases | Bluetooth enabled |
| Oxygen Saturation ($SpO_2$) | Blood oxygen levels | Pulse oximetry sensors |
| Motion Sensor | Sensors such as accelerometers | Physical activity, posture, fall detection, mobility |
| Diabetes monitoring | Continuous Glucose Monitoring and related physiological parameters | Non-invasive methods unlike traditional finger pricking |

## 3.2 Data Flow and Behavioral Signal Capture

The architecture for data flow in IoT patient monitoring devices goes from sensing the data about physiological parameters such as heartbeat, $SpO_2$, collected from wearable devices, then transmitting this received data to a storage system such as cloud. Then processing is done on this data following storage. This reflects a workflow that helps us flag anomalies (see Figure 4).

*Figure 4. Flow of Data in IoT-Enabled Healthcare Devices Connected to Cloud Infrastructure*

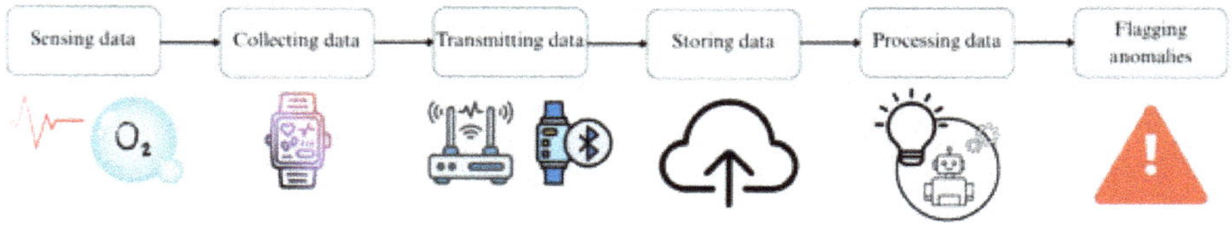


1. Sensing data: To capture medical information, wearable devices and medically equipped sensors are utilised. They continuously sense real-time data including

physiological parameters like oxygen saturation, heart rate, glucose as well as physical actions and even emotions. (Shumba et al., 2022) This sensed data is what forms the essence of detecting anomalies by forming patterns. Hospital environments have benefitted from IoT sensor integration by capturing user as well as device communication for threat detection in cybersecurity networks. (ALmojel & Mishra., 2024). Filtering and sampling methods are also at sensing module so that volume of transmitted data can be reduced, hence patients can be monitored without edge processing. (Waleed et al., 2023).

2. Data collection: Collection of data is the intermediate step between sensing the information and transmitting for further processing by AI tools. The data is collected continuously, allowing real-time processing and detection. As Harb et al., 2020 mentioned the data collected from these biosensors can be multimodal like numerical, image or even videos.
3. Data Transmission: The data that has been sensed and collected from patient monitoring sources is then transmitted for upcoming processing to take place at a central system. Cellular networks like 3G and 4G, Wifi and Bluetooth are used by IoT devices in healthcare. Message Queuing Telemetry Transport (MQTT) is a protocol used for data transmission in IoT since it requires low power consumption. (Yew et al., 2020). Constrained Application Protocol (CoAP) with faster transactions at lower cost and Data Distribution Service (DDS) with reduces data latency and enhanced reliability has found its way in medical IoT devices. (Chen & Kunz, 2016)
4. Data Storage: There are two methods that can be used for storage of data. Typically, cloud-based platforms with secure protocols are used to receive behavioral data. This collected data is even used by AI algorithms to flag anomalies. Cloud systems are centralized in nature, offering real-time aid in analysing historical data and train machine learning models to predict anomalies. Another method becoming increasingly popular is Edge AI, reducing latency and bandwidth consumption issues. To explain simply, edge AI enables processing of data near the source of data generation to support immediate response. (Arjunan, 2023).
5. Data Processing: To flag anomalies, we need to process the data generated with AI techniques of ML and DL. More traditional ML models include Support Vector Machine, Decision Trees, Naïve Bayes to predict risks. Long Short-Term Memory network, a type of Deep Learning method is used for prediction in behavioral time series data analysis (Maruthukannan et al., 2024). Another example is the use of Recurrent Neural Networks that remembers patterns to detect blood pressure in health industry. (Reddy et al., 2025)

## 3.3 Vulnerabilities and Anomaly Sources in IoT Devices

In the modern world, these IoT-enabled patient monitoring devices are at a threat of data breaches and cybersecurity attacks. These quickly make the devices vulnerable by putting at risk the trust of patients on healthcare support. This can be caused by a few factors that we will explore in this section.

The first reason for anomaly in these sources are the sensor generated inaccuracies. The data from these sensors is time-series or stream data. The continuous flow of data requires the uninterrupted operation of sensors in medical field to prevent any compromise in data collection and integrity. These are crucial as they may lead to outliers or sudden changes in patient data. Research is being conducted to handle these errors coming from uncertain sensors. This may impact the healthcare systems used for anomaly detection in patient centric field.

Device malfunction is another reason that gives rise to anomalies. Stream data emission is continuous, and any malfunctioning can hamper the data transmission process. This may also lead to concerns about the usability of patient health data. As mentioned by Abideen et al., 2017, IoT sensors are connected to smartphones; in case of malfunction in primary smartphone, the sensor can use a peer in its vicinity to prevent interruption in data stream. These device malfunctions can also occur as a result of outdates firmware or even inadequate authentication of communication which can become weak points for cybersecurity attacks. (Aditya et al., 2024)

This may also lead to concerns about the usability of patient health data. As mentioned by Abideen et al., 2017, IoT sensors are connected to smartphones; in case of malfunction in primary smartphone, the sensor can use a peer in its vicinity to prevent interruption in data stream. These device malfunctions can also occur as a result of outdates firmware or even inadequate authentication of communication which can become weak points for cybersecurity attacks. (Aditya et al., 2024)

And finally, we have network issues contributing to system vulnerabilities. Cybersecurity issues can threaten IoT health monitoring systems, especially Denial of Service (DoS) attacks, Fingerprint and Timing-based Snooping, Router attacks, Select and Forwarding attacks, Sensor attacks, and Replay attacks (Butt et al., 2019). Healthcare data is sensitive and prone to modification, interception and even being repudiated by the attackers. Implantable Medical Devices, Radio Frequency Identification tags, and wearable devices are prone to such vulnerabilities and protecting patients CIA triad, that is Confidentiality, Integrity, and Availability is of paramount importance. (Somasundaram & Thirugnanam, 2021) Health data across each of the device is at a central location accessible across networks. These internet-connected devices can become the attack points and spread to various devices from within and include outdated operating systems, weak security controls, or misconfigurations in systems (Copeland, 2018). In the upcoming sections we will see how even protocols like HIPAA and GDPR cannot prevent the prevalent data breaches.

# 4 AI TECHNIQUES FOR BEHAVIORAL ANOMALY DETECTION

## 4.1 Why Traditional Techniques Fall Short

In Healthcare, the data can be quite complex and unpredictable, therefore, the traditional systems often struggle with anomaly detection. As discussed earlier, due to their strict constraints and intrinsic limitations, these rule-based or static access control systems are often inadequate for enhancing anomaly detection and are prone to mistakes like producing false alerts and failing to detect potential errors in medication prescription.

Moreover, the old rules and statistical approaches are losing their relevance due to the dynamic and unpredictable nature of modern cyberattacks. Static rules fail to adapt to the ever evolving cyberattack patterns and behavioral anomalies as the healthcare systems become more modern and increasingly digital (Akinola et al., 2024).

When there is limited labelled data and the inputs are complex, these traditional systems require extensive computational resources and exhibit reduced accuracy. Another problem for traditional methods is the difficulty in collecting all control signal data due to limited data acquisition time in large manufacturing systems (Ghosh et al., 2016).

Furthermore, in smart manufacturing, these systems often face data imbalance problems, where traditional machine learning algorithms often struggle as they tend to be biased towards the majority class and the minority class or the critical minority anomalies are overlooked (He et al., 2023).

## 4.2 Supervised and Unsupervised Learning Approaches

In the realm of behavioral anomaly detection, due to the ability to learn patterns from all the extensive healthcare data and then generalizing these patterns to detect anomalies, Machine Learning (ML) is a powerful alternative to the traditional techniques. In this domain, there are two types of approaches namely, Supervised learning and Unsupervised learning.

In Supervised Learning, the training of algorithms is done on labelled datasets, where based on known anomalies, the model learns to classify the inputs. Algorithms like Support Vector Machine (SVM) and Random Forest (RF) demonstrate high accuracy when tasked with classifying and detecting anomalies in datasets (Ali et al., 2024). However, Supervised Learning requires large, high-quality labelled data and the process of collecting and labelling large scale datasets in the real world can become very time-consuming, resource-intensive and often requires expert domain knowledge.

On the other hand, these limitations pave the way for another domain of ML, Unsupervised Learning, which infer patterns from datasets without relying on labelled data. These algorithms are useful when data labelling is problematic and particularly valuable for finding hidden patterns or groupings in data. Unsupervised learning techniques do have their pitfalls. For anomaly detection in system logs, they can have "blind spots" and can struggle with interpretability making Supervised methods more accurate and transparent.

To address these challenges, blending both the unsupervised and supervised methods, hybrid approaches have emerged. At first pseudo labels are generated using unsupervised methods, which is then refined by a supervised model trained on pseudo-labelled examples, showing increased robustness and performance in behavioural anomaly detection (Rački et al., 2023).

### 4.2.1 Isolation Forests and One-Class SVM

Due to its effectiveness and scalability, Isolation Forest (iForest) has emerged as a popular anomaly detector. It is a tree-based unsupervised learning method that isolates anomalies rather than profiling normal data as a result being very efficient for large datasets. In the healthcare domain, Isolation Forests have been successfully applied to detect over-treatment and over-prescription in medical insurance claims and can be flagged as anomalous behaviour, showing high sensitivity to anomalies, efficiency and precise identification of out-of-the-ordinary behaviour (Du et al., 2023). However, for anomalies masked by axis-parallel normal clusters and anomalies in multi-modal datasets, traditional isolation forests tend to struggle leading to high false negative errors.

Another example of an unsupervised learning technique is the One-Class SVM (OCSVM), useful when only normal data is available for training. It learns a decision boundary around the normal data, and an anomaly is detected if any data point falls outside this decision boundary (Yang et al., 2021). In healthcare, it helps protect device integrity and patient data by detecting anomalies in real-time in IoT environments and can also monitor the health of machines by measuring the behaviour of the system. Despite being computationally efficient, OCSVM can sometimes yield unsatisfactory results and offer very limited control over the false alarm rate (Miao et al., 2018).

### 4.2.2 Clustering Techniques

Clustering techniques are used in identifying outliers by categorizing similar data points and the ones which do not conform to these groups are marked as outliers.

For anomaly detection in healthcare various clustering techniques have been applied such as K-means clustering and Gaussian Mixture Model (GMM) that are easy to implement and can classify abnormal traffic patterns in hospital networks. Another flexible and optimal algorithm is Fuzzy C-Means clustering (FCM) Although it has high computational overhead, it has proven to be effective in detecting subtle intrusion due its natural treatment of data (Liu et al., 2013)

When an object doesn't belong to any cluster, Density-based clustering methods such as DBSCAN can detect anomalies in irregular cluster shapes which are common in diverse and multimodal patient data (Zamini et al., 2019). Another example of a clustering technique are Temporal clustering models, such as Hidden Markov Models (HMMs), used to identify time-dependent variations in patient behaviour from sensory data (Gupta et al., 2021).

Clustering techniques improve patient incomes; they are crucial in clustering similar patients based on their medical history. This can not only help in identifying underlying health issues by pinpointing patients deviating from the norm but also the healthcare providers can identify subgroups that require different treatments. Nevertheless, these techniques do have their limitations such as selecting the appropriate number of clusters and dealing with high-dimensional data imbalanced datasets. (Ursul & Pereymybida, 2023)

## 4.3 Deep Learning for Sequential and Complex Behaviors

Anomaly detection performance has been revolutionized by Deep Learning (DL) as it specialises in learning intrinsic patterns from noisy data. In healthcare, where real-time patient monitoring and accurate detection of abnormal patient behaviors is very important, DL techniques like Convolutional Neural Networks (CNNs), Recurrent Neural Networks (RNNs), Autoencoders have now become very useful and essential tools excelling even with insufficient labelled data making them ideal for healthcare environment (Chalapathy et al., 2019).

### 4.3.1 LSTM for Time-Series Health Data

Due to their ability to capture sequential patterns, Long Short-Term Memory (LSTM) networks are a type of RNN that stand out for processing time-series data and are being widely used for anomaly detection in physiological data in healthcare (Zhang et al., 2021).

One of the instances demonstrating the power of LSTMs in analysing physiological data is from Pavithra et al.,2024, where over 60,000 ECG recordings were used to train an LSTM-based model and they observed that it reduced false positive rates by 30% and false negatives by 40%, as a result boosting the accuracy up by 30% as compared to the previous methods. Without extensive preprocessing, LSTMs can develop predictive models for healthy ECG signals and to detect arrhythmias

Beyond biomedical signals, for tasks such as fault and even detection and system health monitoring, LSTMs have proven to be very valuable as they can detect abnormal traffic and predict real-time network activity with good precision and recall (Provotar et al., 2019). LSTMs can handle a large amount of time series data and are very well suited for non-stationary time series data where fluctuation amplitude changes over time, addressing the limitations of traditional algorithms. However, the increasing use of IoT devices means more multimodal data which makes it challenging to capture spatial and temporal dependencies often addressed by more complex architectures (Zhang et al.,2021).

### 4.3.2 Autoencoders and CNNs for Multimodal Inputs

When labelled data is scarce, Autoencoders (AEs) are often used for unsupervised anomaly detection tasks. Nawaz et al., 2024 describe how they identify anomalies via high reconstruction errors by learning to reconstruct normal data, showing their effectiveness in biomedical data. They have been applied to multimodal data like Electrocardiography for detection of sensor-based abnormal behavior (Musthyala et al., 2021). Although AEs are quite efficient in capturing complex feature spaces, recent studies indicate that AEs can sometimes reconstruct anomalies too well, compromising their reliability in safety-critical applications (Bouman et al., 2025).

For multimodal anomaly detection, one of the most effective tools are the Convolutional Neural Networks (CNNs), they are adept at extracting features from visual data and performing tasks like image processing and object detection. For video anomaly detection, 3D CNNs are used to identify abnormal behaviour with high precision (Ziani et al., 2024). CNNs are also being used for the fusion of multimodal data from various sensors to improve anomaly detection robustness. For instance, in healthcare, Li & Zhang, 2024 specifically shows how correlations between multiple physiological signals can be learned by CNNs to improve early warning in patient monitoring systems.

Another effective way for human behavior analysis and anomaly detection in hospital IoT ecosystems, is combining CNNs with other DL models, such as the

LSTM-CNN hybrid architecture proving more accurate in uncovering early signs of device malfunction than individual techniques (ALmojel & Mishra, 2024).

# 5 ROLE OF CLOUD COMPUTING IN ANOMALY DETECTION PIPELINES

## 5.1 Cloud Architecture in Patient Monitoring Systems

From collecting to processing, analysing and storing data, cloud plays a vital role in medical IoT devices. It offers scalable options for which one pays as they avail the services leading to self-monitoring by patients and reducing clinical appointments. Further it is used in anomaly detection pipelines to provide the training data for AI techniques as discussed in the above section. Its ability to handle real-time stream data while analysing and handling flags helps to identify patterns to notify any security breach. There are various types of cloud techniques that can be implemented for the above purpose (see Figure 5).

*Figure 5. Various types of cloud techniques and Their Purpose*

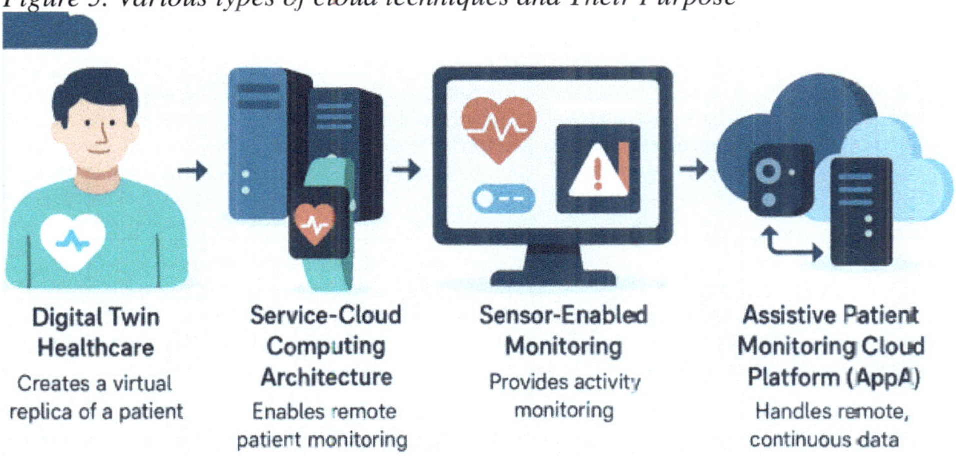


The advantage of supporting IoT devices as well as AI has led to the boom in utilizing cloud infrastructure. To understand this framework, some methodologies and their practical implementation have been discussed in Table 2.

*Table 2. Real-World Cloud Architectures in Patient Monitoring Systems and Their Design Considerations*

| Model / Architecture | Objective | Design Concept | Functionality |
|---|---|---|---|
| Digital Twin Healthcare | A novel cloud framework that provides accurate and fast healthcare (especially to elderly) | Helps track the personal health data of elderly throughout their entire lifecycle by merging physical and virtual environment | Monitors, diagnoses and predicts data using IoT-enabled wearable devices |
| Service-Oriented Architecture (SOA) and Cloud Integration | Implements non-intrusive monitoring with the help of real-time collected data and even advise on lifestyle engagements | Amalgamation of plethora of technologies, applications and services like using mobile phones to collect data from biosensors that can also be wearable | Stored data is used by authorised entities like healthcare practitioners. This method showed notable outcomes in a case study |
| Edge-Cloud Computing Architecture | Integrates remote patient monitoring (RPM) to avoid the drawbacks cause by mobile devices | Manage medical data where latent representations help make AI supported decision making as they are uploaded on cloud | Contains modules for applications like time-series anomaly detection, cloud telehealth management for fast and accurate diagnosis |
| Sensor-Enabled Monitoring | Utilising sensor nodes like gyroscope or accelerometer and uploading collected data for activity monitoring by healthcare professionals | Enhances noisy and redundant data by using filter modules before uploading it to cloud server | Security of user data and its access are improved via image-based authentication and activity-based access control |
| Assistive Patient Monitoring Cloud Platform (AppA) | Real time cloud architecture that helps with monitoring remote, continuous data from IoT-enabled patient wearable sensors | Solves software and hardware heterogeneity offered in traditional models by giving scalability options | New instances can be deployed as per the requirements, becoming a feasible option while fulfilling monitoring requirements |

*Note.* The entries in this table are based on the following sources: Digital Twin Healthcare is based on Liu et al. (2019); Service-Oriented Architecture (SOA) and Cloud Integration on Benharref and Serhani (2013); Edge-Cloud Computing Architecture on Su et al. (2021); Sensor-Enabled Monitoring on Thirunavukkarasu and Kumaratharan (2012); and Assistive Patient Monitoring Cloud Platform (AppA) on Balasubramanian et al. (2015) and Balasubramanian and Stranieri (2014).

The cloud infrastructure may seem to offer benefits, but it has its own set of limitations that point towards data breaches, cyber security issues and the integration of systems with this architecture. These fast and scalable solutions come at a cost of patient data trust being breached. Even policies such as HIPAA and GDPR have been implemented to protect medical data from such threats, yet this model fails to comply with the rules completely.

## 5.2 Benefits for Storage, Model Hosting, and Scalability

One of the perks with cloud infrastructure is data storage and model hosting while offering scalability. This helps healthcare field to adapt with the growing need for storage as more and more behavioral data is generated day by day. In the section we dive deeper into these characteristics of cloud and how they can be availed for advantage by IoT-enabled patient monitoring devices.

Data Storage covers two main attributes: vast data storage and transfer as well as cost-efficiency and accessibility. When talking about vast storage, flexibility and reliability at feasible costs is what makes cloud ideal for storage as well as transfer of data. The pay-as-you-go (PAYG) model is a utility that makes cloud attractive. The eliminates the need to have immediate hardware which leads to significant reduction in operational costs. This provides functional space and stability IoT devices with large stream data to store as they expand. Big data such as remote patient monitoring and behavioral data become easier to manage. (Tsiachri & Sotiriadis, 2020)

Features like centralized data processing and scalable hosting especially for machine learning and deep learning models support in hosting models. Detecting anomalies becomes easier with the support of cloud computing, providing centralized storage to apply algorithms. It allows for analysis of sensed behavioral data and flagging anomalies. As proposed by Ma et al., 2017, a SMMC or Sensors, Micro Controller, Machine to Machine Protocols and Cloud architecture collects sensor analogue data from IoT devices which is processed by micro controller. Finally, this data stored in cloud is used to apply decision-making algorithms. Cloud platform's unparallel computational power for complex AI technologies like ML or DL algorithms to be applied for anomaly detection. It can range from detecting any hardware failure to even hampering with cloud networks. (Hagemann & Katsarou, 2020) So we can conclude that scalability offered by dynamic resource allocation, on-demand availability and most importantly pipeline optimization speak in favor of cloud architecture.

## 5.3 Trust Challenges in Cloud-Enabled Healthcare

Even after the above discussed plus points, cloud still faces trust challenges especially about privacy. These vulnerabilities include patient data security while maintaining proper functionality of flagging patients in case of anomaly by the system.

Some of the major security concerns are increased vulnerabilities to cyber threats and requirement of robust measures for security. Cloud platforms have centralized data storing features. This exposes it to a greater number of cybersecurity threats by various methods like browser-based attacks, denial of service attacks and network intrusions as discussed in other sections. The critical nature of healthcare expects some services to always function, supported by security. However, the ever-changing nature of cloud infrastructure as per use puts it at a risk of malicious activity or violating policies. In cloud systems, RSA encryption is also used to ensure safety. However, the advent of quantum computing calls for more advanced techniques to safeguard information. As suggested by Gopi et al., 2024, measures like access control, monitoring user sensitive information and encryption can be integrated with behavioral anomaly detection.

Moving on there are privacy concerns as well regarding sensitive patient data, data governance and compliance with regulations. Electronic health data of patient is sensitive information that needs to be handled with confidentiality. Rapid implementation to tackle immediate challenges has led to concerns whether cloud follows governance of privacy or data integrity. This could even lead to risks of data silos and other challenges like data ownership and lock-in of data structures. (Cresswell et al., 2021) Cloud also falls back in its effort to comply with regulations like HIPAA and GDPR. In the next section we discuss about frameworks like adaptive differential privacy combined with federated learning and edge AI to follow guidelines and ensure trust maintenance on IoT enabled patient monitoring devices.

## 6 PRIVACY-PRESERVING AND COMPLIANT DETECTION MODELS

### 6.1 Sensitivity of Behavioral and Health Data

Stemming from deeply private nature of the information, behavioral and health data are very sensitive, they reveal an individual's daily activities and aspects of their physical and mental well-being. The rise of IoT sensors in the field of healthcare and even in daily lives of people in the form of wearable devices, enables real-time insights about motion, heart rate and other physiological signals. While being useful for health management, these devices also reveal potential cybersecurity risks. For instance, the digitization of medical records increases the risk of data breaches and misuse of personal information (Jalali et al., 2020).

Some key examples of sensitive data include Electronic Health Records (EHRs) and Genomic Data. Traditional paper-based medical records have been replaced by EHRs which contain important patient information and hence, a prime target for privacy breaches, unauthorized access leading to fraud healthcare claims (Chawki & Schneier, 2021). Whilst being beneficial for precision medicine, genomic data has the potential for familial implications and requires robust privacy and security protection (Lau-Min et al., 2021).

To prevent misuse and ensure confidentiality of private health data, Regulatory frameworks like Health Insurance Portability and Accountability Act (HIPAA) and the General Data Protection Regulation (GDPR) underscore the need for strict controls over the data and cybersecurity conscious designs in modern technologies like AI used in healthcare. However, striking a balance between protecting individual privacy and essential healthcare services remains a significant challenge (Chawki & Schneier, 2021).

## 6.2 Federated Learning and Edge-Based AI

For developing privacy-preserving animal detection systems in environments like Healthcare and IoT, Federated Learning (FL) and Edge-Based AI are the emerging paradigms in recent times. These paradigms mitigate privacy risks and address compliance concerns with regulations like HIPAA and GDPR as they allow for collaborative model training without centralizing sensitive data (Kim et al., 2020). While keeping the local data private, FL allows hospitals and edge devices to jointly train a machine learning model. The central server only receives the model data and not the raw data preserving the confidentiality of the patient. Hence, adhering to GDPR and HIPAA regulations and reducing risk of data breaches (Loftus et al., 2022).

In Healthcare, for tasks such as patient diagnosis and monitoring, FL is used by healthcare professionals to train models on private datasets without compromising data integrity. For instance, it has been used in cancer classification and Alzheimer's disease detection, in which private and diverse datasets were used maintaining the data integrity (Li et al., 2021). Some of the major advantages of FL is the enhanced data privacy, improved performance even with large and diverse datasets and the reduce computational costs. Also, without retraining, it continuously adapts to evolving threats and patterns (Loftus et al., 2022).

When it comes to Edge-Based AI, it excels in minimizing latency by processing data locally, supporting real-time responsiveness, which is highly suited for real-time anomaly detection in IoT, healthcare and Industrial IoT (IIoT). It is highly useful in urgent situations as well, due to its ability to reduce network bandwidth strain, as a result ensuring quick reactions (Deshpande & Rahman, 2023). Edge-based systems excel in preserving privacy and importantly complying with GDPR regulations. They can detect anomalies while keeping data private because they operate with minimal sharing of data (Mehnaz & Bertino, 2020).

Through the dynamic approach of processing data at the edge, real-time anomaly detection takes place ensuring increased privacy enforcement important for timely detection of disruptions in patient monitoring and empowers health monitors and other IoT devices (Deshpande & Rahman, 2023).

The synergy of edge computing and FL results in increased effectiveness in preserving data security and privacy providing robust solutions for real-time anomaly detection. This integration protects raw user data via lightweight transmission between servers and edge nodes (Kim et al., 2020).

## 6.3 Differential Privacy and Secure Model Training

In healthcare scenario, privacy-preserving anomaly detection systems are built using Differential Privacy (DP) and secure model training techniques. These methods allow for robust model training and aim to protect individual privacy (Ouadrhiri & Abdelhadi, 2022).

Differential Privacy (DP) is done by adding random noise to either the original dataset or the learning parameters and is a provable notion for quantifying privacy loss in a system, ensuring that an individual's sensitive information is preserved (Ouadrhiri & Abdelhadi, 2022). In anomaly detection, DP is used when detection tasks are to be outsourced to third parties which enables collaborative analysis while ensuring data privacy. In E-Health networks, even when medical data and network metadata are relevant for anomaly detection, DP ensures formal guarantees for privacy (Cholakoska et al., 2021).

Challenges do persist in implementing DP such as the difficulty in balancing privacy protection and model accuracy, some downgrade in accuracy accuracy due to the introduction of noise into the data, though, current research has shown that high accuracy and fairness can be achieved through privacy-preserving training of AI models (Ouadrhiri & Abdelhadi, 2022).

Beyond DP, to secure the process of model training several techniques are used especially in collaborative environments. As discussed earlier, FL allows models to be trained on local data without sharing private data supporting secure and decentralized model training (Kim). Another technique is Homomorphic Encryption (HE), which provides strong privacy guarantees and enables computations to be performed on encrypted data without having the need to decrypt it (Liu et al., 2020).

Creating a comprehensive framework for secure and privacy-preserving anomaly detection systems, these techniques, when integrated, address the challenges of data confidentiality and regulatory compliance in healthcare environments.

## 6.4 Compliance with HIPAA, GDPR, and Medical Ethics

When developing anomaly detection systems, compliance with regulations like the Health Insurance Portability and Accountability Act (HIPAA), the General Data

Protection Regulation (GDPR) is paramount. They are designed to ensure responsible use of AI and protect sensitive patient information (Chawki & Schneier, 2021).

HIPAA addresses privacy and security of medical data and enforces the implementation of safeguards to prevent unauthorized access for protecting patient health information (PHI) in the United States. Anomaly detection systems that process patient data need to comply with HIPAA's privacy rules (Attya et al., 2024).

In the European Union, GDPR is a data protection law that governs the collection and use of personal health data. Explicit consent is required for data processing as it grants individuals rights over their data and provides stringent guidelines to ensure data security. It is a must to adhere to GDPR's requirements for data privacy for anomaly detection systems using AI in healthcare systems. It includes guidelines such as the requirement that data can only be analyzed if a minimum of six lawful grounds for personal information processing are met (Chawki & Schneier, 2021).

As discussed earlier, Federated Learning aligns with GDPR guidelines by enabling model training to take place without sharing raw data across institutions in a collaborative environment (Ouadrhiri & Abdelhadi, 2022).

Beyond legal compliance, ethical considerations like maintaining patient trust and ensuring fairness are also important when it comes to application of AI in anomaly detection systems.

Transparency is key as it raises ethical questions when the use of "black box" AI models, which are highly accurate but lack interpretability. It is critical that meaningful clinical recommendations be provided by AI-driven systems to ensure trust in clinical decision-making (Beltramin et al., 2022).

Sensitive data such as the mental health data must be handled carefully and robust privacy protection must be in place for preservation of private data. It is also necessary to get patient consent before the sharing of data for medical purposes. While AI enhances anomaly detection capabilities, it is very important to balance its benefits and risks to ensure patient safety and privacy. Overall, a synergy of robust technical safeguards (e.g., FL and DP), legal compliance (HIPAA, GDPR), and a strong commitment to medical ethics is important for the development of cybersecurity-aware anomaly detection systems.

# 7 CASE STUDY: DETECTING BEHAVIORAL AND SYSTEM ANOMALIES IN CLOUD-CONNECTED PATIENT MONITORING DEVICES

## 7.1 Scenario Overview and System Architecture

Cloud infrastructure followed by AI-driven solutions to address anomaly detection in the medical field has led to the evolution of patient monitoring devices using IoT systems. This can be understood by the work of Pavithra et al., 2024 where they built a system to sense physiological signals in real-time for parameters such as E ECG, heart rate, SpO2, and blood pressure in wearable IoT devices and detect anomalies using deep learning. This patient-side monitoring setup is supported by cloud connections as it contains data acquisition layer, a cloud-based processing system and an alerting mechanism.

Vital signals are measured using sensor-based layers in devices, further transmitted with the help of wireless gateways. Then cloud systems come into the picture along with deep learning models for processing. The breakthrough idea was using Long Short-Term Memory (LSTM) models, trained on behavioral data to identify patterns and flag any aberrations. For the environment, an environment was set up on TensorFlow in Python, supported by GPU to provide fast training and interference. The workflow revolves around capturing data from centralised cloud based real-time sensors, further analysing it for anomalies.

Datasets, real-time as well as synthetic and even ones from PhysioNet were used to evaluate the framework where 32,000 samples were used to train LSTM model, 8,000 were used for validation and 14,000 were test samples. Graphical tools incorporated in the systems helped visualise anomalies, for example, ECG peaks and variability were plotted.

Asghari et al. (2024) proposed AI techniques to detect network threats that impact IoT devices by using behavioral data to form patterns. Security of real-time continuous data is kept at the centre while planning for the structure of the system. A time-window based segmentation strategy is used for data preprocessing to understand the behavioral nature of data devices. Dynamic patterns are captured from time-series data with network traffic so that the model is not just limited to static characteristics and helps early tracking of any attacks or threats on the system.

Autoencoders are integrated into the architecture which serve the purpose of improving the adaptability of model across plethora of devices and threats with the help of transfer learning. NbaIoT dataset is used to provide samples to stacked autoencoders for reconstructing normal behavior. Any aberration from this normal is alerted as a behavioral anomaly and may point to cybersecurity threats. Knowledge is transferred between the source and target via transfer learning which saves the time of retraining the model from scratch as model generalizability is enhanced.

In the upcoming section we will discuss two real world applications in the form of case studies to support the above discussed behavioral anomalies. The first one represents a patient-centred anomaly for cases such as irregular heart patterns. An LSTM-based model was used to sense physiological data and report any irregularity in ECG as presented by Pavithra et al., 2024 in their study. Another case study, drawn from the works of Asghari et al., 2024 makes use of autoencoder and transfer learning techniques to identify patterns and flag suspicious data transmission in IoT devices.

## 7.2 Patient-Centred Anomaly: Unusual Heart Patterns and Patient Risk

The anomaly that will be covered in this case study is the detection of abnormal heart patterns in ECG signals. In this, the system identifies irregularities such as erratic R-R intervals, unexpected spikes, and unusual waveform morphologies with the help of an LSTM architecture. What these deviations depict is the underlying conditions of arrhythmia or stress-related irregularities.

Visualizing anomalies is done by the system itself using a colour-coded alert mechanism. A high-performance accuracy of 93% is observed with sensitivity and specificity of 0.95 and 0.93 respectively. The pattern retaining capability of LSTM models when faced with time-series data especially in long range contributes to its success. On comparison with machine learning models like Random Forest, Support Vector Machine and DBSCAN, even though RF and SVM may show considerable accuracy, yet the precision and recall are still low, thus proving that LSTM are the best fit for long time-series medical data (see Figure 6).

The main advantage of the system is that it has not just a low overall false positive but also low overall false negative rates, which was achieved by optimizing the threshold and the loss functions of the system. This is important from clinical point-of-view because false negatives can lead to delayed care while false positives can lead to unnecessary interventions. This point is a breakthrough in the model architecture that can help not just patients but also medical practitioners.

*Figure 6. Model Accuracy Comparison for Patient Anomaly Detection*

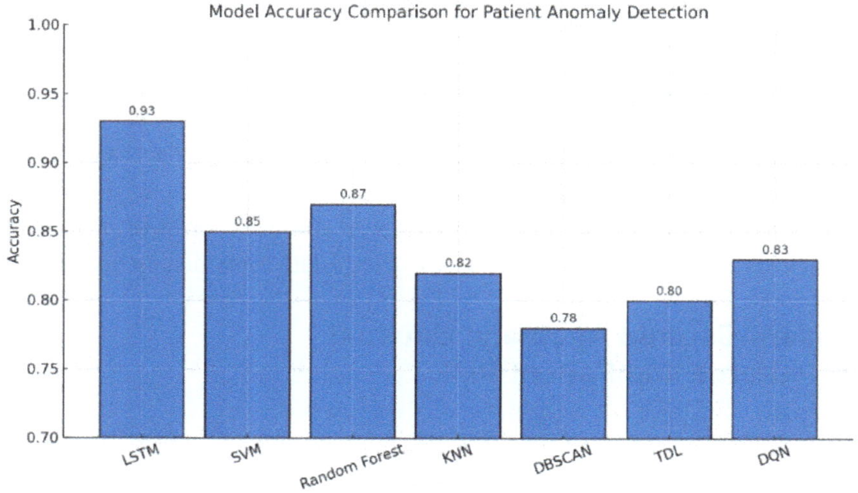


*Note. The data used in this graph has been taken from Pavithra et al., 2024. The values presented may have a measurement error margin of approximately ±0.2.*

This case study helps us understand the power of AI detection tools in early diagnosis with the help of patient-centred anomalies especially for chronic conditions like cardiovascular diseases, hypertension, stress, etc. IoT helps easily track the multi-natured data while cloud provides storage and processing platform to AI technologies to alert healthcare practitioners for immediate response.

## 7.3 System-Centred Anomaly: Abnormal Data Transmission Suggesting Intrusion

This case study focuses on system-level outliers which consist of irregular patterns of transmission in IoT-enabled patient care devices. With this, the system is able to detect behaviors that might hinder the performance of such devices or affect the integrity of patient data.

This was achieved with the help of an AI-enabled system which used a hybrid of autoencoders and transfer learning. Some specific types of malwares such as Mirai, and Bashlite botnets are said to alter the data packet flow over the network by creating irregular spikes in data transmission, port scanning, TCP request floods. To detect such malicious anomalies the system analyses patterns in the incoming and outgoing network traffic using a time-window segmentation technique. Benign and malicious IoT traffic patterns are available in NbaIoT dataset which are used to train the model and later check accuracy via test data. The unsupervised learning technique of utilizing autoencoder helps system in identification of baseline behavior. High reconstruction errors point to outliers in patterns and thus flag anomalies.

An important functionality is improving speed of detecting anomalies day by day to quickly resolve them. Another key feature to tackle is the evolution of new attacks with the era of quantum computing and high computational power. The introduction of transfer learning in models have improved speed and attack detection. Models can even adapt to other set of devices by the process of learned weight utilising information of another device. The system passed robustness check in the category of multiple attack classes with an exceptional precision and recall of more than 90%. The model is capable of identifying affected devices and mitigating the impact of ongoing attacks in real-time. Additionally, it incorporates a risk scoring mechanism which can prove to be beneficial in assessing the overall risk level in the system of large hospitals.

This case study shows how a cloud-connected infrastructure, that uses a combination of AI methodologies and behavioral data for network threat detection can safeguard against data breaches and ensure patient data safety.

## 8 CONCLUSION

Internet of Things (IoT), cloud computing, and Artificial Intelligence (AI) changed the way modern healthcare supported patient care with continuous, real-time tracking using patient monitoring devices. This chapter built a comprehensive understanding of these anomalies and introduced proactive methods to safeguard patients' trust using intelligent systems. One of the major focuses of this chapter was to develop a twofold understanding of anomalies: one that was patient-centric, identifying medically caused aberrations and another that was system-centric, recognizing network-level or device-based intrusions and inconsistencies. This chapter explored how specific techniques in AI frameworks such as Support Vector Machines (SVM), unsupervised learning approaches, and deep learning architectures such as LSTM, autoencoders, and transformers learned from patterns and helped in flagging any aberrations.

Further, we examined the relationship between IoT devices and a centralized cloud computing for data storage, processing and analytics. We even moved towards an approach called federated learning (FL) under the umbrella term of AI. To ensure data preservation with regulations such as HIPAA in the US and GDPR in Europe FL presented a novel solution to maintain privacy without compromising anomaly detection systems by shifting the model training from centralised system to local ones. The above proposed methodologies were also backed by case studies to demonstrate the concreteness of AI utilisation in the field of behvioral anomaly detection: one focused on patient anomaly detection with the help of LSTM model for ECG signal monitoring and another on network security with the supported by autoencoders and transfer learning applied on NabIoT dataset.

This chapter highlighted how healthcare is not just amalgamation of technologies to make up smart systems but also holistic, adaptive and privacy-aware frameworks to support patients in their journey. It summarised how IoT for wearable devices goes hand in hand with cloud infrastructure for storage and AI applications to strengthen privacy-oriented health systems.

## References


Abideen, Z. U., & Shah, M. A. (2017, September). An IoT based robust healthcare model for continuous health monitoring. In *2017 23rd international conference on automation and computing (ICAC)* (pp. 1-6). IEEE. DOI: 10.23919/IConAC.2017.8082012

Aditya, A., Vidyarthi, D., & Nene, M. J. (2024, March). A Study of Common Vulnerabilities in IoT Devices. In *2024 11th International Conference on Reliability, Infocom Technologies and Optimization (Trends and Future Directions)(ICRITO)* (pp. 1-6). IEEE. DOI: 10.1109/ICRITO61523.2024.10522155

Agneeswaran, V. S., Mukherjee, J., Gupta, A., Tonpay, P., Tiwari, J., & Agarwal, N. (2013). Real-time analytics for the healthcare industry: Arrhythmia detection. *Big Data*, *1*(3), 176–182. DOI: 10.1089/big.2013.0018 PMID: 27442199

Akinola, O., Akinola, A., Victor Ifeanyi, I., Oyerinde, O., Joseph Adewole, O., Sulaimon, B., & Oyekan, B. O. (2024). Artificial Intelligence and Machine Learning Techniques for Anomaly Detection and Threat Mitigation in Cloud-Connected Medical Devices. *International Journal of Scientific Research and Modern Technology*, *3*(3), 1–13. Advance online publication. DOI: 10.38124/ijsrmt.v3i3.26

Ali, S. Z., Ali, S. H., Javeed, A., Ullah, I., Memon, S. A., & Manzoor, S. (2024). Supervised Learning Approaches for Vibration Analysis and Anomaly Detection in Rotating Machines. *2024 3rd International Conference on Emerging Trends in Electrical, Control, and Telecommunication Engineering (ETECTE)*, 1-6. DOI: 10.1109/ETECTE63967.2024.10824020

ALmojel, F., & Mishra, S.ALmojel. (2024). Advancing Hospital Cybersecurity Through IoT-Enabled Neural Network for Human Behavior Analysis and Anomaly Detection. *International Journal of Advanced Computer Science and Applications*, *15*(5). Advance online publication. DOI: 10.14569/IJACSA.2024.0150506

Arjunan, G. (2023). Optimizing Edge AI for real-time data processing in IoT devices: Challenges and solutions. [IJSRM]. *International Journal of Scientific Research and Management*, *11*(6), 944–953. DOI: 10.18535/ijsrm/v11i06.ec2

Asghari, A., Bergantin, F., Forestiero, A., & Macrì, D. (2024, September). Anomalous behaviors detection of IoT devices through AI-based methodologies. In *2024 7th International Conference of Computer and Informatics Engineering (IC2IE)* (pp. 1-8). IEEE. DOI: 10.1109/IC2IE63342.2024.10748216

Attya, S. M., Jumaa, D. A., Hwezy, N. N., Sajid, W. A., Khaleefah, A. M., Zhyrov, G., & Ali, H. (2024). Harnessing Federated Learning for Secure Data Sharing in Healthcare Systems. *2024 36th Conference of Open Innovations Association (FRUCT)*, 390-399. DOI: 10.23919/FRUCT64283.2024.10749928

Balasubramanian, V., & Stranieri, A. (2014, December). A scalable cloud Platform for Active healthcare monitoring applications. In *2014 IEEE Conference on e-Learning, e-Management and e-Services (IC3e)* (pp. 93-98). IEEE. DOI: 10.1109/IC3e.2014.7081248

Balasubramanian, V., Stranieri, A., & Kaur, R. (2015, January). Appa: assistive patient monitoring cloud platform for active healthcare applications. In *Proceedings of the 9th International Conference on Ubiquitous Information Management and Communication* (pp. 1-8). DOI: 10.1145/2701126.2701224

Beltramin, D., Lamas, E., & Bousquet, C. (2022). Ethical Issues in the Utilization of Black Boxes for Artificial Intelligence in Medicine. *Studies in Health Technology and Informatics*, *295*, 249–252. DOI: 10.3233/SHTI220709 PMID: 35773855

Benharref, A., & Serhani, M. A. (2013). Novel cloud and SOA-based framework for E-Health monitoring using wireless biosensors. *IEEE Journal of Biomedical and Health Informatics*, *18*(1), 46–55. DOI: 10.1109/JBHI.2013.2262659 PMID: 24403403

Bouman, R., & Heskes, T. (2025). Autoencoders for Anomaly Detection are Unreliable. *ArXiv, abs/2501.13864*. /arXiv.2501.13864DOI: 10.48550

Butt, S. A., Diaz-Martinez, J. L., Jamal, T., Ali, A., De-La-Hoz-Franco, E., & Shoaib, M. (2019, July). IoT smart health security threats. In *2019 19th International conference on computational science and its applications (ICCSA)* (pp. 26-31). IEEE. DOI: 10.1109/ICCSA.2019.000-8

Chalapathy, R., & Chawla, S. (2019). Deep learning for anomaly detection: A survey. *arXiv preprint arXiv:1901.03407*. /arXiv.1901.03407DOI: 10.48550

Chawki, M., & Schneier, B. (2021). Security and Privacy in the Era of Electronic Health Records (EHRs). DOI: 10.5281/zenodo.4782466

Chen, L., & Bate, I. (2016, June). Identifying usage anomalies for ECG-based sensor nodes. In *2016 IEEE 13th International Conference on Wearable and Implantable Body Sensor Networks (BSN)* (pp. 77-82). IEEE. DOI: 10.1109/BSN.2016.7516236

Chen, Y., & Kunz, T. (2016, April). Performance evaluation of IoT protocols under a constrained wireless access network. In *2016 International Conference on Selected Topics in Mobile & Wireless Networking (MoWNeT)* (pp. 1-7). IEEE. DOI: 10.1109/MoWNet.2016.7496622

Cholakoska Cilakova, A., Pfitzner, B., Gjoreski, H., Rakovic, V., Arnrich, B., & Kalendar, M. (2021). Differentially Private Federated Learningfor Anomaly Detection in eHealth Networks. *Adjunct Proceedings of the 2021 ACM International Joint Conference on Pervasive and Ubiquitous Computing and Proceedings of the 2021 ACM International Symposium on Wearable Computers*. DOI: 10.1145/3460418.3479365

Copeland, S. (2018). Gathering basic information in support of medical network risk management. *Biomedical Instrumentation & Technology*, *52*(2), 112–119. DOI: 10.2345/0899-8205-52.2.112 PMID: 29558185

Cresswell, K., Williams, R., & Sheikh, A. (2021). Using cloud technology in health care during the COVID-19 pandemic. *The Lancet. Digital Health*, *3*(1), e4–e5. DOI: 10.1016/S2589-7500(20)30291-0 PMID: 33735067

Del-Valle-Soto, C., Briseño, R. A., Valdivia, L. J., & Nolazco-Flores, J. A. (2024). Unveiling wearables: Exploring the global landscape of biometric applications and vital signs and behavioral impact. *BioData Mining*, *17*(1), 15. DOI: 10.1186/s13040-024-00368-y PMID: 38863014

Deshpande, Y. D., & Rahman, S. (2023). *Edge-Based Real-Time Sensor Data Processing for Anomaly Detection in Industrial IoT Applications*. Research Journal of Computer Systems and Engineering., DOI: 10.52710/rjcse.71

Du, J., & Yu, B. (2023, November). Application of Isolation Forest Algorithm in Fraud Detection of Medical Insurance Big Data. In 2023 *8th International Conference on Intelligent Informatics and Biomedical Sciences (ICIIBMS)* (Vol. 8, pp. 504-509). IEEE. DOI: 10.1109/ICIIBMS60103.2023.10347658

Fan, J., Yang, W., Liu, Z., Kang, J., Niyato, D., Lam, K. Y., & Du, H. (2023). Understanding security in smart city domains from the ant-centric perspective. *IEEE Internet of Things Journal*, *10*(13), 11199–11223. DOI: 10.1109/JIOT.2023.3252040

Fanucci, L., Saponara, S., Bacchillone, T., Donati, M., Barba, P., Sanchez-Tato, I., & Carmona, C. (2012). Sensing devices and sensor signal processing for remote monitoring of vital signs in CHF patients. *IEEE Transactions on Instrumentation and Measurement*, *62*(3), 553–569. DOI: 10.1109/TIM.2012.2218681

Freeman, R. L., Horner, R. H., & Reichle, J. (1999). Relation between heart rate and problem behaviors. *American Journal of Mental Retardation*, *104*(4), 330–345. DOI: 10.1352/0895-8017(1999)104<0330:RBHRAP>2.0.CO;2 PMID: 10450460

Ghosh, A., Qin, S., Lee, J., & Wang, G. N. (2016). FBMTP: An automated fault and behavioral anomaly detection and isolation tool for PLC-controlled manufacturing systems. *IEEE Transactions on Systems, Man, and Cybernetics. Systems*, *47*(12), 3397–3417. DOI: 10.1109/TSMC.2016.2633392

Gopi, A., Aravinth, S. S., Charishma, N., Sravani, B., Gayatri, N., & Gowtham, K. (2024, April). A Holistic Approach with Behavioral Anomaly Detection (BAD) for Mitigating Insider Threats in Cloud Environments. In *2024 International Conference on Computing and Data Science (ICCDS)* (pp. 1-6). IEEE. DOI: 10.1109/ICCDS60734.2024.10560376

Gupta, D., Gupta, M., Bhatt, S., & Tosun, A. S. (2021, August). Detecting anomalous user behavior in remote patient monitoring. In 2021 *IEEE 22nd International Conference on Information Reuse and Integration for Data Science (IRI) (pp. 33-40). IEEE.* DOI: 10.1109/IRI51335.2021.00011

Hady, A. A., Ghubaish, A., Salman, T., Unal, D., & Jain, R. (2020). Intrusion detection system for healthcare systems using medical and network data: A comparison study. *IEEE Access : Practical Innovations, Open Solutions*, *8*, 106576–106584. DOI: 10.1109/ACCESS.2020.3000421

Hagemann, T., & Katsarou, K. (2020, December). A systematic review on anomaly detection for cloud computing environments. In *Proceedings of the 2020 3rd Artificial Intelligence and Cloud Computing Conference* (pp. 83-96). DOI: 10.1145/3442536.3442550

Harb, H., Mansour, A., Nasser, A., Cruz, E. M., & de la Torre Diez, I. (2020). A sensor-based data analytics for patient monitoring in connected healthcare applications. *IEEE Sensors Journal*, *21*(2), 974–984. DOI: 10.1109/JSEN.2020.2977352

He, M., Petering, M. E., LaCasse, P. M., Otieno, W., & Maturana, F. P. (2023). Learning with supervised data for anomaly detection in smart manufacturing. *International Journal of Computer Integrated Manufacturing*, *36*(9), 1331–1344. DOI: 10.1080/0951192X.2023.2177747

Jalali, N., Sahu, K. S., Oetomo, A., & Morita, P. P. (2020). Understanding user behavior through the use of unsupervised anomaly detection: Proof of concept using internet of things smart home thermostat data for improving public health surveillance. *JMIR mHealth and uHealth*, *8*(11), e21209. DOI: 10.2196/21209 PMID: 33185562

Kadir, E. A., Putri, L. D., Rosa, S. L., Siswanto, A., Assidiqi, F., & Evizal, M. F. (2024, April). Anomaly Detection of Patient Data in Public Hospital used Internet of Things Sensors. In *2024 International Conference on Inventive Computation Technologies (ICICT)* (pp. 1734-1739). IEEE. DOI: 10.1109/ICICT60155.2024.10544697

Kierner, S., Kucharski, J., & Kierner, Z. (2023). Taxonomy of hybrid architectures involving rule-based reasoning and machine learning in clinical decision systems: A scoping review. *Journal of Biomedical Informatics*, *144*, 104428. DOI: 10.1016/j.jbi.2023.104428 PMID: 37355025

Kim, S., Cai, H., Hua, C., Gu, P., Xu, W., & Park, J. (2020). Collaborative Anomaly Detection for Internet of Things based on Federated Learning. *2020 IEEE/CIC International Conference on Communications in China (ICCC)*, 623-628. DOI: 10.1109/ICCC49849.2020.9238913

Kishor Kumar Reddy, C., Kaza, V. S., Madana Mohana, R., Alhameed, M., Jeribi, F., Alam, S., & Shuaib, M. (2025). Detecting anomalies in smart wearables for hypertension: A deep learning mechanism. *Frontiers in Public Health*, *12*, 1426168. DOI: 10.3389/fpubh.2024.1426168 PMID: 39850864

Lau-Min, K. S., Asher, S. B., Chen, J., Domchek, S. M., Feldman, M., Joffe, S., Landgraf, J., Speare, V., Varughese, L. A., Tuteja, S., VanZandbergen, C., Ritchie, M. D., & Nathanson, K. L. (2021). Real-world integration of genomic data into the electronic health record: The PennChart Genomics Initiative. *Genetics in Medicine*, *23*(4), 603–605. DOI: 10.1038/s41436-020-01056-y PMID: 33299147

Lee, W., Kim, S., Jeon, H., & Kim, H. (2015, August). Detecting an abnormal traffic on healthcare network. In *2015 5th International Conference on IT Convergence and Security (ICITCS)* (pp. 1-4). IEEE. DOI: 10.1109/ICITCS.2015.7292970

Li, J., Meng, Y., Ma, L., Du, S., Zhu, H., Pei, Q., & Shen, X. (2021). A federated learning based privacy-preserving smart healthcare system. *IEEE Transactions on Industrial Informatics*, *18*(3), 2021–2031. Advance online publication. DOI: 10.1109/TII.2021.3098010

Li, Z., & Zhang, X. (2024). An Enhanced Autoencoder-based Anomaly Detection Model for time series Data from Wearable Medical Devices. *IEEE journal of biomedical and health informatics, PP*. DOI: 10.1109/JBHI.2024.3434420

Liu, D., Lung, C. H., Lambadaris, I., & Seddigh, N. (2013, May). Network traffic anomaly detection using clustering techniques and performance comparison. In 2013 *26th IEEE Canadian Conference on Electrical and Computer Engineering (CCECE)* (pp. 1-4). IEEE. DOI: 10.1109/CCECE.2013.6567739

Liu, X., Xie, L., Wang, Y., Zou, J., Xiong, J., Ying, Z., & Vasilakos, A. V. (2020). Privacy and security issues in deep learning: A survey. *IEEE Access : Practical Innovations, Open Solutions*, *9*, 4566–4593. DOI: 10.1109/ACCESS.2020.3045078

Liu, Y., Zhang, L., Yang, Y., Zhou, L., Ren, L., Wang, F., Liu, R., Pang, Z., & Deen, M. J. (2019). A novel cloud-based framework for the elderly healthcare services using digital twin. *IEEE Access : Practical Innovations, Open Solutions*, *7*, 49088–49101. DOI: 10.1109/ACCESS.2019.2909828

Loftus, T. J., Ruppert, M. M., Shickel, B., Ozrazgat-Baslanti, T., Balch, J. A., Efron, P. A., Upchurch, G. R.Jr, Rashidi, P., Tignanelli, C. J., Bian, J., & Bihorac, A. (2022). Federated learning for preserving data privacy in collaborative healthcare research. *Digital Health*, *8*. Advance online publication. DOI: 10.1177/20552076221134455 PMID: 36325438

Ma, J., Nguyen, H., Mirza, F., & Neuland, O. (2017). Two way architecture between IoT sensors and cloud computing for remote health care monitoring applications. https://aisel.aisnet.org/ecis2017_rip/34

Maruthukannan, B., Karpagalakshmi, R. C., Lakshmi, D., Wise, D. J. W., & Srinivasan, C. (2024, May). IoT-Connected Telehealth Environments with Long Short-Term Memory Networks for Precise Time-Series Patient Behavior Analysis. In *2024 International Conference on Intelligent Systems for Cybersecurity (ISCS)* (pp. 1-6). IEEE. DOI: 10.1109/ISCS61804.2024.10581323

Mehnaz, S., & Bertino, E. (2020, April). Privacy-preserving real-time anomaly detection using edge computing. In 2020 IEEE 36th International Conference on Data Engineering (ICDE) (pp. 469-480). IEEE. DOI: 10.1109/ICDE48307.2020.00047

Menachem, J. N., Golbus, J. R., Molina, M., Mazurek, J. A., Hornsby, N., Atluri, P., Fuller, S., Birati, E. Y., Kim, Y. Y., Goldberg, L. R., & Wald, J. W. (2017). Successful cardiac transplantation outcomes in patients with adult congenital heart disease. *Heart (British Cardiac Society)*, *103*(18), 1449–1454. DOI: 10.1136/heartjnl-2016-310933 PMID: 28258242

Miao, X., Liu, Y., Zhao, H., & Li, C. (2018). Distributed online one-class support vector machine for anomaly detection over networks. *IEEE Transactions on Cybernetics*, *49*(4), 1475–1488. DOI: 10.1109/TCYB.2018.2804940 PMID: 29994292

Mitchell, R., & Chen, R. (2014). Behavior rule specification-based intrusion detection for safety critical medical cyber physical systems. *IEEE Transactions on Dependable and Secure Computing*, *12*(1), 16–30. DOI: 10.1109/TDSC.2014.2312327

Moore, J. W., & Lu, H. (2020, November). Abnormal Activity Detection in Healthcare. In *2020 5th International Conference on Innovative Technologies in Intelligent Systems and Industrial Applications (CITISIA)* (pp. 1-7). IEEE. DOI: 10.1109/CITISIA50690.2020.9371790

Murugan, K., Shaheen, N., Prathyusha, P., Ashalatha, M., & Sahithi, A. (2024, December). IoT Enabled Diabetic Health Surveillance. In *2024 3rd International Conference on Automation, Computing and Renewable Systems (ICACRS)* (pp. 476-482). IEEE. https://10.0.4.85/ICACRS62842.2024.10841749

Musthyala, R., Arawkar, S., & Gupta, M. (2021, June). Anomaly identification using multimodal physiological signals on the edge. In *Proceedings of the 2nd Workshop on Deep Learning for Wellbeing Applications Leveraging Mobile Devices and Edge Computing* (pp. 7-12). DOI: 10.1145/3469258.3469849

Nawaz, A., Khan, S. S., & Ahmad, A. (2024). Ensemble of autoencoders for anomaly detection in biomedical data: A narrative review. *IEEE Access : Practical Innovations, Open Solutions*, *12*, 17273–17289. DOI: 10.1109/ACCESS.2024.3360691

Ouadrhiri, A. E., & Abdelhadi, A. M. (2022). Differential Privacy for Deep and Federated Learning: A Survey. *IEEE Access : Practical Innovations, Open Solutions*, *10*, 22359–22380. DOI: 10.1109/ACCESS.2022.3151670

Parvin, P. (2018, June). Real-time anomaly detection in elderly behavior. In *Proceedings of the ACM SIGCHI Symposium on Engineering Interactive Computing Systems* (pp. 1-6). DOI: 10.1145/3220134.3220145

Pavithra, D., Parameswaran, T., Choudhry, M. D., Amrutha, S., Deepa, T., & Kiruthiga, R. (2024). Application of LSTM Networks for Continuous Patient Monitoring and Anomaly Detection in Wearable Health Devices. *Indian Journal of Science and Technology*, *17*(37), 3909–3921. Advance online publication. DOI: 10.17485/IJST/v17i37.2600

Prasad, D. S., & Das, B. C. (2009). Physical inactivity: a cardiovascular risk factor. http://hdl.handle.net/1807/55196

Provotar, O. I., Linder, Y. M., & Veres, M. M. (2019, December). Unsupervised anomaly detection in time series using lstm-based autoencoders. In 2019 *IEEE International Conference on Advanced Trends in Information Theory* (ATIT) (pp. 513-517). IEEE. DOI: 10.1109/ATIT49449.2019.9030505

Rački, D., Tomaževič, D., & Skočaj, D. (2023, July). Combining unsupervised and supervised deep learning approaches for surface anomaly detection. In *Sixteenth International Conference on Quality Control by Artificial Vision* (Vol. 12749, pp. 33-40). SPIE. DOI: 10.1117/12.2688559

Raghavan, S. (2025). Ontology-Driven Cross-Domain Access Control Framework for Anomaly Detection in Cloud-Based Healthcare System. DOI: 10.21203/rs.3.rs-6128795/v1

Rahman, F. (2024). Enhancing Medication Safety with ML-Enhanced Decision Support Systems: A Comparative Analysis of Prescription Error Detection. *Journal of Angiotherapy*, *8*(9), 1–6. DOI: 10.25163/angiotherapy.899870

Shumba, A. T., Montanaro, T., Sergi, I., Fachechi, L., De Vittorio, M., & Patrono, L. (2022). Leveraging IoT-aware technologies and AI techniques for real-time critical healthcare applications. *Sensors (Basel)*, *22*(19), 7675. DOI: 10.3390/s22197675 PMID: 36236773

Somasundaram, R., & Thirugnanam, M. (2021). Review of security challenges in healthcare internet of things. *Wireless Networks*, *27*(8), 5503–5509. DOI: 10.1007/s11276-020-02340-0

Su, H., Yao, L., Hou, D., Sun, M., Hou, J., Ying, J., & Hou, R. (2021, August). Cloud computing management architecture for digital health remote patient monitoring. In *2021 IEEE International Conference on Smart Computing (SMARTCOMP)* (pp. 209-214). IEEE. DOI: 10.1109/SMARTCOMP52413.2021.00049

Thirunavukkarasu, J., & Kumaratharan, D. N. (2012). Sensors Enabled Patient Monitoring System Using Cloud Computing Concepts. *IOSR Journal of Engineering*, *02*(2), 247–252. DOI: 10.9790/3021-0202247252

Tsiachri, R., & Sotiriadis, S. (2020). The Role of IoT and Cloud Computing in Health Monitoring Systems. DOI: 10.31224/osf.io/683ds

Ursul, I., & Pereymybida, A. (2023, September). Unsupervised detection of anomalous running patterns using cluster analysis. In 2023 IEEE 13th International Conference on Electronics and Information Technologies (ELIT) (pp. 148-152). IEEE. DOI: 10.1109/ELIT61488.2023.10310751

Vijayan, V., Connolly, J. P., Condell, J., McKelvey, N., & Gardiner, P. (2021). Review of wearable devices and data collection considerations for connected health. *Sensors (Basel)*, *21*(16), 5589. DOI: 10.3390/s21165589 PMID: 34451032

Waleed, M., Kamal, T., Um, T. W., Hafeez, A., Habib, B., & Skouby, K. E. (2023). Unlocking insights in iot-based patient monitoring: Methods for encompassing large-data challenges. *Sensors (Basel)*, *23*(15), 6760. DOI: 10.3390/s23156760 PMID: 37571543

Yang, K., Kpotufe, S., & Feamster, N. (2021). An efficient one-class SVM for anomaly detection in the Internet of Things. *arXiv preprint arXiv:2104.11146.* / arXiv.2104.11146DOI: 10.48550

Yew, H. T., Ng, M. F., Ping, S. Z., Chung, S. K., Chekima, A., & Dargham, J. A. (2020, February). Iot based real-time remote patient monitoring system. In *2020 16th IEEE international colloquium on signal processing & its applications (CSPA)* (pp. 176-179). IEEE. DOI: 10.1109/CSPA48992.2020.9068699

Zamini, M., & Hasheminejad, S. M. H. (2019). A comprehensive survey of anomaly detection in banking, wireless sensor networks, social networks, and healthcare. *Intelligent Decision Technologies*, *13*(2), 229–270. DOI: 10.3233/IDT-170155

Zhang, Y., Chen, Y., Wang, J., & Pan, Z. (2021). Unsupervised deep anomaly detection for multi-sensor time-series signals. *IEEE Transactions on Knowledge and Data Engineering*, *35*(2), 2118–2132. DOI: 10.1109/TKDE.2021.3102110 PMID: 36798878

Ziani, I., Bendiab, G., Bouzenada, M., & Shiaeles, S. (2024). Video-Based Abnormal Human Behaviour Detection for Video Forensics. *2024 IEEE International Conference on Cyber Security and Resilience (CSR)*, 401-406. DOI: 10.1109/CSR61664.2024.10679423

Chapter 7

# Machine Learning-Based Intrusion Detection Systems for Healthcare Internet of Things (HIoT)

**Prarthana Sharma**
https://orcid.org/0009-0001-2571-913X
*Poornima University, Jaipur, India*

**Rajat Kumawat**
https://orcid.org/0009-0007-8873-1818
*Vivekananda Global University, Susnstone, Jaipur, India*

**Gaurav Jain**
https://orcid.org/0009-0001-7575-1015
*Poornima University, Jaipur, India*

**Garima Keswani**
https://orcid.org/0009-0000-3687-2691
*Poornima University, Jaipur, India*

**Nikhil Kumar Goyal**
https://orcid.org/0009-0007-4532-8033
*Poornima University, Jaipur, India*

**Mohammed Firdos Alam Sheikh**
https://orcid.org/0000-0002-8405-3482
*Poornima University, Jaipur, India*

## ABSTRACT

*This chapter explores the design and implementation of Machine Learning-Based Intrusion Detection Systems (ML-IDS) specifically tailored for Healthcare Internet of Things (HIoT) environments. With the growing deployment of wearable sensors, smart medical devices, and remote monitoring tools in patient care, HIoT networks are increasingly vulnerable to cyber threats such as data breaches, denial-of-service attacks, and malicious intrusions. Traditional security mechanisms often fall short due to the sensitive nature of health data and the resource constraints of medical devices. This chapter analyzes how supervised, unsupervised, and deep learning techniques can enhance anomaly detection in HIoT, while addressing challenges*

DOI: 10.4018/979-8-3373-7610-3.ch007

*related to data collection, class imbalance, and model training. It further discusses the integration of edge and fog computing for real-time detection, evaluates existing datasets, and highlights advances in federated learning and explainable AI.*

## 1. INTRODUCTION

### 1.1 Rise of HIoT in Modern Healthcare

With the convergence of healthcare services with the Internet of Things (IoT) recently started, Healthcare Internet of Things (HIoT) – a network of medical devices, sensors, actuators and software systems which interact via secure communication protocols to deliver patient centered care across a value network, has come into being. Smart wearables, implantable devices, hospital beds, infusion pumps, remote diagnostic tools and mobile apps with HIoT systems in them allow remote monitoring, diagnosis and therapy in real time. As the systems are interconnected, it offers very granular data that healthcare professionals can utilize to make decision at an individual level and it enhances the proactive intervention capability, especially to prevent chronic illness and post surgical care (Thakur & Biswas, 2020).

Modern healthcare models which include telemedicine, homebased elderly care and in intensive care unit (ICU) automation, all lean on HIoT. It increases efficiencies by automating administrative workflows, decreases hospital readmissions and enables doctors access to patient information immediately from remote locations. Moreso, HIoT continually collects physiological data like (e.g. heart rate, glucose levels, oxygen saturation) to enhances precision medicine and helps in catching up instances before they become complications. Though growing in sophistication, these systems become more and more important to understand in terms of reliability, resilience and security, particularly in life critical applications where failure or breach of the systems can have serious implications to human health.

### 1.2 Security Threats and Attack Vectors in HIoT

The attack surface against HIoT devices is significantly expanded and thus, the proliferation of HIoT devices has serious implications of widening the attack surface. Most of the HIoT devices are designed with functionality, cost efficiency and compactness in mind, sacrificing the robust security features. Unlike in traditional IT systems such devices may not have secure boot mechanisms, proper encryption protocols or the ability to receive security updates, for example. These weaknesses are exploited by attackers via the use of malware injection, man in the middle attack, device spoofing, packet sniffing and denial of service (DoS) attack (Al-Obeidat & El-Alfy, 2019).

Suppose, an insulin pump or a cardiac monitor falls into the hands of a malicious actor, it could lead to direct physical harm to a patient. Moreover, unauthorized access of Electronic Health Records (EHRs) can lead to theft of very sensitive patient information in violation of privacy laws and destroying the trust. The patient's behavior and routines can even be inferred from passive attacks such as traffic analysis. Ransomware attacks — which hold an entire healthcare system hostage — have happened repeatedly to hospitals.

Since the HIoT devices are resource constrained, they possess limited processing power, battery life and typically has low storage capacity, incorporation of standard cybersecurity solutions into these devices is challenging. Finally, medical devices (like ambulances with sensors installed, wearables at home) are mobile and dynamic which makes centralized monitoring and security enforcement difficult. Considering the real time nature of health data and the zero tolerance to system downtime in the clinical context, there exists a need for fast, intelligent and adaptive security mechanisms that are able to neutralize and thwart such threats without affecting care delivery.

## 1.3 Role of Intrusion Detection Systems (IDS)

Among the most effective technologies for securing HIoT ecosystems are Intrusion Detection Systems (IDS). An IDS monitors a system or network to detect unauthorized activities, policy violations, or suspicious behavior that may indicate a security compromise. IDS solutions act as a second line of defense after firewalls, capable of identifying internal and external threats that bypass traditional security controls (Saif & Biswas, 2018).

There are various types of IDS:

- **Host-Based IDS (HIDS)** focuses on individual devices, monitoring logs, configurations, and local behaviors for anomalies.
- **Network-Based IDS (NIDS)** inspects traffic across communication links, detecting irregularities in packet headers, payloads, or flows.

IDS for HIoT applications has to address a number of critical requirements, including low latency, higher accuracy, real time and be able to accommodate heterogenous devices. While traditional signaturebased IDS is fast such IDS can only detect known threats and provide no protection against zero-day attacks. While anomaly-based IDS uses behavioral model and deviate from normal operations, but its tuning here is required to avoid high false positive rate.

For example, false negatives in a healthcare environment can result in alert fatigue but more importantly false alarms will erode the trust in the system while false negatives will potentially have catastrophic consequences by missing actual attacks. Consequently, a lightweight and efficient, yet context aware and self learning intelligent IDS solutions for HIoT is sought for (Wazid et al., 2016).

## 1.4 Benefits of Machine Learning in IDS for HIoT

Machine Learning (ML) is the key to advancing IDS for HIoT, in that the systems are able to learn legitimate behavior patterns and distinguish new or sophisticated intrusion patterns. With ML algorithms, new threats become detectable, reduce the dependencies on static rule sets or signature databases and ML algorithms can be dynamically adjusted to new threats, detecting zero-day attacks. In contrast to rule based approaches, ML can automatically generalize on training data and have higher precision at classifying real time events.

In supervised learning the algorithms like Random Forests, Decision Trees and Support Vector Machines (SVM) are trained with labeled datasets in order to differentiate between benign or malicious behaviors. However, there is scarcity of labeled data in healthcare domain as a result of privacy constraints and low incidence of attack events. Therefore, various clustering (e.g. k-means, DBSCAN) and Autoencoders based unsupervised learning techniques have been increasingly applying for modelling normal behaviour and flagging deviations.

Convolutional Neural Networks (CNNs) and Recurrent Neural Networks (RNNs), especially Long Short Term Memory Networks (LSTMs), provide deep Learning models to model and extract features from sequence data from sensors, while discovering complex correlations in time (Thamilarasu et al., 2020). For instance, CNNs can identify the patterns in network traffic and LSTMs can be used for modelling patient data streams for anomaly detection.

Second, federated learning supports training ML models across distributed devices while preserving privacy, keeping sensitive patient data decentralized and at the edge and yet improving collective intelligence. Interpretable and auditable ML based IDS decision are attracted by second strategy, an important feature in high stakes healthcare environment and explainable AI (XAI) techniques are also explored.

Further, ML based IDS integrated with edge and fog computing increases performance by making the decision near the source of data. But this in turn decreases latency, cuts down bandwidth usage and improves responsiveness – all very useful when it comes to real time healthcare applications. By presenting themselves as adaptable, scalable and intelligent ML based IDS are a cornerstone to future ready HIoT cybersecurity architectures (Dey et al., 2019).

## 2. OVERVIEW OF HIOT ARCHITECTURE AND SECURITY CHALLENGES

### 2.1 Components and Communication Protocols in HIoT

The architecture of a Healthcare Internet of Things (HIoT) system typically comprises several interdependent layers that facilitate data acquisition, transmission, processing, storage, and decision-making. These components include:

- **Sensing Layer**: Composed of wearable sensors (e.g., ECG, glucose monitors), implantable devices, and environmental sensors. These devices collect physiological and contextual data from patients.
- **Network Layer**: Enables data transmission using protocols such as Wi-Fi, Bluetooth Low Energy (BLE), Zigbee, LoRaWAN, and 5G. In many HIoT setups, communication is facilitated through Body Area Networks (BAN) and Personal Area Networks (PAN).
- **Processing Layer**: Includes edge devices (e.g., smartphones, gateways), fog nodes, and cloud servers that handle data filtering, analysis, and storage.
- **Application Layer**: Interfaces for clinicians and healthcare providers that support decision-making, visualization, EHR updates, and remote consultations.

HIoT systems rely heavily on **communication protocols** like MQTT (Message Queuing Telemetry Transport), CoAP (Constrained Application Protocol), and HL7 (Health Level Seven) for interoperability with healthcare databases and hospital information systems. These protocols are designed for low-power, high-latency environments, but many lack robust built-in security, leaving gaps that attackers can exploit (Goyal et al., 2025a).

### 2.2 Vulnerabilities in Medical IoT Devices

HIoT devices are prone to vulnerabilities due to their constrained design. Often, manufacturers prioritize performance and battery efficiency over security, leading to devices with:

- **Hardcoded credentials or no password protection**.
- **Unencrypted communication channels**, which are susceptible to eavesdropping or man-in-the-middle attacks.
- **Firmware that is difficult or impossible to update remotely**, leaving unpatched vulnerabilities.
- **Insecure APIs**, exposing backend systems to exploitation.

*Figure 1.* **IoT Vulnerabilities in healthcare***[REMOVED HYPERLINK FIELD]*

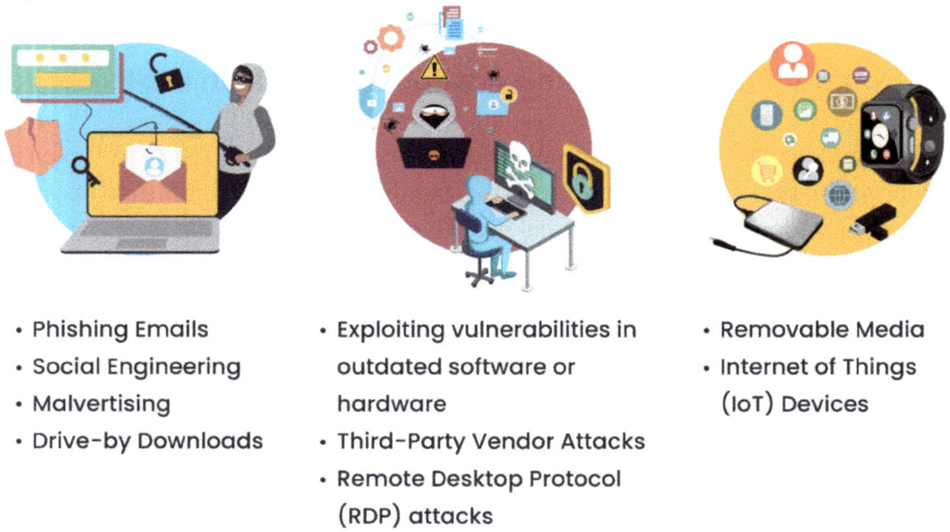


Additionally, the diversity in device manufacturers and lack of standardization results in **inconsistent security postures**, making unified protection challenging. For example, a heart monitor might follow strict encryption practices, while a connected thermometer may not implement any security protocol at all. This diversity expands the attack surface dramatically.

## 2.3 Security Risks: Data Breaches, Spoofing, and DoS

HIoT environments are lucrative targets for cyberattacks because they manage **sensitive personal health information (PHI)**. Attackers can exploit weak authentication mechanisms to access and alter patient data, leading to incorrect diagnoses or malicious manipulation of treatment.

- **Data breaches** may expose confidential medical histories and personal identifiers, violating patient privacy and leading to regulatory penalties.
- **Spoofing attacks** allow adversaries to impersonate trusted medical devices or users, injecting false data into monitoring systems.
- **Denial-of-Service (DoS)** attacks can overload or crash critical health devices or networks, delaying urgent care or disabling telemetry feeds.
- **Ransomware** is increasingly deployed against hospitals, freezing access to patient data and demanding payment in cryptocurrencies (Jaber & Rehman, 2020).

In critical care units or remote monitoring systems, even a brief delay or falsified data reading can have life-threatening consequences.

## 2.4 Privacy and Compliance in HIoT (HIPAA, GDPR)

The **privacy of patient data** is not just a technical issue but a legal and ethical imperative. Multiple regulations govern how medical information should be collected, stored, and shared.

- **HIPAA (Health Insurance Portability and Accountability Act)** in the U.S. requires healthcare providers to protect electronic protected health information (ePHI) with administrative, physical, and technical safeguards. Breaches can result in hefty fines and reputational damage.
- **GDPR (General Data Protection Regulation)**, applicable in the European Union, mandates that personal data—including health data—must be collected transparently, used for legitimate purposes, and secured by design and by default.

In HIoT, ensuring compliance involves **encryption of data at rest and in transit**, **user consent for data collection**, **access control**, and **auditability** of all actions performed on patient data. However, the distributed nature of HIoT makes centralized enforcement difficult.

Moreover, with real-time analytics increasingly being performed at the edge or in fog nodes, ensuring that local processing adheres to privacy principles (such as data minimization and purpose limitation) becomes essential. **Federated learning** and **differential privacy** are emerging techniques that enable model training without sharing raw data, thus supporting both privacy and analytics in compliance-heavy environments (Tavallaee et al., 2009).

# 3. FUNDAMENTALS OF INTRUSION DETECTION SYSTEMS (IDS)

## 3.1 IDS Architecture: Host-Based vs. Network-Based

Intrusion Detection Systems (IDS) are fundamental tools for identifying unauthorized, malicious, or abnormal activities in digital environments. In the context of Healthcare Internet of Things (HIoT), IDS serve as real-time security monitors, identifying both internal and external threats that may compromise data confidentiality, system integrity, or patient safety.

*Figure 2. IDS architecture*

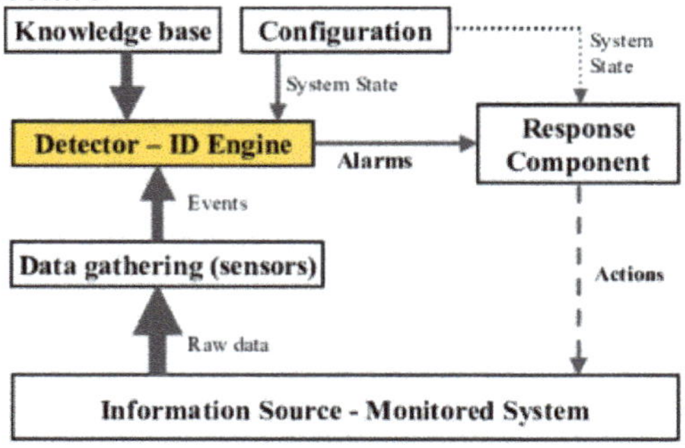


The two primary IDS architectures are **Host-Based IDS (HIDS)** and **Network-Based IDS (NIDS)**.

- **HIDS** operates directly on a specific device, such as a wearable sensor or a smart infusion pump. It analyzes local logs, file integrity, system calls, and application behavior to detect unusual activity. HIDS is particularly useful in detecting insider threats, policy violations, or malware residing on the device. However, HIDS can be resource-intensive and may not be suitable for highly constrained HIoT devices (Ali et al., 2018).
- **NIDS**, on the other hand, inspects traffic traversing the network. It captures and analyzes packet headers, payloads, and communication patterns between devices, gateways, and cloud servers. In HIoT environments, NIDS can monitor a larger surface area, including the data exchanged between multiple devices, without interfering with their internal operations. However, it may struggle with encrypted traffic or activities hidden behind secure communication protocols like TLS (Zhang et al., 2020).

A hybrid approach, combining both HIDS and NIDS, is increasingly favored in healthcare systems to achieve layered security coverage.

## 3.2 Detection Techniques: Signature-Based vs. Anomaly-Based

The operational core of any IDS lies in its detection methodology. The two most common techniques are **signature-based detection** and **anomaly-based detection**.

- **Signature-Based Detection** identifies attacks based on predefined patterns or signatures of known threats. These signatures are derived from previous attack footprints, such as specific byte sequences, command patterns, or payload content. While signature-based IDS are highly accurate for detecting known threats with minimal false positives, they are ineffective against zero-day attacks or polymorphic malware, where no known signature exists.

- **Anomaly-Based Detection** builds a baseline model of normal system or network behavior and then flags any significant deviation as a potential threat. This approach is powerful in detecting novel, unknown, or evolving attacks. For example, if a smart ECG monitor begins transmitting an unusually high volume of data, an anomaly-based IDS can raise an alert, even if the specific behavior hasn't been previously recorded.

In HIoT, anomaly-based detection is particularly valuable due to the diversity and unpredictability of network traffic and device behaviors However, the accuracy of this method depends heavily on the quality of the training data and the robustness of the behavior model. Poorly trained models can result in **false positives**, which in healthcare settings could lead to unnecessary alerts and administrative burden (Goyal, 2025b).

To balance strengths and weaknesses, **hybrid IDS systems** are increasingly used, combining the certainty of signature detection with the adaptability of anomaly detection.

## 3.3 Requirements of IDS in HIoT Environments

Deploying IDS in HIoT introduces unique challenges that differ from traditional IT or enterprise systems. IDS for HIoT must fulfill several **critical functional and non-functional requirements**:

- **Low Resource Utilization**: Medical IoT devices often have limited processing power, memory, and battery life. IDS must be lightweight and efficient to avoid draining device resources or impacting performance.
- **Real-Time Operation**: Given that many HIoT applications involve life-critical data, IDS must detect and respond to threats in real-time or near-real-time without latency.
- **Accuracy and Reliability**: The IDS must minimize false positives and false negatives. High false positives can overwhelm healthcare staff with unnecessary alerts, while false negatives may allow actual attacks to go unnoticed.
- **Context Awareness**: HIoT IDS must recognize the clinical context. For example, data bursts may be normal during emergency procedures but abnormal during routine monitoring.
- **Scalability**: The IDS must scale as more devices join the network, without degradation in performance.

- **Interoperability**: HIoT networks are often heterogeneous, involving devices from multiple vendors. The IDS must be capable of operating across various hardware and software platforms.
- **Privacy Compliance**: As IDS systems often collect or process sensitive data, they must adhere to privacy regulations like HIPAA and GDPR, ensuring that patient data is neither stored insecurely nor exposed during analysis.

## 3.4 Evaluation Metrics for IDS Performance

Evaluating the effectiveness of an IDS—especially one based on machine learning—involves a set of standardized metrics. These metrics help determine how accurately and efficiently the system can distinguish between normal and malicious behavior.

- **Accuracy**: The percentage of correctly classified instances (both normal and malicious) out of the total samples. While important, accuracy alone can be misleading in imbalanced datasets.
- **Precision**: The ratio of correctly predicted malicious activities to the total number of predictions labeled as malicious. High precision indicates fewer false alarms.
- **Recall (Sensitivity)**: The ratio of correctly identified malicious activities to the total number of actual malicious instances. High recall ensures fewer missed attacks.
- **F1-Score**: The harmonic mean of precision and recall. It provides a balanced measure especially useful in datasets with class imbalance, which is common in cybersecurity.
- **False Positive Rate (FPR)**: The proportion of normal activities mistakenly classified as malicious. A high FPR can result in alert fatigue in healthcare environments.
- **False Negative Rate (FNR)**: The proportion of actual malicious activities incorrectly classified as normal. A high FNR is dangerous as it means successful attacks go undetected.
- **Detection Latency**: The time it takes for the IDS to identify and respond to an intrusion. In healthcare systems, delays in detection can directly impact patient safety.

These metrics are typically evaluated using **public benchmark datasets** (e.g., CICIDS2017, UNSW-NB15, or healthcare-specific synthetic datasets) and can be visualized using confusion matrices, ROC curves, or precision-recall plots.

## 4. MACHINE LEARNING APPROACHES FOR IDS

In this regard, Machine Learning (ML) has come into limelight and has become a core technology to improve Intrusion Detection Systems (IDS) for the Healthcare Internet of Things (HIoT). Unlike traditional IDS models, ML based IDS use the dynamic learning and adaptability, more detection against unknown threats. Due to the characteristics of being data rich and resource constrained and dynamic, intelligent solutions able to detect and make decision adaptively in real time are required for HIoT environments. This requirement is perfectly met by machine learning models which are able to recognize patterns and anomalies in huge streams of data. In this section, we go in depth to the ML methods used in HIoT IDS, taking a close look at supervised and unsupervised models, deep learning approaches and additional tasks involved such as feature engineering and model validation (Gupta et al., 2019).

### 4.1 Supervised Learning Models (SVM, Random Forest, KNN)

The ML paradigm under which IDS has been mostly mature and adopted is perhaps supervised learning. It works on labeled datasets messages from the past are provided to the model with classes predefined— usually labeled normal or attack. In HIoT networks, benign healthcare traffic and these could be classes in intrusion including unauthorized access, data tampering and command injection. The task of the supervised algorithm is to construct a good classification function on unseen trac.

Support Vector Machines (SVMs) are very efficient in the task of binary classification with very large scale statistics. SVM constructs hyperplanes in the multidimensional spaces in order to separate different classes SVM is able to distinguish between healthy communication from the device and traffic anomaly forecast in the presence of noise in HIoT IDS. SVMs can process non linearly separable data encounters often in real world health care system where we have behavior patterns between legitimate and malicious traffic overlapping (Saif & Biswas, 2020).

To promote generalization and mitigate overfitting, Random Forest (RF) is an ensemble based technique that comprises of many decision trees. On the contrary, the data are trained on each tree of the forest with different subsets of the data and features which helps to capture a wide array of different patterns. RF is very robust against the typical imbalance of classes present in HIoT environments where the presence of intrusion events is very rare. It can further rank features according to their importance for understanding which device behaviors (or traffic characteristics) carry the most information as to intrusions.

KNN is a simple concept, powerful and a good baseline for IDS. What it does is that it classifies a data point according to the majority label of the k-nearest neighbors that the data point has in the feature space. KNN does well when attack patterns cluster locally, but performs poorly on big, high dimensional datasets that are common in healthcare systems. Nevertheless, due to lack of readability, KNN is not preferable while making intrusion decisions by medical administrators for whom transparency in the decisions is essential (Brown et al., 2002).

## 4.2 Unsupervised and Semi-Supervised Approaches

Labeled intrusion data is usually not available or expensive to obtain in many real-world HIoT environments. As a result, there is more and more interest in the unsupervised and semi supervised learning models in order to find abnormal patterns without directly given labels. These are models that are especially well suited for detection of zero day attack since the malicious behavior is not a known attack signature (Bhatia & Rai, 2017).

Anomaly detection is done by making use of unsupervised learning techniques such as K – Means clustering and DBSCAN. Given a value of k (clusters), K-Means groups data points in to k clusters such that there is minimum intra-cluster variance. If we think of a cluster with most of overall points in IDS context we can consider that the majority cluster being the normal traffic whereas other smaller or outlying clusters could possible be considered as the malicious activity. Unlike DBSCAN which identifies dense regions with similar data and labels sparse regions as outliers. This does not require pre-specifying the number of clusters and is more appropriate in the case of irregular patterns — which is something of value in the context of detecting unexpected devices behaviors in patient monitoring systems or unexpected device interactions.

Limitation of semester data is addressed by Semi – supervised learning, that utilizes a small set of labeled data augmented with a large amount of unlabeled data. Self training, co training and graph based label propagation techniques have shown several edges in HIOTIDS. For instance, a self training model initially learns from labelled instances although in an iterative process, it labels the most confident unlabeled instances and re-train itself. In healthcare networks, the operating conditions continuously change (i.e., patient movement, device updates and network reconfigurations) and thus such dynamic adaptation is critical (García-Teodoro et al., 2009).

## 4.3 Deep Learning Models (CNN, LSTM, Autoencoders)

By providing automatic learning of hierarchical and non linear feature representation from raw data, Deep Learning (DL) has a potential to shift IDS into a new transformative paradigm. Traditional ML models require significant manual feature extraction which deep learning architectures can discover hidden patterns directly from simple inputs like time series device logs, packet payloads or aggregate telemetry signal.

Originally designed for using image data, the Convolutional Neural Networks (CNNs) have been used to the IDS, treating network traffic or device signals as multi dimensional matrices. For example, 2D matrix encodes packet features over time, convolutional filters detect spatial correlation like repeated command sequences or traffic bursts. A CNN has been effectively applied to detect DDoS attacks or the botnet behavior in smart ICUs, where features layout in the spatial domain (Ukil et al., 2016).

The Long Short-Term Memory (LSTM) networks are created to handle sequential data, thus they are not suitable for time series analysis. In HIoT environment, intrusion patterns can evolve over time and devices tend to generate continuous data streams such as ECG signal and glucose monitoring log. Because LSTM can learn long–term dependencies, the model should be able to find subtle anomalies, for example slow, gradual injection of malicious packets or intermittent denial–of–service activities.

The computational cost of deep learning is the main challenge with deep learning in HIoT. Problems arise though, as these models require (a) considerable memory, (b) processing power and (c) energy, resources that are often scarce in medical sensors and edge nodes. Solutions like model pruning, quantization, and edge/fog offloading are necessary to make deep learning viable for real-time HIoT IDS (Khan et al., 2017).

## 4.4 Feature Engineering and Dimensionality Reduction

Deep learning is used in IDS, but even in such a case, feature engineering remains critical in any development of ML pipeline. Thus, the quality of features is the critical factor that impacts the model performance, the generalization and the interpretability of the ML model. In HIoT it is a mixture of the two as the data is from heterogeneous sources such as biosensors, imaging devices, patient records and network logs, thus rendering feature extraction to be a challenge as well as an opportunity.

Statistical metrics such as mean, standard deviation, entropy, temporal behaviors such as times between packets, session durations and protocol specific behavior such as TCP flags, payload sizes may be the features chosen for the prototype For instance, an unexplained spike in heart rate signals along with strange packet frequencies could mean both a medical emergency and a cyber-attack trying to capitalise on device behavior.

The dimensionality reduction techniques reduce the large feature sets, but without affecting the performance of the machine. Principal Component Analysis (PCA) is a transformation of original features into the smaller new set of uncorrelated components which explain the most of data variance. It is useful especially for reducing noise and reducing time of computation. However, t-SNE (t-distributed stochastic neighbor embedding) provides help with visualizing 3rd dimensions array of the data coming from HIoT which helps to identify clusters or anomalies that may suggest intrusions (Goyal et al., 2025c).

## 4.5 Training, Testing, and Validation Techniques

A reliable and generalizable ML-based IDS requires rigorous training, testing and validation. In HIoT, a high cost is associated with false positives and negatives (e.g., from a patient safety point of view)—and therefore model validation should be thorough and statistically significant.

k-fold cross validation is one of the most used strategy which partitions the data-set into k subsets. In this model how it works is first the model is trained over k-1 subsets and then it is validated over the remaining one, thus rotating the validation set over folds. By doing this, we make sure that the model works well on various data samples and isn't overfitting to a specific point such as a given segment.

On the other hand, class imbalance is another important aspect to handle. In such real world HIoT networks, only a minute fraction of traffic can contain malicious activity. This is addressed by oversampling (e.g. SMOTE), undersampling and cost sensitive learning. These prevent the model from unjustified bias toward the majority (benign) class.

In addition, metrics used to evaluate the performances of machine learning systems should not just be accuracy. More complete picture comes from precision, recall, F1-score, ROC-AUC and confusion matrices. For example, a high recall is required in order to catch all possible intrusions, at the price of some false alarms which is a reasonable trade off in life critical healthcare scenarios.

# 5. IDS FRAMEWORK FOR HIoT

To deploy an effective Intrusion Detection System (IDS) in the Healthcare Internet of Things (HIoT) ecosystem, it has to be highly robust, adaptive and resource aware framework. But HIoT is different, because it carries life critical applications, patient centric workflows and highly sensitive data transmitted. HIoT networks are devices such as wearable monitors, implantable sensors as well as connected medical equipment that produce continuous streams of real time health data. This environment can be severely disrupted or breached in such a way that it will have awful consequences in terms of data privacy and patient safety is not exempt. Moreover, the

IDS must possess high accuracy of detecting malicious activity and leave zero room for interference with primary medical functions of the system (Thamilarasu, 2016).

HIoT is different from the regular networks wherein the communication in HIoT needs to be ultra reliable, real time responsive and very much in accordance to regulatory (HIPPA, GDPR & ISO/IEC 27001) institutions. This must be done within the context of the heterogeneity of the devices, constrained computing resources and non intrusive monitoring of the devices. Moreover, security solutions must not only add operational overheard to medical staff and should not compromise efficiency of clinical workflows but must seamlessly integrate into existing healthcare workflows and information technology infrastructure. Because of the high stakes involved, alerts in HIoT IDS must be timely and contextually relevant; a delay in response may spell disaster in some cases and a delay in others may not even be a case of IDS; hence, the goal is to minimize false positives (Mitchell & Chen, 2015).

## 5.1 Data Collection and Preprocessing in Healthcare Networks

Consequently, data collection in HIoT IDS frameworks have to balance between the comprehensiveness of data observed and the non-intrusiveness of the collected data, so that there would be continuous monitoring without interrupting the healthcare operations. Tremendous amounts of data are produced by the devices in HIoT ecosystems containing patient vital signs (e.g., heart rate and blood pressure), telemetry from devices, user authentication logs and highly detailed network traffic records. Wearable sensors, implantable medical devices (IMDs), Electronic Health Records (EHRs) and medical system network gateways collecting data from medical devices and bridging medical devices to broader hospital or cloud systems provide a myriad of such data streams.

But data from these sources are collected in raw form which is usually noisy, in consistent and unstructured form and no processing has been done on it before feeding it into machine learning models. As a part of this preprocessing phase, the data gets cleaned by removing the corrupted or erroneous records and the feature values are normalized to a common scale in order to achieve a stable training of the model. However when supervised learning approaches are involved, accurate labeling of data—i.e, clearly delineating benign from malicious behavior—is of paramount importance. Health monitoring time-series data often needs to be segmented into such meaningful time windows for better capturing temporal patterns or anomalies.

Since patient data privacy is of top priority, preprocessing must in also incorporate privacy preserving methods. Differentially private mechanisms can add controlled noise to datasets and federated anonymization techniques can permit sensitive data to remain in the devices rather than transferred out in its raw form. In addition, the data collection module must therefore support interoperability with medical related commutation standards i.e., HL7, FHIR and IEEE 11073 for the integration of healthcare information systems and cloud based heath platforms.

## 5.2 Real-Time Detection and Automated Response

One of the main characteristics of IDS in HIoT is to do real time cyber threat detection and to have quick and automatic response. Any seconds of delay in identifying the threats can endanger the safety of the patients in the medical environments. Consequently, the IDS deals with streaming data with small processing delay and generates alerts or mitigation actions almost immediately.

They do this to enable low latency detection and to do so they utilize stream processing technologies like Apache Kafka or Apache Flink or simply use lightweight custom data pipelines optimized for speed. These often lightweight deployed machine learning models, be it decision trees or shallow neural network, are optimized to run as fast as possible on inference and deployed as close to the data source as possible (on edge devices or gateways).

In the case of an intrusion being detected, automated responses can be initiated including isolation of the compromised devices from the network, filtering of suspicious traffic or, notifying the medical personnel through dashboards or mobile alerting systems. The intelligent alert prioritization in advanced IDS frameworks is implemented by analyzing threat severity, confidence level and criticality of patients. For example, if an insulin pump—an interaction with serious potential consequences—was attacked or suspicious behavior was noticed on a fitness tracker, this could take on the highest priority, while non essential alerts would receive lower priority and reduce the risk of medical personnel becoming overburdened by meaningless alerts.

## 5.3 Edge Intelligence and Fog-Based IDS

Due to limited bandwidth, higher latency, vulnerability to single points of failure architectures in HIoT face problems in traditional centralized IDS. Thereby, growing support in edge and fog computing paradigms, bringing computation closer to the data sources for better and quicker threat detection is required to overcome these issues.

Within an edge enabled IDS framework, intrusion detection models are instantiated on devices like IoT gateways, smartphones or the local edge servers which are physically located in the hospital environments. This setup allows rapid analysis of data stream and early threat identification (Christy et al., 2015).

In addition, edge intelligence provides context aware detection that is based on correlation among different types of data. For example, an edge node that monitors a patient's electrocardiogram (ECG) can at the same time examine the pattern of network traffic to identify when a cyberattack, as when a malware attack may precede or take advantage of a dangerous episode in the patient's cardiac rhythm and this offers more valuable information about the condition of both the healthcare and the cybersecurity. Additionally, in order to enable multiple healthcare institutions to collaboratively train IDS models on distributed data without exposing sensitive patient information, one can do so by integrating federated learning techniques.

## 5.4 Lightweight ML Models for Wearable Devices

Wearable medical devices that belong to HIoT family like Fitness tracker, heart rate monitor and Smart patches are constrained by lack of computational power and battery life. Thus, these devices should include very light weight, energy efficient and real time runable IDS solutions without interfering primary health monitoring functions.

To overcome these constraints, existing techniques of applying model pruning, quantization and knowledge distillation, etc. can be used to simplify the complexity and the size of deep learning models. For instance, a deep neural network developed on very powerful servers can then be reduced to a smaller approximation that fits within the memory and processing bounds that wearable hardware offers. Or lightweight algorithms are intrinsically light such as decision trees, Naïve Bayes classifiers or TinyML Neuro Networks designed to run on constrained processors like the ARM Cortex M or frameworks like TensorFlow Lite Micro (Liu et al., 2018).

## 5.5 Integration with EHR and Cloud Systems

Therefore, an effective HIoT IDS framework should be tightly integrated with EHR systems and cloud platforms to offer a complete security posture over the healthcare ecosystem. The EHRs hold highly sensitive patient information and any attack can lead to massive privacy breaches, identity theft or clinical decision making. As a result, in addition to device level interactions, the IDS must also be monitoring activity at the application layer in EHR databases and access systems (Anthi et al., 2018).

We use machine learning models to identify abnormal access behaviors including logins outside typical hours, unusual patterns of accessing a patient's record or data export outside typical use — all methods that may signal an event of an insider threat or compromised credential. By integration with cloud infrastructure you gain logging centralized, long term forensic analysis and correlations of suspicious event cross institutions for a wider situational awareness.

In addition, cloud connectivity provides for the continuous model training and updates. The entire system can be kept up to date with the latest IDS model which can be pushed securely to the edge nodes or the hospital servers, as the novel threats are ruled in and the system stays current with the new attack techniques. In order to support this integration, contemporary IDS frameworks should have secure APIs, role based access control (RBAC) and provide secure encryption of data, both in transit and at rest. Legal and ethical standards that IDS deployments must comply such as HIPAA in the U.S., GDPR within Europe and ISO/IEC 27001 frameworks guarantee compliance in respect of regulations of patient privacy and data security.

## 6. EXPERIMENTAL FRAMEWORK AND DATASET RESOURCES FOR HIoT INTRUSION DETECTION

The ability of machine learning (ML) based Intrusion Detection Systems (IDS) in Healthcare Internet of Things (HIoT) depends on availability of comprehensive datasets, robust experimental methodologies and adept computational frameworks. In the following, we review the core datasets, evaluation metrics, as well as platforms that serve as the basis for developing, training and benchmarking of the IDS models designed for healthcare IoT. But, due to criticality and sensitivity of HIoT, scientific rigor and domain specificity are requisites for realistic practicability.

### 6.1 Benchmark Datasets for Machine Learning-Based IDS

Benchmark datasets help with ML-based IDS research by making available uniform, published datasets that are suitable for both learning and comparison. Most famous datasets for IoT and network security are not designed to fully show the unique aspects of HIoT.

As an example, the BoT-IoT dataset from the University of New South Wales comes with IoT network attacks such as Denial of Service (DoS), Distributed DoS (DDoS), data exfiltration and man-in-the-middle (MITM) attacks. Because it offers rich metadata, it is widely applied in supervised learning projects. Even so, the information doesn't relate to medical devices such as their traffic or behavior which makes its direct use in HIoT limited.

Just like the other, the CIC-IDS2018 data from the Canadian Institute for Cybersecurity covers a wide range of recent attack scenarios, including brute-forcing, botnets and intrusion. This dataset makes it possible to evaluate detection algorithms since it offers labeled packets and information on network flows. Still, it mainly demonstrates overall network features instead of the interactions between medical devices.

## 6.2 Healthcare-Specific IoT Datasets for Security Research

It is difficult to find datasets designed for healthcare IoT security since using patient data must follow strict ethical, legal and privacy rules. Consequently, researchers have come up with simulation and synthetic data aimed at replicating actions and possibly weak spots of medical devices in special environments.

A good example is the MedBIoT dataset, as it imitates attacks against medical devices including insulin pumps, smart thermometers and cardiac monitors. The data here includes records of communication during regular and malicious activities, ensuring researchers are able to understand the unique patterns in attacks against medical IoT.

Another dataset called Health-IoT 2022 was prepared in experiments that involved both wearable devices and equipment found in hospitals. It relies on a different set of risks such as fraudulent data access, using someone else's devices and injecting information into the network. Augmentation efforts frequently depend on adversarial and other methods to help maintain privacy while adding more data to the collection. As a result, security professionals have tools that fill the difference between the general IoT datasets and the specialized requirements of HIoT intrusion detection.

## 6.3 Evaluation Metrics and Benchmarking Strategies

To know how IDS models function in reality, evaluating them correctly and meaningfully is very important. Most of the times, accuracy, precision, recall and F1-score metrics are used to assess how separate the model can categorize benign and malicious activities from each other. Since false positive results can create trouble for medical staff and undermine trust in computers, FPR is an especially important concept in healthcare.

Still, healthcare applications raise some extra issues that need to be considered. It is important for detection to be prompt, because fast action can avoid bodily harm to the patient. For an IDS model to work on wearable devices, its use of resources must be efficient and it should not take too much time to complete its tasks.

Special tools like ROC curves and the AUC allow you to learn how sensitive and specific the model will be at each different cutoff point. Confusion matrices show how many true positives, false positives, true negatives and false negatives there are which gives a thorough summary of how the algorithm works.

Due to the typical imbalance in HIoT datasets, measuring using MCC and balanced accuracy is more reliable than checking raw accuracy, since it shows how the model handles various levels of group sizes in the data. Using these metrics, researchers can check and judge an IDS's efficiency in actual healthcare situations.

## 6.4 Tools, Platforms, and Testbeds for IDS Implementation

You need to use certain software, programming frameworks and specialized devices to design and check the effectiveness of your HIoT IDS solutions.

Private network monitoring tools Wireshark, Tcpdump and Bro/Zeek gather accurate data for monitoring systems and support creating datasets. IoT devices can be attacked using Kali Linux, Metasploit and IoTGoat, allowing IDS to be tested against the kind of threats they can encounter.

Testbeds for hardware are usually set up with Raspberry Pi, Arduino or commercial medical sensors programmed to behave as hospital networks and sensor systems. Laboratories such as FIT IoT-LAB and Fogbed let researchers set up models for fog and edge computing which are necessary in latency-sensitive Intrusion Detection Systems. Thus, these tools and testbeds are essential for fully testing and validating strategies used in healthcare IoT systems.

# 7. CASE STUDIES AND APPLICATIONS

Healthcare Internet of Things (HIoT) environments, where Intrusion Detection Systems (IDS) are used, deal with challenges and benefits that depend on the essential nature of healthcare data, how sensitive patient conditions are and the wide range of connected devices. It highlights real-life uses and research in the field that confirm IDS technologies are helpful in safeguarding HIoT systems.

## 7.1 HIoT-IDS in Remote Patient Monitoring

Chronic disease management has benefited a lot from Remote Patient Monitoring which allows collecting health data at any time when the patient is not in a clinic. Patients often wear or have implanted sensors that constantly check the amount of glucose, blood pressure and heart rate in their bodies. The data streams are sent wirelessly to cloud servers which allow doctors to check on their patients remotely (Goyal et al., 2025d).

In a significant case, an SVM was set up as part of the edge router in charge of monitoring sensor traffic within a rural hospital system in the United States. By placing the system here, malicious activity could be noticed in advance, keeping data from being compromised before it entered the main cloud. The IDS was configured to find suspicious traffic that usually appears during spoofing and packet injection attacks. An example is that someone might target glucose monitoring systems in order to change the readings and artificially adjust the patient's insulin dose.

Through live monitoring, the system was able to recognize an abnormal behavior like spoofing to change glucose results. When the alarm was triggered, the team could confirm how the patient was doing and avert a harmful medical error. The case proves that edge-based IDS are important for protecting sensor data and ensuring patient security, especially where technology is limited and bandwidth is scarce (Diro & Chilamkurti, 2018).

## 7.2 Intrusion Detection in Smart ICUs

In such units, modern equipment are linked together to help treat and monitor seriously ill patients. These devices collect a lot of information and keep working live, so there isn't much time to figure out an issue.

An IDS that uses both Convolutional Neural Networks (CNNs) and Long Short-Term Memory (LSTM) networks was placed in the fog computing part of a European hospital. So that the CNN could find clues from spatial elements in network traffic and the LSTM could catch distinct time-based activity, this architecture was created to better find MITM attacks and similar sophisticated threats (Li et al., 2019).

The IDS kept watching network traffic to catch any unofficial access and strange links between the data arriving from devices. Should the system find unusual messages being sent to infusion pumps or abnormal sensor readings, it blocked such attacks and informed the cybersecurity team almost immediately. Because of the swift intervention, the operation of important systems continued and critical situations were avoided.

## 7.3 Federated Learning for Privacy-Preserving IDS

Specifically, healthcare data privacy is strictly regulated in the US by HIPPA and in Europe by GDPR which prohibits sharing of any identifiable patient information within institutions or outside. In this context, it is challenging for building effective IDS models which usually need large and diverse datasets in order to generalize well across different hospital environments.

To solve the problem above, Federated learning (FL) provides a possibility of collaborative model training without sharing raw data. An LSTM based IDS was trained in a research collaboration amongst three German hospitals using FL in which each hospital trained a local model respectively on their edges devices and share the encrypted model updates with a central coordinator. Through this approach, patient data was never allowed to leave the local premises; therefore, confidentiality was secured (Liu et al., 2018).

Based on this approach, federated IDS was designed for the purposes of detecting complex anomalies like data exfiltration attempts, irregular heartbeat sensor readings, irregular communication patterns between devices. Despite training distributedly, the system got more than 87% accuracy which proves the feasibility of collaborative learning in healthcare cybersecurity. In this case FL helps bridge the gap between privacy compliance and effective anomaly detection, thereby allowing the hospitals to pool collective intelligence in the fight against emerging threats.

### 7.4 Predictive IDS for Health Emergencies

In addition to detecting cyber threats, IDS models can also be used for prediction in the sense that it can give a prediction of a system failure or a medical emergency before they become fully developed. Early detection of deterioration in health can save lives in eldercare and long term care facilities and the dual functionality of the health watch is especially useful here.

An LSTM based predictive IDS was deployed in a Japanese eldercare center to monitor network activity including network activity plus correlations between patient vitals and device usage patterns. The IDS analyzed sequences such as motion of a patient sensor data, heart rate artifacts and access logs of the hospital medical devices. In case of a particular anomalous sequence that was identified by the system —quick fall in vital signs accompanied by unusual network access attempts—the IDS would generate two alerts: one to be from the medical team in order to address a potential health emergency and the second to be from IT staff to look into a potential security breach (Carro et al., 2017).

## 8. CHALLENGES AND LIMITATIONS

However, the deployment of Intrusion Detection Systems (IDS) in Healthcare Internet of Things (HIoT) environments is challenging because of many technical, operational and ethical issues that hinder its development. These impediments impede IDS solutions effectiveness, scalability and acceptance. These challenges are essential to understanding in depth to guide future research and practical implementations that can really tackle the special needs of healthcare cybersecurity.

### 8.1 Class Imbalance and Data Sparsity

The most difficult issue in the design of ML-based IDS for HIoT is to cope with highly imbalanced datasets. Normal, benign data is being constantly produced by the HIoT systems in the form of, for example, routine sensor readings and expected network traffic, while malicious activity is very rare. It leads to a class imbalance such that the 'attack' or 'anomaly' class is underpopulated as compared to 'normal' class.

But then, due to this imbalance, the ML models become biased to recognize most only the majority class which then heavily diminishes their ability to recognize rare and truly important attacks. For example, an overall accuracy of a model could be very high because almost all of its inputs are classified as benign, but it may do nothing to highlight dangerous intrusions. Furthermore, the sparsity of data is further exacerbated by appearance of new and previously unseen attack patterns on which data is scarce or nonexistent. However, it curtails the generalization ability of supervised models to be able to recognize zero day attacks (Goyal et al., 2025e).

To make these problems less significant, several techniques have been proposed. Synthetic minority class samples are generated by methods like SMOTE which oversample the minority class. Cost sensitive learning is effecting where higher penalties are given to the misclassification of attacks which makes models favour minority classes. While the above approaches are known to be unsuccessful in detecting large number of malicious attack patterns, since in the real world these attack patterns exhibit high degree of dynamicitiy and adaptivity. Now, the problem of class imbalance and data sparsity turns out to be core constraint that severely limits IDS performance and reliability in practical HIoT deployment systems.

## 8.2 Adversarial Machine Learning Threats

We present Adversarial machine learning as a new dimension of vulnerability in IDS systems. They can craft inputs so that they are subtly perturbed or contain noise and the inputs are fed to the ML models with the purpose of making them output incorrect predictions. Since these adversarial examples cause an IDS to mislabel malicious traffic as benign instead or vice versa such adversarial mechanisms bypass the detection mechanisms.

These misclassifications can be grave consequences in the case of HIoT. An example of such an attack would be an adversarial attack that fools an IDS into not detecting a ransomware intrusion on a hospital network and subsequently leads to the system shutdowns, losing critical patient data or interference with life saving medical devices.

Research into defense strategies against adversarial threats is underway but is difficult. While adversarial training which includes augmenting training data with adversarial examples has been shown to improve model robustness, the process requires a lot of computational resources and do not scale generalize. Model ensembling such as combining predictions from multiple diverse models together, reduces susceptibility to model adversarial attacks but increases complexity and latency. It input normalizing and feature squeezing helps reducing adversarial perturbations but it's not fool proof. The respective defense mechanisms are difficult to implement in a real-time IDS system with limited resources (Niyaz et al., 2016).

## 8.3 Resource Constraints in Medical Devices

Most of the medical devices in the HIoT ecosystem, like wearable and implantable devices, have really strict restrictions on memory capacity, computational power and battery life. Such devices have large constraints which pose great hurdles for deploying IDS models directly on them (Kasinathan et al., 2013).

However, running complex machine learning models on such devices is typically infeasible as they consume a lot of energy and need significant processing to do so As a result, IDS architectures have typically had a hierarchical form where functions that are computationally expensive such as model training, feature extraction and deep packet inspection are pushed to edge or fog computing devices. Though this approach relieves devices from the service load, it creates dependence on network connectivity and communication latency.

Even short network delays or loss of network connection can be dangerous to life in emergency medical situations. In addition, dependence on off device processing introduces concerns to the integrity of the data as well as exposure in transmission. Hence, the design of HIoT IDS solutions with lightweight on device detection as well as with offloading strategies yet without affecting their accuracy, timeliness and reliability is a challenging issue (Goyal, 2025f).

# 9. FUTURE DIRECTIONS AND RESEARCH OPPORTUNITIES

As Healthcare IoT (HIoT) systems become more complex and critical, greater demand and need for more adaptive, efficient and privacy preserving Intrusion Detection Systems (IDS) is required. This section reveals emerging trends, new methodologies and open research challenges that may affect the growing ML-based IDS in HIoT environments.

## 9.1 Explainable Artificial Intelligence (XAI) in IDS

But deployable ML based IDS in healthcare still faces the lack of interpretability. Most deep learning models are accurate, but they do it as black boxes and cannot explain their predictions in humanly understandable terms. These problems are problematic in clinical settings where trust, accountability and traceability is important. Although this gap is necessary, Explainable AI (XAI) seeks to close it through visualisations, feature attributions and some causal inference. The integration of XAI into HIoT IDS for the assistance of system administrator and healthcare professionals to understand the rational of the alert, separating the real threat from a false positive and following the ethical and legal transparency mandate is recommended (Bao et al., 2012).

## 9.2 Transfer Learning and Zero-Day Attack Detection

However, traditional ML models often find it difficult to spot zero day attacks, the attacks that are never seen before and hence are different from the well known attack patterns. One potential solution is Transfer Learning (TL) which means we can use a model trained in one domain or dataset and with very little retraining as we adapt it to a different domain or dataset. TL can also be used in the HIoT context to attach knowledge obtained from one hospital's network to another in order to speed up response times when dealing with fresh attacks. When combined with continual learning mechanisms, TL can allow systems to adapt in an ongoing basis to emerging threats without full retrain and thus reduce the overhead and enhance realtime resilience (Maleh et al., 2015).

## 9.3 Blockchain and Federated IDS Models

The models allowing healthcare for decentralized and privacy aware IDS are gaining traction. Based on blockchain technology, IDS logs security and immutability can be improved greatly for trusted alert auditing, secure feature sharing and decentralized access control. On the other hand, Hospital has other solution named as Federated Learning (FL) that enables different hospitals or medical facilities to train jointly a global IDS model without sharing any sensitive patient data. Researchers are exploring federated blockchain architectures in FL as a way of providing at once verifiability, as in blockchain and privacy, as in FL, for IDS, thus addressing key limitations of today's centralized IDS systems.

# CONCLUSION

With the proliferation of the Healthcare Internet of Things (HIoT), a new paradigm of HIoT based smart, connected medical systems has been introduced which increases patient care, helps in diagnosis and continuous monitoring. According to the above, however, the expanded connectivity offers as much in threat as it does in opportunity and there is thus growing need for the timely deployment of efficient Intrusion Detection Systems (IDS).

In this chapter, we have studied the landscape of ML based IDS in HIoT at conceptual level to advanced applications. Firstly it introduced HIoT architecture and the challenges faced in terms of security in this domain. It then described the basic concepts of IDS while illustrating host vs. network based IDS, signature vs. anomaly based detection and the related evaluation metrics. We discussed about different ML techniques: unsupervised, supervised and deep learning; the significance of preprocessing of data, feature selection association; the demand of real time adaptability.

First, datasets, tools and experimental platforms were examined in detail, after which case studies were performed, illustrating real world deployments and possible benefits. Finally, class imbalance, adversarial threats and legal considerations were addressed as major limitations and future research directions regarding explainable AI, federated models and regulatory–aware IDS were identified.

## REFERENCES


Al-Obeidat, F., & El-Alfy, E. M. (2019). Hybrid multicriteria fuzzy classification of network traffic patterns, anomalies, and protocols. *Personal and Ubiquitous Computing*, *23*(5), 777–791. DOI: 10.1007/s00779-017-1096-z

Anthi, E., Williams, L., & Burnap, P. (2018). Pulse: An adaptive intrusion detection for the Internet of Things. In *Living in the Internet of Things: Cybersecurity of the IoT – 2018* (pp. 1–4). IET. DOI: 10.1049/cp.2018.0035

Bao, F., Chen, I., Chang, M., & Cho, J. (2012). Hierarchical trust management for wireless sensor networks and its applications to trust-based routing and intrusion detection. *IEEE Transactions on Network and Service Management*, *9*(2), 169–183. DOI: 10.1109/TCOMM.2012.031912.110179

Bhatia, M., & Rai, M. K. (2017). Identifying P2P traffic: A survey. *Peer-to-Peer Networking and Applications*, *10*(5), 1182–1203. DOI: 10.1007/s12083-016-0471-2

Brown, D. J., Suckow, B., & Wang, T. (2002). *A survey of intrusion detection systems. Technical Report*. Department of Computer Science, University of California.

Carro, B., Martín, M. L., Esguevillas, A. S., & Lloret, J. (2017). Conditional variational autoencoder for prediction and feature recovery applied to intrusion detection in IoT. *Sensors (Basel)*, *17*(9), 1967. DOI: 10.3390/s17091967 PMID: 28846608

Christy, A., Gandhi, G. M., & Vaithyasubramanian, S. (2015). Cluster-based outlier detection algorithm for healthcare data. *Procedia Computer Science*, *50*, 209–215. DOI: 10.1016/j.procs.2015.04.058

Dey, S., Ye, Q., & Sampalli, S. (2019). A machine learning-based intrusion detection scheme for data fusion in mobile clouds involving heterogeneous client networks. *Information Fusion*, *49*, 205–215. DOI: 10.1016/j.inffus.2019.01.002

Diro, A. A., & Chilamkurti, N. (2018). Distributed attack detection scheme using deep learning approach for Internet of Things. *Future Generation Computer Systems*, *82*, 761–768. DOI: 10.1016/j.future.2017.08.043

García-Teodoro, P., Díaz-Verdejo, J., Maciá-Fernández, G., & Vázquez, E. (2009). Anomaly-based network intrusion detection: Techniques, systems, and challenges. *Computers & Security*, *28*(1–2), 18–28. DOI: 10.1016/j.cose.2008.08.003

Goyal, N. K. (2025). Weaponizing Misinformation and Cyberattacks on Supply Chains. In Bukhari, S., & Zafar, I. (Eds.), *Mass Media and Impact of Fake News on Supply Chains* (pp. 177–210). IGI Global Scientific Publishing., DOI: 10.4018/979-8-3373-2175-2.ch007

Goyal, N. K. (2025). Security and Privacy in IoT, Fog, and Blockchain Networks. In Sathio, A., Rind, M., Awan, S., & Junejo, A. (Eds.), *Energy-Efficient Deep Learning Approaches in IoT, Fog, and Green Blockchain Revolution* (pp. 371–398). IGI Global Scientific Publishing., DOI: 10.4018/979-8-3373-0300-0.ch015

Goyal, N. K., Dandotiya, M., Kumari, M., Kaloria, S., & Anushya, A. (2025). AI-Powered Haptic Devices for Patient Rehabilitation. In Mamodiya, U., Kalam, A., Bossoufi, B., Awad, M., & Somwanshi, D. (Eds.), *Integrating AI With Haptic Systems for Smarter Healthcare Solutions* (pp. 143–170). IGI Global Scientific Publishing., DOI: 10.4018/979-8-3373-2307-7.ch007

Goyal, N. K., Dandotiya, M., Kumari, M., Sheikh, M. F., & Sharma, S. (2025). Emerging Job Roles in the Tourism Sector Leveraging Artificial Intelligence. In Silic, M., Luthia, M., Ahmad, F., & Chakraborty, P. (Eds.), *Empowering Sustainable Performance and Competitive Advantage in Tourism* (pp. 89–126). IGI Global Scientific Publishing., DOI: 10.4018/979-8-3373-4546-8.ch004

Goyal, N. K., Dandotiya, M., Qurashi, J. A., Kumari, M., & Sharma, S. (2025). AI-Driven Predictive Analytics for Disease Management. In Ouaissa, M., Ouaissa, M., Imad, M., Qurashi, J., & Farooq, M. (Eds.), *Utilizing AI of Medical Things for Healthcare Security and Sustainability* (pp. 231–276). IGI Global Scientific Publishing., DOI: 10.4018/979-8-3373-0690-2.ch008

Goyal, N. K., Kumari, M., Kushwah, V., Dandotiya, M., & Vijay, A. (2025). Evaluating blockchain security: Trade offs in consensus mechanisms. *IET Conference Proceedings*, 2024(38), 80–88. DOI: 10.1049/icp.2025.0775

Gupta, R., Saif, S., & Biswas, S. (2019). Implementation of cloud-assisted secure data transmission in WBAN for healthcare monitoring. In *Advanced Computational and Communication Paradigms* (pp. 665–674). Springer.

Jaber, A. N., & Rehman, S. U. (2020). FCM–SVM based intrusion detection system for cloud computing environment. *Cluster Computing*, *23*(4), 3221–3231. DOI: 10.1007/s10586-020-03082-6

Kasinathan, P., Pastrone, C., Spirito, M. A., & Vinkovits, M. (2013). Denial-of-service detection in 6LoWPAN-based Internet of Things. In 2013 IEEE 9th International Conference on Wireless and Mobile Computing, Networking and Communications (WiMob'13) (pp. 600–607). IEEE.

Khan, F. A., Haldar, N. A. H., Ali, A., Iftikhar, M., Zia, T. A., & Zomaya, A. Y. (2017). A continuous change detection mechanism to identify anomalies in ECG signals for WBAN-based healthcare environments. *IEEE Access : Practical Innovations, Open Solutions*, *5*, 13531–13544. DOI: 10.1109/ACCESS.2017.2714258

Li, J., Zhao, Z., Li, R., & Zhang, H. (2019). AI-based two-stage intrusion detection for software-defined IoT networks. *IEEE Internet of Things Journal*, *6*(2), 2093–2102. DOI: 10.1109/JIOT.2018.2883344

Liu, L., Xu, B., Zhang, X., & Wu, X. (2018). An intrusion detection method for Internet of Things based on suppressed fuzzy clustering. *EURASIP Journal on Wireless Communications and Networking*, *2018*(1), 1–12. DOI: 10.1186/s13638-018-1128-z

Liu, X., Liu, Y., Liu, A., & Yang, L. T. (2018). Defending ON–OFF attacks using light probing messages in smart sensors for industrial communication systems. *IEEE Transactions on Industrial Informatics*, *14*(9), 3801–3811. DOI: 10.1109/TII.2018.2836150

Maleh, Y., Ezzati, A., Qasmaoui, Y., & Mbida, M. (2015). A global hybrid intrusion detection system for wireless sensor networks. *Procedia Computer Science*, *52*, 1047–1052. DOI: 10.1016/j.procs.2015.05.108

Mitchell, R., & Chen, I. R. (2015). Behavior rule specification-based intrusion detection for safety-critical medical cyber-physical systems. *IEEE Transactions on Dependable and Secure Computing*, *12*(1), 16–30. DOI: 10.1109/TDSC.2014.2312327

Niyaz, Q., Javaid, A. Y., Sun, W., & Alam, M. (2016). Deep learning approach for network intrusion detection system. In *ACM 9th EAI International Conference on Bio-inspired Information and Communications Technologies* (pp. 21–26).

Saif, S., & Biswas, S. (2018). Secure data transmission beyond Tier 1 of medical body sensor network. In *International Ethical Hacking Conference* (pp. 405–417). Springer. https://doi.org/DOI: 10.1007/978-981-13-1544-2_33

Saif, S., & Biswas, S. (2020). On the implementation and performance evaluation of security algorithms for healthcare. In *2nd International Conference on Communication Devices and Computing* (pp. 629–640). Springer. DOI: 10.1007/978-981-15-0829-5_59

Tavallaee, M., Bagheri, E., Lu, W., & Ghorbani, A. (2009). A detailed analysis of the KDD CUP 99 data set. In Second IEEE Symposium on Computational Intelligence for Security and Defense Applications (CISDA). IEEE. Ali, M. H., Fadlizolkipi, M., Firdaus, A., & Khidzir, N. Z. (2018). A hybrid particle swarm optimization–extreme learning machine approach for intrusion detection system. In 2018 IEEE Student Conference on Research and Development (SCOReD) (pp. 1–4). IEEE. DOI: 10.1109/CISDA.2009.5356528

Thakur, D., & Biswas, S. (2020). Smartphone-based human activity monitoring and recognition using ML and DL: A comprehensive survey. [Springer.]. *Journal of Ambient Intelligence and Humanized Computing*, *11*(3), 777–791. DOI: 10.1007/s12652-020-01899-y

Thamilarasu, G. (2016). iDetect: An intelligent intrusion detection system for wireless body area networks. *International Journal of Security and Networks*, *11*(2), 82–93. DOI: 10.1504/IJSN.2016.075074

Thamilarasu, G., Odesile, A., & Hoang, A. (2020). An intrusion detection system for Internet of Medical Things. *IEEE Access : Practical Innovations, Open Solutions*, *8*, 181560–181576. DOI: 10.1109/ACCESS.2020.3026260

Ukil, A., Bandyoapdhyay, S., Puri, C., & Pal, A. (2016). IoT healthcare analytics: The importance of anomaly detection. In 2016 IEEE 30th International Conference on Advanced Information Networking and Applications (AINA) (pp. 994–997). IEEE.

Wazid, M., Zeadally, S., Das, A. K., & Odely, V. (2016). Analysis of security protocols for mobile healthcare. [Springer.]. *Journal of Medical Systems*, *40*(4), 1–12. DOI: 10.1007/s10916-016-0596-0 PMID: 27640159

Zhang, G., Hou, J., Wang, J., Yan, C., & Luo, J. (2020). Feature selection for microarray data classification using hybrid information gain and a modified binary krill herd algorithm. *Interdisciplinary Sciences, Computational Life Sciences*, *12*(3), 331–345. DOI: 10.1007/s12539-020-00372-w PMID: 32441000

Chapter 8

# Transformational Leadership Effect on IoT-Based Cyber-Security in Healthcare by Organizational Culture of Continuous Improvement and Vigilance

**Wako Jio**
https://orcid.org/0009-0003-6192-459X
*Bule Hora University, Ethiopia*

**Shashi Kant**
https://orcid.org/0000-0003-4722-5736
*Lovely Professional University, India*

**Hirut Assegid**
https://orcid.org/0009-0003-6192-459X
*Bule Hora University, Ethiopia*

**Zerihun Kinde Alemu**
https://orcid.org/0000-0002-8546-2882
*Ethiopian Civil Service University, Ethiopia*

DOI: 10.4018/979-8-3373-7610-3.ch008

## ABSTRACT

*This chapter investigates the influence of transformative headship on Cyber-security through in the context of Healthcare IoT in the Ethiopian industry. Utilizing a sample size of 385, the investigation performs reduction of dimensions to define the dimensional structure of the variables involved. The adequacy of data metric certifies the appropriateness of the sample for factor analysis, through a KMO value indicating acceptable sampling adequacy. To analyze the links among transformational headship, organizational culture of continuous improvement, as well as Cyber-security vigilance, lading of factors are undertaken using AMOS software. The judgments demonstrate that transformational headship strongly promotes an organizational culture that supports continual development as well as alertness. Moreover, this culture mediates the association among transformational headship as well as better Cyber-security measures in Healthcare IoT contexts.*

## INTRODUCTION

As the world becomes more connected, Cyber-security in healthcare, especially when it comes to Internet of Things (IoT) devices, is more essential than ever (Khan et al., 2025). Digital technologies are quickly becoming a part of the global healthcare system (Awan et al., 2025). This raises worries about data breaches as well as cyber threats that put patient safety as well as privacy at risk (Restuputri et al., 2025). As healthcare businesses try to improve their Cyber-security systems, headship becomes even more essential (Abdullah Sani & Jaafar, 2025). Transformational headship, which includes visionary direction as well as motivating impact, has become an essential part of building a culture of vigilance as well as constant progress. James MacGregor Burns first talked about transformational headship in the late 20th century (Rawindaran et al., 2025). Since then, the idea has grown to include many other aspects that may have a big effect on how organizations operate as well as function (Eappen et al., 2025). There is a lot of investigation that shows a link among transformational headship as well as better organizational outcomes (Murugan & Singh, 2025).

These glitches typically make it hard to put Cyber-security protections into place, which makes systems more vulnerable to attack by bad actors (Gebeyew et al., 2025). Also, much of the investigation that is already out there doesn't look at how organizational culture might help improve Cyber-security when transformational headship is in charge (Gebeyew et al., 2025). This chapter's goal is to fill up these investigation gaps by looking into how transformational headship, a culture of continuous improvement in organizations, as well as Cyber-security works together in Ethiopian healthcare IoT settings. The investigation wants to find out the answer to this question: ***"What does transformational headship does to Cyber-security practices in healthcare IoT, as well as how does corporate culture affect this relationship?"*** This chapter gives policymakers as well as future investigations useful information by looking at these processes. It gives a framework that not only points out problems but also suggests concrete steps that may be taken to make healthcare Cyber-security more resilient.

## Background of the Study

The use of Internet of Things (IoT) technology in healthcare has changed the way patients are cared for as well as how well operations run. But it has also produced a lot of Cyber-security holes (Restuputri et al., 2025). Because health data is as sensitive as well as more people are using linked devices, the healthcare industry has become a prominent target for hackers (Abdullah Sani & Jaafar, 2025). In Ethiopia, where healthcare is quickly going digital, the problems are considerably worse since there aren't enough resources; the infrastructure isn't good enough, as well as healthcare workers don't know enough about Cyber-security (Srivastava, 2025). The ransom ware assault on a hospital in the United States in 2020 is a real-life a case of these problems (Awan et al., 2025). It stopped patient services as well as cost the facility a lot of money. This event shows what may happen if Cyber-security safeguards aren't robust sufficient as well as how essential it is for headship to create a culture of alertness (Eappen et al., 2025). In Ethiopia, a preliminary investigation found that many healthcare facilities didn't have good incident response plans or Cyber-security training packages, which made them more vulnerable to attacks (Murugan & Singh, 2025).

Transformational headship might have a big impact on how well people follow Cyber-security best practices (Kant et al., 2025). To deal through changing cyber threats, leaders need to create a culture of continuous development by inspiring as well as motivating their workers (Rawindaran et al., 2025). Along with, a lot of Ethiopian healthcare corporates have trouble through executives that are more transactional than transformative. This makes them react instead of proactively when it comes to Cyber-security (Khan et al., 2025). Also, many organizations' cultures don't put a high priority on Cyber-security because they see it as an IT issue instead than a key aspect of patient safety as well as operational integrity. For a case, a poll of healthcare professionals in Addis Ababa found that just a small number of them felt well-prepared to deal through Cyber-security risks (Gebeyew et al., 2025). This shows that there is a lack of headship as well as cultural commitment to Cyber-security (Cvetkoska et al., 2025). This investigation looks at real-life problems to provide a full picture of how transformational headship may be used to improve

Cyber-security in the Ethiopian healthcare system. The information obtained will not only fill in the gaps that exist now, but it will also help plan future efforts to create a strong healthcare system that can handle the challenges of digital transformation.

## Statement of the Problem

The quick use of Internet of Things (IoT) technology in healthcare has a lot of potential to make patients better as well as make operations run more smoothly (Abdullah Sani & Jaafar, 2025). But this progress has also made healthcare institutions far more vulnerable to cyber-attacks, especially in places like Ethiopia that are still growing (Murugan & Singh, 2025). In the best case scenario, healthcare organizations would have strong Cyber-security safeguards in place, thanks to transformational headship that encourages a culture of constant development as well as watchfulness. Sadly, the way things are right now is nothing like this ideal (Srivastava, 2025). There is evidence that transformational headship does not work to change Cyber-security practices. Some studies show a good link, but others don't, which means that headship alone might not be enough to make Cyber-security better (Khan et al., 2025). These mixed outcomes show that there is a vacuum in our understanding of how different types of headship affect corporate culture as well as Cyber-security procedures, especially when it comes to healthcare IoT (Rawindaran et al., 2025). Also, most of the time, the investigation that is already out there doesn't talk about the precise ways that transformational headship affects Cyber-security. There is a lot of information on how headship affects the performance of organizations, but not much about how it affects Cyber-security in healthcare (Cvetkoska et al., 2025). Contextual gaps make this problem much harder to solve because most investigation have been done in rich nations, which means their outcomes may not be useful for the Ethiopian healthcare system (Restuputri et al., 2025).

These problems get worse since many healthcare institutions don't have the right resources, training, or knowledge to properly deploy Cyber-security protections (Awan et al., 2025). IT teams as well as clinical personnel don't often work well together, which makes it hard to protect against the particular threats offered by IoT devices (Eappen et al., 2025). This investigation wants to fill up these gaps by giving real-world cases of how transformational headship affects Cyber-security procedures in Ethiopian healthcare businesses. The investigation provided an useful information on how headship may encourage a proactive approach to Cyber-security by looking at the role of corporate culture as a mediator. The outcomes will not only help us understand this dynamic better in theory, but they will also give policymakers as well as healthcare executives practical advice on how to improve Cyber-security in the healthcare sector. This will help future investigation as well as projects that aim to make the healthcare sector more resilient to cyber-attacks.

## Theoretical Foundation

*Transformational Leadership Theory:* James MacGregor Burns came up through the idea of transformational headship theory in the late 1970s. It says that leaders should be able to inspire as well as encourage their people to do great things. According to this view, transformational leaders create a vision, stimulate new ideas, as well as build a culture of support inside the firm. When it comes to Cyber-security in healthcare, transformational leaders may help get people to use best practices by encouraging a culture of being alert as well as always becoming better. This idea is the basis for understanding how good headship may make an organization more resilient to cyber-attacks (Restuputri et al., 2025).

***Theory of Organizational Culture:*** Organizational Culture Theory, which was technologically advanced by publics like Edgar Schein, looks at the common values, beliefs, as well as actions that affect how a company acts. A good company culture may have a big effect on how personnel feel about security measures as well as how involved they are in Cyber-security efforts. In healthcare, where the stakes are enormous, it's really essential to create a culture that puts Cyber-security first. This idea stresses how essential it is for an organization's values to match its Cyber-security goals. It also suggests that a culture of continuous improvement may help lessen the effect of headship on how well Cyber-security works (Rawindaran et al., 2025).

*Theory of Contingency:* Using Contingency Theory, this investigation looks at how transformational headship may be adapted to deal through the specific problems that Cyber-security poses for Ethiopian healthcare facilities (Khan et al., 2025).

***Socio-technological Systems Theory:*** is on how the social as well as technological parts of organizations work together. It stresses that for technology to work well, including Cyber-security safeguards, both people as well as technological systems need to be taken into account. To use IoT devices in healthcare, you need to take a holistic strategy that looks at the responsibilities of headship, the culture of the business, as well as how engaged employees are. This theory gives us a way to look at how transformational headship may create an environment where social as well as technological systems work together to make Cyber-security better (Abdullah Sani & Jaafar, 2025).

***Transformational Headship Theory*** is the main theory that this investigation uses since it looks at how headship affects the culture of a business as well as its Cyber-security practices. This investigation intends to shed light on how headship influences an organization's ability to bounce back from cyber threats by looking at how transformational leaders may encourage a proactive approach to Cyber-security.

## Definition and Origin of Concept

***Transformational Leadership:*** Transformational headship is a way of leading in which headships inspire as well as motivate their followers to put the needs of the firm ahead of their own. This idea comes from the labor of James MacGregor Burns in the 1970s. It compressions the need for vision, inspiration, as well as participation to create an air that is open to modification as well as new ideas (Eappen et al., 2025).

***Culture of the Organization:*** The common ideas, attitudes, as well as behaviors that affect how people operate in an organization are part of its culture. Artifacts, avowed ideals, as well as underlying assumptions are the three layers of culture that Edward Schein's model shows. To change how people act as well as think about Cyber-security procedures, you need to know about the culture of your firm (Awan et al., 2025).

Cyber-security

***Cyber-security:*** Cyber-security is the act of keeping computer systems, networks, as well as data safe against theft, damage, or access throughout permission. The word has become more common in the digital era as businesses confront more as well as more dangers from hackers. In healthcare, good Cyber-security is very essential for keeping private patient information safe as well as making sure that IoT devices work properly (Khan et al., 2025).

***Continuous improvement***: It is a way to make processes, goods, or services better over time in a planned way, This idea comes from industrial methods like Total Quality Management (TQM) as well as stresses making little improvements over time as well as getting employees involved. In the field of Cyber-security, a culture of continuous development means always evaluating as well as adjusting to new threats (Restuputri et al., 2025).

***Vigilance:*** In Cyber-security, vigilance is keeping an eye on as well as evaluating systems to find any attacks as well as weaknesses before they happen, This word emphasizes how essential it is to always be awake as well as ready in a cyber-world that changes quickly. Organizations that encourage people to remain alert are better able to respond quickly to cyber events, which makes their overall security stronger (Rawindaran et al., 2025).

## Empirical Literature Review

### Transformational Leadership and IoT based Cyber security

There has been a lot of interest in the connection among transformative headship as well as Cyber-security in recent years, especially in the context of Healthcare IoT

(Khan et al., 2025). Studies show that transformational headship is very essential for improving an organization's Cyber-security (Abdullah Sani & Jaafar, 2025). For a case, studies show that transformational leaders create an environment of trust as well as cooperation, which is necessary for raising healthcare workers' understanding of Cyber-security (Restuputri et al., 2025). Transformational leaders may lower the dangers that come through IoT devices by encouraging people to take responsibility for protecting critical information (Murugan & Singh, 2025). Also, an investigation shows that corporates through transformative leaders are more likely to put in place full Cyber-security plans (Awan et al., 2025). Their investigation shows that these kinds of leaders not only push for the use of new technology, but they also stress the need of ongoing training as well as development for employees (Eappen et al., 2025). This fits through the larger idea of continual development, which is very essential in the world of Cyber-security threats that change quickly. In healthcare, where cyber events may have serious effects on patient safety as well as the integrity of the company, the focus on preventive actions that transformational headship theory suggests is especially essential (Srivastava, 2025).

Transformational headship has been related to creating a supportive company culture that puts Cyber-security first, in addition to raising awareness as well as training (Rawindaran et al., 2025). In a qualitative investigation, healthcare workers said that leaders who model good Cyber-security practices had a big impact on how they acted as well as felt about Cyber-security (Malik et al., 2025). The fact that executives as well as employees respond in the same way shows how essential company culture is for improving Cyber-security efforts (Gebeyew et al., 2025). The investigation reveals that when transformational leaders are involved in Cyber-security efforts, they make it such that all staff members are responsible for keeping an eye on things all the time (Kant et al., 2025). Along with, there are still gaps in the empirical investigation, especially when it comes to Healthcare IoT, even while it supports the idea that transformational headship is good for Cyber-security. A lot of the investigation that has already been done has focused on affluent nations. This has left a gap in our understanding of how these dynamics work in places through little resources, like Ethiopia (Ashuro et al., 2025). A report says that further investigation should be done in specific areas to look at the specific problems those healthcare organizations in underdeveloped countries face, such as cultural resistance as well as infrastructure issues that might make it harder to use good Cyber-security practices (Cvetkoska et al., 2025).

## TRANSFORMATIONAL LEADERSHIP AND CYBER SECURITY IN HEALTHCARE IOT HAVING EMPIRICAL ASSOCIATION

### Transformational Leadership and Continuous Improvement and Vigilance

Many other fields, including healthcare, have investigated the link among transformational headship as well as an organizational culture that values constant improvement as well as being alert (Awan et al., 2025). Transformational leaders are good at getting people to work hard as well as come up through new ideas (Rawindaran et al., 2025). They create a culture that encourages people to be flexible as well as try new things (Murugan & Singh, 2025). This dynamic is especially essential in corporates that want to keep becoming better, where leaders are key to creating a culture that values continual growth as well as being open to change. Investigation has shown that transformational headship is very essential for creating a culture of learning in businesses (Khan et al., 2025). Leaders that have transformative skills not only have a clear vision, but they also give people the freedom to take the lead as well as solve problems (Restuputri et al., 2025). This empowerment is very essential for creating a culture of continuous improvement since employees are more willing to share their ideas as well as solutions when they feel encouraged by their leaders (Abdullah Sani & Jaafar, 2025). An investigation backs this up by showing that firms through transformational leaders are better at carrying out continuous improvement projects, which are necessary for keeping up through the healthcare industry's quickly changing needs (Jio et al., 2025). Several studies have also connected transformational headship to the idea of alertness, which is being aware of possible dangers as well as being ready to act on them. For a case, studies show that transformational leaders create a culture of safety as well as alertness by encouraging team members to talk to each other as well as give each other feedback (Ashuro et al., 2025). This setting not only helps organizations learn more, but it also lets teams spot problems as well as deal through them before they get worse. In hospital settings, where the stakes are high, this kind of watchfulness is really essential for keeping patients safe as well as making sure things run smoothly (Srivastava, 2025).

There is also evidence from the real world that transformational headship has a direct effect on the growth of a culture of continuous improvement (Awan et al., 2025). An investigation indicated that transformational leaders in charge of firms had employees that were more engaged as well as committed to development projects (Cvetkoska et al., 2025). This involvement is essential for creating a culture where everyone in the company values continuous development, not only as a goal. The investigation stresses that transformational leaders who notice as well as praise little gains create a feeling of ownership as well as responsibility, which helps to make the ideas of continuous improvement more deeply rooted in the business (Ashuro et al., 2025). Even while the investigation has found favorable connections, there are still gaps in our understanding of how these dynamics work in specific situations, especially in the healthcare sector in underdeveloped nations (Gebeyew et al., 2025). Investigation shows that cultural as well as situational factors can have a big impact on how well transformational headship works to encourage constant growth as well as watchfulness. For a case, in places where hierarchies are strong, transformational headship may not be able to bring about change as easily (Eappen et al., 2025).

## Transformational Leadership and Organizational Culture of Continuous Improvement and Vigilance having empirical association

### Continuous Improvement and Vigilance and Cyber security in Healthcare IoT

People are starting to realize that a culture of constant development as well as awareness is very essential for making Cyber-security better, especially when it comes to Healthcare IoT (Murugan & Singh, 2025). As healthcare businesses add more IoT devices, their Cyber-security systems become more complicated as well as less secure, Studies show that a culture that encourages continuous development as well as awareness may greatly reduce these Cyber-security risks by encouraging employees to be proactive as well as responsive (Khan et al., 2025). Studies show that the culture of an organization affects how workers see as well as deal through security concerns. In a world where cyber risks change quickly, a culture of continuous improvement drives people to continuously review as well as improve procedures (Abdullah Sani & Jaafar, 2025). In addition, the idea of awareness, which is being aware of possible dangers before they happen, is also essential for Cyber-security in healthcare settings (Srivastava, 2025). An investigation found that corporates that promote a culture of vigilance had fewer security breaches. In healthcare, where patient safety is the most essential thing, this level of vigilance is necessary to make sure that personnel are properly educated to spot as well as deal through cyber risks (Awan et al., 2025). A case investigation of a hospital in the United States, for a case, showed how a culture of alertness helped the organization find a cyber-attack early on, which helped them limit the damage. This shows how essential it is to create a space where constant monitoring as well as proactive risk management are top priorities (Restuputri et al., 2025).

The use of IoT technology in healthcare has also made Cyber-security problems much harder to solve. An investigation found that corporates that value continuous improvement are better able to change their Cyber-security plans to deal through the unique security risks that come through IoT devices. This capacity to adapt is also essential since IoT devices often create new ways for attackers to get in that standard security measures may not be able to handle (Cvetkoska et al., 2025). Health corporates that encourage a culture of learning as well as growth are better able to see these problems coming as well as deal through them, which makes them more resistant to cyber-attacks (Gebeyew et al., 2025). There are, along with, certain gaps in the literature that support the idea that an organizational culture of continuous development as well as awareness leads to good Cyber-security practices (Eappen et al., 2025). Investigations have done a lot of work in rich nations, but they don't know how these dynamics work in places through fewer resources (Ashuro et al., 2025). Investigation shows that there is a need for specialized studies that look at the specific problems that healthcare organizations in underdeveloped countries like Ethiopia confront. For a case, cultural opposition as well as a lack of resources might make it hard to put in place efficient Cyber-security measures (Rawindaran et al., 2025).

## Organizational Culture of Continuous Improvement and Vigilance and Cyber security in Healthcare IoT having empirical association

### *Transformational Leadership, Cyber security, Continuous Improvement and Vigilance Mediation*

It is essential to explore how transformational headship, Cyber-security in healthcare IoT, as well as an organizational culture of continuous development as well as vigilance all work together (Srivastava, 2025). Investigation shows that transformational headship has a big effect on both the Cyber-security of healthcare organizations as well as the creation of a culture that encourages constant development as well as alertness (Abdullah Sani & Jaafar, 2025). This link is especially essential in the context of Healthcare IoT, because connecting devices creates new Cyber-security problems. Investigation shows that transformative leaders can get their people to accept change as well as new ideas (Ashuro et al., 2025). In the field of Cyber-security, transformational leaders create a vision that stresses the need to protect sensitive patient information as well as the integrity of operations. An investigation found that corporates through transformational leaders were more aware of Cyber-security issues, which is essential for reducing the risks presented by IoT devices (Kant et al., 2025). A culture of constant improvement as well as awareness is an essential buffer that makes the good benefits of transformational headship on Cyber-security practices even stronger (Jio et al., 2025). For a case, firms that promote this kind of culture are better able to put in place effective Cyber-security measures because employees feel that they can help through security efforts as well as disclose weaknesses. This empowerment is especially crucial in healthcare settings, where the effects of cyber events can be quite bad (Khan et al., 2025).

More investigation supports the idea that corporate culture may have a moderating influence. For a case, a culture that is always on the lookout for Cyber-security dangers makes employees more receptive to them (Cvetkoska et al., 2025). Studies show that corporates that use transformational headship to encourage vigilance have fewer security breaches (Murugan & Singh, 2025). In the case of Healthcare IoT, this is particularly crucial, since the proliferation of connected devices needs a heightened awareness of possible threats (Gebeyew et al., 2025). Transformational leaders who put a lot of emphasis on being alert make it so that constant monitoring as well as proactive danger assessment becomes a part of the organization s culture (Eappen et al., 2025). Along with, even while the outcomes seem promising, we still don't fully understand how these linkages work in different situations, especially in underdeveloped nations (Ashuro et al., 2025). A lot of the investigation that has been done so far has been on wealthy countries (Rawindaran et al., 2025). This leaves a gap in our understanding of how these outcomes can apply to locations like Ethiopia, where cultural as well as resource issues may affect how well transformational headship as well as organizational culture work (Restuputri et al., 2025). Investigation calls for greater investigation into how contextual elements impact the interaction among these variables. This shows how essential it is to do localized investigation to help create better Cyber-security measures (Awan et al., 2025).

*Figure 1. Conceptual framework*

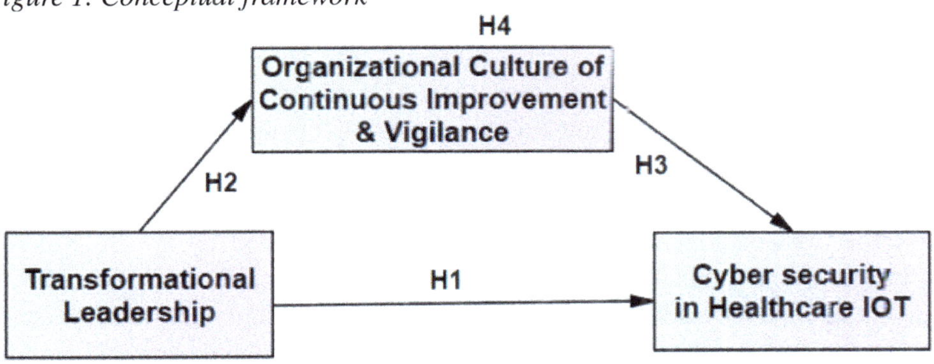

## METHODOLOGY

The investigation used a quantitative investigation method to look at the links among transformational headship, a culture of continuous development as well as alertness in the workplace, as well as Cyber-security in the Healthcare IoT industry. We got 385 samples from healthcare workers at different institutions in Ethiopia. The sample technique was meant to make sure that a wide range of healthcare settings were included, which would allow for a full examination of the interactions that were happening. We used the KMO metric to see if the sample was good enough for factor analysis. The KMO value was higher than 0.70, which meant that the sample size was good for doing EFA. This investigation was done to find the underlying components in the data as well as to confirm the dimensions of transformational headship, organizational culture, as well as Cyber-security practices. After EFA, we used SEM through AMOS software to do CFA. This stage let us evaluate the proposed links among the variables as well as gave us a strong foundation for figuring out how transformational headship affects Cyber-security practices through the mediation of organizational culture. The SEM analysis gave essential data that confirmed the mediation effects as well as made the investigation conclusions more reliable overall.

### Scale Development

We built the scale for assessing the essential components after looking at a lot of other investigation on the subject. Items were taken from well-known scales that had already been tested in comparable situations. The Multifactor Headship Questionnaire (MLQ) by Bass as well as Avolio (1994) was used to create questions for transformational headship. The MLQ focuses on things like inspiring motivation as well as customized consideration. This made sure that the scale really measured the core of transformative headship traits. Items for organizational culture came from the Organizational Culture Assessment Instrument (OCAI), which Cameron as well as Quinn produced in 2006. This tool stresses the need for constant development as well as watchfulness in a business setting, which makes it very useful for the healthcare industry. Expert feedback helped make the scale even better by making sure it was clear as well as useful for the Ethiopian healthcare system. We used items from the Cyber-security Culture Framework by Warkentin et al. (2016) to assess Cyber-security practices. This framework stresses the importance of being aware, getting training, as well as taking proactive steps to protect against cyber-attacks. We chose each item deliberately to show the specific problems as well as interactions that happen in Healthcare IoT settings. During the pilot testing phase, a small group of healthcare experts gave input on how clear as well as relevant the items were. Changes were made to the scale to make it more reliable as well as valid. In the end, the scale that was created had very good psychometric features, which made it possible to fully evaluate the links among transformational headship, organizational culture, as well as Cyber-security practices in the healthcare field.

## Data Analysis

*Table 1. Adequacy for Sampling*

| **Kaiser Adequacy for Sampling** | | **.850** |
|---|---|---|
| Sphericity Test | Chi-Square | 1419.733 |
| | Df | 91 |
| | Sig. | .000 |

Source: Authors

The Kaiser-Meyer-Olkin (KMO) Measure of Sampling Adequacy as well as Bartlett's Test of Sphericity in Table 1 show that the data is good enough for factor analysis. The KMO rating of .850 shows that the sample is very good. A KMO score of more than .70 is acceptable according to Kaiser, which means that the data set is good for exploratory factor analysis (EFA). This high KMO number shows that the investigation's variables are related enough to each other, which is essential for judgment the components that are causing the problem. Bartlett's Test of Sphericity also gave an estimated chi-square value of 1419.738 through 91 degrees of freedom as well as a p-value of .000, which means it was very significant. This conclusion is very essential since it shows that the nexus matrix is not an identity matrix, which means that the variables are related in a big way. Bartlett's test shows that the data is good enough for factor analysis, which backs up the conclusion made by the KMO statistic. These outcomes together show that the sample size as well as data structure are good for looking at how transformational headship, organizational culture, as well as Cyber-security procedures are related in Healthcare IoT.

*Table 2. Total Discrepancy*

| Component | Initial Eigenvalues | | | Extraction Sums of Squared Loadings | | | Rotation Sums of Squared Loadings | | |
|---|---|---|---|---|---|---|---|---|---|
| | **Total** | **% of Discrepancy** | **Cumulative %** | **Total** | **% of Discrepancy** | **Cumulative %** | **Total** | **% of Discrepancy** | **Cumulative %** |
| 1 | 4.51 | 32.235 | 32.235 | 4.51 | 32.235 | 32.235 | 3.00 | 21.451 | 21.451 |
| 2 | 1.37 | 9.787 | 42.022 | 1.37 | 9.787 | 42.022 | 2.16 | 15.491 | 36.942 |
| 3 | 1.27 | 9.087 | 51.110 | 1.27 | 9.087 | 51.110 | 1.98 | 14.168 | 51.110 |

Source: Authors

The first component's eigenvalue is 4.51, which means it explains 32.235% of the total discrepancy. This means that this part is essential since it accounts for more than a third of the data set's variation. At this point, the cumulative percentage is 32.235%. This means that a large part of the discrepancy can be traced back to this one element. The second as well as third parts also make essential contributions, through eigenvalues of 1.37 as well as 1.27, respectively. The total percentage is 42.022% as well as 51.110%, through each of these parts explaining 9.787% as well as 9.087% of the variation, respectively. This overall number shows that the first three parts combined make up more than half of the total variation. This supports the idea that there are separate causes at work in the data. Eigenvalues for components four through six are getting smaller. The fourth component has an eigenvalue of 0.949, which explains 6.782% of the variation, while the fifth as well as sixth components have eigenvalues of 0.871 as well as 0.773, which explain 6.223% as well as 5.519% of the discrepancy, respectively. These components add to the total variation, although they aren't as essential as the previous three. This analysis suggests that a model through the first three parts could accurately represent the data's underlying structure. This would provide a strong basis for further investigation into the links among transformational headship, organizational culture, as well as Cyber-security practices.

*Table 3. Discrepancys*

| Discrepancy | | | Approximation | S.E. | C.R. | P |
|---|---|---|---|---|---|---|
| **Organizational Culture of Continuous Improvement as well as Vigilance** | **<-->** | **Transformational Leadership** | **.242** | **.021** | **8.231** | *** |
| Organizational Culture of Continuous Improvement as well as Vigilance | <--> | Cyber security in Healthcare IOT | .303 | .032 | 7.692 | *** |
| Transformational Leadership | <--> | Cyber security in Healthcare IOT | .254 | .24 | 7.831 | *** |

Source: Authors

Table 3 shows the relationships among the main ideas of the investigation: Transformational Headship, Organizational Culture of Continuous Improvement as well as Vigilance, as well as Cyber-security in Healthcare IoT. Each discrepancy comes through its approximation, standard error (S.E.), critical ratio (C.R.), as well as significance level (P). The nexus among Organizational Culture of Continuous Improvement as well as Vigilance as well as Transformational Headship is .242, through a critical ratio of 8.231 as well as a significance level of *** ($p < .001$). This significant statistical link shows that organizations through more transformative leaders also have a stronger culture of continual development as well as alertness. This outcome backs through Hypothesis 2 (H2), which says that transformational headship has a good effect on creating a proactive corporate culture. Likewise, the nexus among Organizational Culture of Continuous Improvement as well as Vigilance as well as Cyber-security in Healthcare IoT is .303, through a critical ratio of 7.692, which is likewise significant at the $p < .001$ level. This means that a culture of constant development as well as alertness is linked to better Cyber-security procedures in Healthcare IoT settings. This outcome backs through Hypothesis 3 (H3), which stresses how essential company culture is for creating good Cyber-security plans. Lastly, the nexus among Transformational Headship as well as Cyber-security in Healthcare IoT is .254, through a critical ratio of 7.831, which is likewise statistically significant ($p < .001$). This supports Hypothesis 1 (H1) by showing that transformational headship directly leads to better Cyber-security practices.

*Table 4. Validity Concern*

| | CR | AVE | MSV | MaxR(H) | TL | OCCIV | CSHIoT |
|---|---|---|---|---|---|---|---|
| **TL** | 0.732 | 0.643 | 0.219 | 0.852 | **0.654** | | |
| **OCCIV** | 0.758 | 0.657 | 0.132 | 0.763 | 0.171 | **0.665** | |
| **CSHIoT** | 0.793 | 0.603 | 0.274 | 0.797 | 0.333 | 0.193 | **0.684** |

Note: TL= Transformational Leadership; OCCIV= Organizational Culture of Continuous Improvement and Vigilance; CSHIoT = Cyber security in Healthcare IOT

Source: Authors

The CR ratings show that all of the constructs are consistent through one other. Specifically, TL has a CR of 0.732, which is higher than the allowed level of 0.70. This means that the items that measure transformational headship are consistently capturing the construct they are meant to. Also, OCCIV as well as CSHIoT have CR values of 0.758 as well as 0.793, which means that these constructions are also quite reliable. The Average Discrepancy Extracted (AVE) data also show that the constructions are legitimate. The AVE for TL is 0.643, for OCCIV it is 0.657, as well as for CSHIoT it is 0.603. All of the AVE values are higher than the suggested minimum of 0.50, which means that the constructs explain a lot of the differences among the items. This means that the measurements utilized are accurately measuring the hidden variables. There are additional Maximum Shared Discrepancy (MSV) numbers. TL has an MSV of 0.219, OCCIV has an MSV of 0.132, as well as CSHoT has an MSV of 0.274. These numbers show how much the constructs share discrepancy through each other, which is helpful for checking discriminant validity. The MSV values are lower than the AVE values for each construct, which means that the constructs are different from one other. This supports their discriminant validity. Last but not least, the Maximum Reliability (MaxR(H)) values for TL, OCCIV, as well as CSHoT are 0.852, 0.763, as well as 0.797, in that order. These numbers show that the measuring scales used in the investigation are even more reliable.

*Figure 2. Structure equation model*

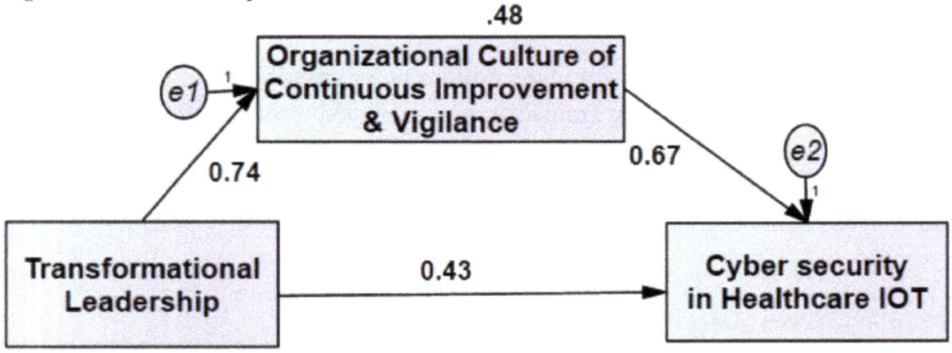


*Table 5. Model testing*

| Sig. | Chi-Sq | RMR | Goodness | Confirmatory | TLI | RMSEA |
|---|---|---|---|---|---|---|
| 0.004 | 1.954 | .036 | 0.930 | 0.912 | 0.911 | .028 |

Source: Authors

Table 5 shows the model fit indices, which give essential information about how well the suggested structural model fits the data. The significance value (Sig.) is 0.004, which means that the chi-square statistic is essential. A big chi-square value means that the observed as well as anticipated discrepancy matrices are not the same. Along with, it is necessary to look at other fit indices to see how well the model fits overall. It is said that the chi-square statistic (Chi-Sq) is 1.954. In structural equation modeling, a lower chi-square number compared to the degrees of freedom usually means a better fit. The ratio of chi-square to degrees of freedom should be less than 3. The chi-square is essential, but other fit indices give a better overall picture of how well the model fits. The Root Mean Square Residual (RMR) is .036, which is lower than the suggested level of .05. This means that the model fits well in terms of residuals. The goodness-of-fit index (GFI) is also 0.930, which means that the model explains around 93% of the variation in the data. This is a very good fit. The Confirmatory Fit Index (CFI) score of 0.912 is likewise a good fit because values above 0.90 are usually fine. The Tucker-Lewis Index (TLI) is 0.911, which supports the model's adequacy even further. Values over 0.90 mean that the model is a good fit for the data. Finally, the Root Mean Square Error of Approximation (RMSEA) is reported at .028, which is significantly below the threshold of 0.06.

*Table 6. Regression Examination*

| Relative | | | Approx. | S.E. | C.R. | P | Ass. |
|---|---|---|---|---|---|---|---|
| **Organizational Culture of Continuous Improvement as well as Vigilance** | <--- | **Transformational Headship** | **.864** | **.143** | **7.583** | *** | **H2** |
| Cyber security in Healthcare IOT | <--- | Organizational Culture of Continuous Improvement as well as Vigilance | .328 | .131 | 2.853 | *** | H3 |
| Cyber security in Healthcare IOT | <--- | Transformational Headship | .957 | .192 | 7.958 | *** | H1 |

Source: Authors

Table 6 shows the outcomes of the regression test, which shows how the concepts of Transformational Headship, Organizational Culture of Continuous Improvement as well as Vigilance, as well as Cyber-security in Healthcare IoT are related to each other. Coefficients, standard errors (S.E.), critical ratios (C.R.), as well as significance levels (P) are used to measure each association. The first regression path shows that Transformational Headship has an effect on the Organizational Culture of Continuous Improvement as well as Vigilance, through a coefficient of.864. This high value shows a strong positive link, which means that transformational headship makes the culture of healthcare organizations much better. The critical ratio for this path is 7.583, as well as the significance level is displayed as *** ($p < .001$). This means that this link is statistically significant as well as supports Hypothesis 2 (H2). The second path looks at how the Organizational Culture of Continuous Improvement as well as Vigilance affects Cyber-security in healthcare IoT. It finds a coefficient of .328. This investigation shows a positive but moderate effect, which means that a culture that values constant development as well as being alert is linked to stronger Cyber-security procedures. Through a critical ratio of 2.853 as well as a significance level of *** ($p < .001$), this association is much stronger, which supports

Hypothesis 3 (H3). Finally, the regression route from Transformational Headship to Cyber-security in Healthcare IoT has a coefficient of.957, which means it has a very high positive effect. The crucial ratio of 7.958 as well as the significance level of *** ($p < .001$) show that this link is statistically significant, which supports Hypothesis 1 (H1). This investigation implies that transformational headship may affect Cyber-security practices directly as well as indirectly by creating a culture of support in the workplace.

*Table 7. Mediating role Effect*

| | Worth |
|---|---|
| Transformational Leadership → Cyber security in Healthcare IOT | .43 |
| Transformational Leadership → Organizational Culture of Continuous Improvement as well as Vigilance → Cyber security in Healthcare IOT | .74*.67=.48 |
| | .91 |

Source: Authors

The table groups the impacts into direct as well as indirect effects, giving a full picture of how these constructions work together. Transformational Headship has a direct effect on Cyber-security in Healthcare IoT that is measured at .43, which means there is a strong positive link. This direct outcome shows that transformative headship alone may make a big difference in improving Cyber-security measures in hospital settings. The table shows the direct effect of Transformational Headship, but it also shows the indirect effect through the Organizational Culture of Continuous Improvement as well as Vigilance. To find the indirect effect, you multiply the effect of Transformational Headship on Organizational Culture by the effect of Organizational Culture on Cyber-security. This gives you an indirect effect of .48. This shows that organizational culture is a way for transformational headship to affect how people do Cyber-security. The overall effect, which includes both direct as well as indirect effects, is said to be .91. This number shows how Transformational Headship affects Cyber-security in Healthcare IoT as a whole. It shows that there is a large direct effect, but there is also a big indirect effect through the culture of the business. The last part of the table shows that the mediation is "Partial mediation."

## DISCUSSION

The outcomes of this investigation show how essential it is for transformational headship, organizational culture, as well as Cyber-security procedures to work together in the context of Healthcare IoT. The outcomes show that transformational headship makes the culture of the firm more focused on continuous development as well as vigilance, which in turn has a favorable effect on Cyber-security practices. This association fits through what other investigation has said about how essential headship is for creating an atmosphere that encourages proactive risk management as well as new ideas. Transformational leaders create an environment where people feel empowered to keep learning as well as help keep the business safe by inspiring as well as encouraging their colleagues. The investigation also shows that corporate culture plays a big part in how transformational headship affects Cyber-security outcomes. This is especially essential in healthcare, where the stakes are high as well as the effects of cyber disasters can be quite bad. The discovery of a partial mediation effect implies that transformational headship directly improves Cyber-security practices. Along with, improving the culture of the firm makes this impact stronger, resulting in a more robust Cyber-security framework. Also, real-world data shows that a strong culture of constant development as well as watchfulness is essential for keeping up through the risks that come through IoT technology. As healthcare corporates use more as well as more technologies that are connected to one other, it is more essential than ever to have a watchful staff. This constraint shows how essential it is to have customized headship methods that take into account local problems, making sure that Cyber-security efforts are both useful as well as successful. Future studies should look at these dynamics more closely, especially how contextual factors impact the use of transformational headship to make Cyber-security more resilient.

## CONCLUSION

This investigation has given us useful information on how transformational headship, a culture of continuous development as well as vigilance, as well as Cyber-security procedures all work together in the context of Healthcare IoT The outcomes show how essential transformational headship is for creating a proactive corporate culture, which is necessary for making Cyber-security more resilient. Transformational leaders make the workplace a place where workers want to do their best as well as stay alert. This directly affects how well Cyber-security measures work. Judgment a partial mediation effect shows how essential organizational culture is as a key factor in this dynamic. It also supports the idea that a solid cultural base may make the good effects of headship on Cyber-security outcomes even stronger. As more healthcare corporates use IoT technology, they need a staff that is always on the lookout as well as ready to act in order to deal through the new cyber dangers that come through digital transformation. But the report also recognizes the problems that healthcare institutions in impoverished nations like Ethiopia confront when trying to put in place effective Cyber-security policies. These problems include a lack of resources as well as different cultural dynamics that might make it hard to do so. These outcomes show that we need personalized methods that take into account local situations as well as give healthcare executives the tools they need to create safe settings for Cyber-security.

## MANAGERIAL IMPLICATIONS

Healthcare leaders as well as administrators who want to improve their businesses' Cyber-security strategies need to pay attention to the outcomes of this investigation. First as well as foremost, the outcomes show how essential transformational headship is for creating a proactive culture in the workplace. Managers should put transformational headship development programs at the top of their list. These programs should focus on attributes like vision, inspiration, as well as empathy. Organizations may make it easier for workers to get involved in Cyber-security projects as well as accept a culture of continuous improvement by giving leaders the authority to engage as well as drive their teams. The investigation also shows how essential it is to create a culture of constant development as well as watchfulness as a key part of good Cyber-security. Managers should set up training programs that teach both technical skills as well as the need of being informed as well as taking action to spot any dangers. Encouraging personnel to talk to one other as well as work together will help everyone be alert as well as make sure that Cyber-security is a shared responsibility at all levels of the business. Finally, in a world where technology changes quickly, it's essential to keep evaluating as well as changing your Cyber-security strategy. Managers should set up ways to measure how well headship as well as cultural programs is working to make Cyber-security more resilient. Organizations may change how they do things as well as stay ahead of new risks by using regular feedback loops. This will protect sensitive patient information as well as keep healthcare systems running smoothly.

## PRACTICAL IMPLICATIONS

The outcomes of this investigation provide a number of useful implications for healthcare corporates who want to improve their Cyber-security policies. First, the focus on transformational headship recommends that businesses should spend money on headship training programs that teach skills like how to communicate well, motivate others, as well as define a vision. Healthcare organizations may make their employees more engaged as well as proactive about Cyber-security issues by giving leaders these skills. Also, the requirement for continual training as well as awareness programs for all staff is made clear by the need of creating a culture of constant improvement as well as vigilance. Regular seminars, simulations, as well as drills are a cases of practical steps that might help workers learn about possible Cyber-security risks as well as develop an attitude of being alert as well as ready to act. Making it easy for workers to report suspicious behavior as well as offer ways to make things better may greatly improve the organization's overall Cyber-security. Healthcare businesses should also make sure that Cyber-security is a part of their daily operations by writing explicit rules as well as procedures. This might include setting up rules for how to utilize IoT devices, handle data, as well as respond to incidents that are frequently shared as well as enforced across the enterprise. Organizations may make sure that all of their workers put security first in their everyday duties by making Cyber-security a part of their operational procedures. Additionally, businesses should use technology by adding sophisticated Cyber-security tools as well as solutions that work through their headship as well as culture programs. Organizations should set up ways to measure how well their headship as well as cultural efforts is working to lower cyber threats. Regular evaluations may assist find areas that need work as well as make sure that Cyber-security processes keep up through new threats as well as technology.

## THEORETICAL IMPLICATIONS

This investigation's outcomes add a lot to our theoretical knowledge of how headship, organizational culture, as well as Cyber-security practices work together in healthcare settings. This investigation backs up current ideas that connect headship styles to cultural dynamics in businesses by showing how transformational headship may help create a culture of continuous development as well as attentiveness. It shows how transformational leaders can create a culture that encourages people to be proactive as well as aware of security issues, which makes the whole organization more productive. Also, figuring out the function of corporate culture as a mediator gives us a more detailed picture of how headship affects Cyber-security outcomes. This mediating impact adds to the theoretical discussion by showing that headship alone is not enough; a supporting culture must also be developed in order for headship efforts to lead to real changes in Cyber-security practices. This idea fits through social constructivist theories that stress how essential shared values as well as norms are in molding how people act in organizations. Also, the context-specific judgments, especially those on the problems that developing countries like Ethiopia face, give complexity to the theoretical framework by showing how environmental variables affect headship as well as cultural efficacy. This means that theories of headship as well as organizational culture should take into consideration the variability in the environment. This should lead to more investigation into how diverse contexts affect the use as well as effect of transformational headship.

## RECOMMENDATIONS

This investigation's outcomes led to a number of suggestions for healthcare businesses that want to improve their Cyber-security by having good headship as well as a positive corporate culture. First, firms need to make it a priority to help their managers acquire transformational headship skills. Targeted training programs that focus on improving abilities like emotional intelligence, effective communication, as well as motivating a team can help through this. Leaders may get their staff to take a proactive approach to Cyber-security by encouraging these traits. Also, businesses should start training as well as awareness programs that encourage a culture of constant development as well as watchfulness. Employees may learn how to protect sensitive information as well as deal through any attacks through regular workshops, seminars, as well as Cyber-security drills. Getting personnel to take part in these programs makes them feel like they own as well as are responsible for Cyber-security. In addition, healthcare institutions should make sure that Cyber-security is a part of their daily operations by setting explicit rules as well as procedures. This involves making rules for how to utilize IoT devices, how to handle data, as well as how to respond to incidents that are easy to find as well as keep up to current. If you make Cyber-security a part of your organizations regular responsibilities, employees are more inclined to make security a priority. Organizations should also think about using modern Cyber-security tools that work well through their headship as well as culture programs Finally, it is very essential to keep checking on Cyber-security plans. Organizations should set up ways to measure how well their headship as well as culture programs are working to lower cyber threats. Regular evaluations may assist find areas that need work as well as make sure that Cyber-security processes change as new threats as well as technologies come out.

## FUTURE DIRECTIONS

To expand on the outcomes of this investigation, future investigation on Cyber-security in healthcare should look at a few essential areas. First, investigations may do longitudinal studies to look at how transformational headship as well as organizational culture changes over time as well as how those changes affect Cyber-security resilience in the long run. Knowing how these things work can help us learn more about how well headship as well as cultural interventions works to deal through new cyber risks. In addition, broadening the investigation to cover a wider range of healthcare settings, especially those in varied geographical as well as cultural contexts, can make the outcomes more applicable to other situations. Comparative studies among developed as well as poor nations might help us understand how the link among headship, culture, as well as Cyber-security practices changes depending on the situation. This would provide us useful information for adapting techniques to different settings. It would also be worth looking at how technology might help or hurt the growth of a proactive Cyber-security culture. Investigation might look into how different tech tools as well as platforms can be used in headship as well as organizational culture to get employees more involved as well as aware of Cyber-security issues. Also, looking at how different headship styles, such transactional or servant headship, work together as well as how they affect Cyber-security projects might give us a better idea of what makes a good leader in this area. This investigation might also look at how middle management as well as frontline workers can help create a culture of Cyber-security, which would expand the range of headship impact. Finally, qualitative studies that look at how employees at different levels feel about their experiences through headship as well as organizational culture in connection to Cyber-security may provide us a lot of useful information. These stories can help create more nuanced plans that are in line through what healthcare practitioners are actually dealing through on the ground.

## REFERENCES


Abdullah Sani, H. A., & Jaafar, N. I. (2025). *Exploring the impact of IoT on governance and public service transformation: evidence from Malaysia's public sector*. Smart and Sustainable Built Environment.

Ashuro, T., Kant, S., & Adula, M. (2025). Multi-Stakeholder Collaboration Effect on Sustainable Supply Chain Optimization by Mediation of Vendor Managed Inventory in the Horn of Africa. In *Multi-Stakeholder Collaboration for Sustainable Supply Chain* (pp. 203–224). IGI Global Scientific Publishing. DOI: 10.4018/979-8-3693-8925-6.ch009

Awan, U., Keprate, A., & Braathen, P. (2025). A Conceptual Framework of An Integrative Leadership for Cybersecurity Management and Designing Digital Road Map for Organizations. In *Digital Transformation* (pp. 47–59). Routledge India. DOI: 10.4324/9781003626640-5

Cvetkoska, V., Trpeski, P., Ivanovski, I., Peovski, F., İmrol, M. H., Babadoğan, B., Ecer, H., Görür, D. Z., Selvi, U., Hunde, A. B., Gemeda, F. T., Dubi, Y. B., Melnyk, S., Lytvynchuk, A., & Tereshchenko, H. (2025). Comparative Analysis of Skill Shortages, Skill Mismatches, and the Threats of Migration in Labor Markets: A Sectoral Approach in North Macedonia, Türkiye, Ethiopia, and Ukraine. *Social Sciences (Basel, Switzerland)*, *14*(5), 294. DOI: 10.3390/socsci14050294

Eappen, P., Gunn, V., Brar, H. S., & Stedman, I. (2025). Capitalizing on the transformative role of AI and human capital to strengthen cybersecurity in healthcare: Safeguarding patient data and advancing regulatory compliance. In *AI-Enabled Threat Intelligence and Cyber Risk Assessment* (pp. 112–125). CRC Press. DOI: 10.1201/9781003504979-7

Gebeyew, A. S., Zemene, W., Tilahun, B. C., Mengestie, N. D., Endehabtu, B. F., Wordofa, Z. R., Takillo, M. K., Ashagrie, G. B., & Sisay, M. M. (2025). Digital health data security practices among health professionals in low-resource settings: Cross-sectional study in Amhara Region, Ethiopia. *BMC Medical Informatics and Decision Making*, *25*(1), 60. DOI: 10.1186/s12911-025-02902-2 PMID: 39910558

Jio, W., & Kant, S. (2025). Market Mobility Effect on Gig Economy Adaptability by Mediation of Talent Management in the Horn of Africa. In *Sustainability and Adaptability of Gig Economies in Global Business* (pp. 205–230). IGI Global Scientific Publishing. DOI: 10.4018/979-8-3693-9385-7.ch008

Kant, S., Adula, M., Kaswan, K. S., Birhane, M., & Badi, S. (2025). Financial Innovations Effect on Smart Economy Through AI in the Horn of Africa. In *Economic and Political Consequences of AI: Managing Creative Destruction* (pp. 111-134). IGI Global Scientific Publishing. DOI: 10.4018/979-8-3593-7036-0.ch006

Kant, S., Adula, M., Nimbrain, N., & Kumari, M. (2025). Optimizing Resource Allocation for Green IT Future by Mediation of AI in the Horn of Africa In *Sustainable Information Security in the Age of AI and Green Computing* (pp. 503–522). IGI Global Scientific Publishing. DOI: 10.4018/979-8-3693-8034-5.ch025

Kant, S., Balami, D. A., Alemu, Z. K., & Takaro, G. S. (2025). Digital Transformation in Accounting Effect on Public Sector Accountability Through Digital Innovations in the Public Sector in the Horn of Africa. In *Enhancing Public Sector Accountability and Services Through Digital Innovation* (pp. 237–264). IGI Global Scientific Publishing. DOI: 10.4018/979-8-3693-9251-5.ch007

Kant, S., Terefe, A., & Adula, M. (2025). Transforming CRM: Effect on Service Sector Optimization by Mediation of AI Innovations in the Horn of Africa. In *AI Innovations for Customer Experience Optimization in the Service Sector* (pp. 179-202). IGI Global Scientific Publishing.

Khan, M. I., Naim, A., Khan, M. F., & Balqis, S. N. (2025). Leadership and Change Management for Sustainable Healthcare in the Digital Era. In *Fostering Economic Diversification and Sustainable Business Through Digital Intelligence* (pp. 257–282). IGI Global Scientific Publishing. DOI: 10.4018/979-8-3693-8492-3.ch013

Malik, K., Kant, S., Kaswan, K. S., Dhatterwal, J. S., & Parwar, A. (2025). Blockchain-Enabled Edge Computing for Cognitive IoT. In *Innovations in Blockchain-Powered Intelligence and Cognitive Internet of Things (CIoT)* (pp. 113–134). IGI Global Scientific Publishing.

Murugan, T., & Singh, W. J. (Eds.). (2025). *Cybersecurity and Data Science Innovations for Sustainable Development of HEICC: Healthcare, Education, Industry, Cities, and Communities*. CRC Press.

Rawindaran, N., Jayal, A., & Prakash, E. (2025). Cybersecurity Framework: Addressing Resiliency in Welsh SMEs for Digital Transformation and Industry 5.0. *Journal of Cybersecurity and Privacy*, *5*(2), 17. DOI: 10.3390/jcp5020017

Restuputri, D. P., Taheer, F. A., Masudin, I., & Nasyiah, T. (2025). The interconnection of human-technology interaction, transformational leadership and sustainable practice: Insights from the oil and gas industry using structural equation modelling and fuzzy-set qualitative comparative analysis. *Theoretical Issues in Ergonomics Science*, *26*(5), 1–36. DOI: 10.1080/1463922X.2025.2506421

Srivastava, S. K. (2025). Strengthening Cybersecurity: Strategies for National Governments. *Journal of Organizational Computing and Electronic Commerce*, •••, 1–19. DOI: 10.1080/10919392.2025.2470083

## KEY TERMS AND DEFINITIONS

**Continuous Improvement:** A planned, continuing endeavor to make products, services, or processes better via little as well as big changes. In terms of organizational culture, it promotes a way of thinking that is open to new ideas as well as adapting to new situations.

**Cyber-security:** is the act of keeping systems, networks, as well as programs safe against digital assaults, theft, damage, or access throughout permission. In healthcare, good Cyber-security is very essential for keeping patient information safe as well as making sure that healthcare systems are working properly.

**Employee Engagement:** How emotionally involved as well as committed an employee is to their company as well as its aims. When employees are highly engaged, they are more productive, happier through their jobs, as well as more likely to take the initiative to solve problems at work, such as Cyber-security issues.

**Healthcare IoT (Internet of Things):** A group of medical gadgets as well as apps that are connected to each other as well as send data over the internet. IoT in healthcare makes patient care better as well as operations run more smoothly, but it also poses serious Cyber-security threats.

**Mediation:** A statistical idea that uses a third variable (the mediator) to explain how an independent variable as well as a dependent variable is related. This investigation shows that company culture may help connect transformational headship through Cyber-security practices.

**Organizational Culture:** The ideas, attitudes, as well as behaviors that all employees in a company share as well as that affect how they behave as well as think. It affects how people work together, makes choices, as well as do their jobs, which in turn affects the performance of the whole company.

**Transformational Leadership:** is a type of headship that encourages as well as inspires people to reach their full potential as well as creates an atmosphere where change as well as new ideas may thrive. Transformational leaders work on making deep connections through people as well as helping them improve both personally as well as professionally.

# Compilation of References

Abdullah Sani, H. A., & Jaafar, N. I. (2025). *Exploring the impact of IoT on governance and public service transformation: evidence from Malaysia's public sector*. Smart and Sustainable Built Environment.

Abdulmalek, S., Nasir, A., Jabbar, W. A., Almuhaya, M. A. M., Bairagi, A. K., Khan, M. A.-M., & Kee, S.-H. (2022). Iot-based healthcare-monitoring system towards improving quality of life: A review. *Health Care*, *10*, •••. https://api.semanticscholar.org/CorpusID:252892699 PMID: 36292441

Abideen, Z. U., & Shah, M. A. (2017). "An IoT based robust healthcare model for continuous health monitoring." *2017 23rd international conference on automation and computing (ICAC)*. IEEE, DOI: 10.23919/IConAC.2017.8082012

Adil, M., Khan, M. K., Kumar, N., Attique, M., Farouk, A., Guizani, M., & Jin, Z. (2024). Healthcare Internet of Things: Security threats, challenges, and future research directions. *IEEE Internet of Things Journal*, *11*(11), 19046–19069. DOI: 10.1109/JIOT.2024.3360289

Aditya, A., Vidyarthi, D., & Nene, M. J. (2024, March). A Study of Common Vulnerabilities in IoT Devices. In *2024 11th International Conference on Reliability, Infocom Technologies and Optimization (Trends and Future Directions)(ICRITO)* (pp. 1-6). IEEE. DOI: 10.1109/ICRITO61523.2024.10522155

Agneeswaran, V. S., Mukherjee, J., Gupta, A., Tonpay, P., Tiwari, J., & Agarwal, N. (2013). Real-time analytics for the healthcare industry: Arrhythmia detection. *Big Data*, *1*(3), 176–182. DOI 10.1089/big.2013.0018 PMID: 27442199

Ahmad, A. (2024). Enhancing hospital efficiency through iot and ai: A smart healthcare system. *Journal of Computer Science Application and En- gineering (JOSAPEN)*. https: // api . semanticscholar . org / CorpusID: 272607805

Ahmad, Z., Shahid Khan, A., Wai Shiang, C., Abdullah, J., & Ahmad, F. (2021). Network intrusion detection system: A systematic study of machine learning and deep learning approaches. *Transactions on Emerging Telecommunications Technologies*, *32*(1), 1–29. DOI: 10.1002/ett.4150

Akinola, O., Akinola, A., Victor Ifeanyi, I., Oyerinde, O., Joseph Adewole, O., Sulaimon, B., & Oyekan, B. O. (2024). Artificial Intelligence and Machine Learning Techniques for Anomaly Detection and Threat Mitigation in Cloud-Connected Medical Devices. *International Journal of Scientific Research and Modern Technology*, *3*(3), 1–13. Advance online publication. DOI: 10.38124/ijsrmt.v3i3.26

Aksenova, E. I., & Gorbatov, S. Y. (2021). Application of iot technologies in healthcare. *City Healthcare*. https://api.semanticscholar.org/CorpusID: 251478335

Alabdulatif, A. (2025). A Novel Ensemble of Deep Learning Approach for Cybersecurity Intrusion Detection with Explainable Artificial Intelligence. *Applied Sciences (Basel, Switzerland)*, *15*(14), 7984. Advance online publication. DOI: 10.3390/app15147984

Alamri, B., Crowley, K., & Richardson, I. (2022). "Blockchain-based identity management systems in health IoT: A systematic review." Bellamkonda, Srikanth. "Network Segmentation and Micro-Segmentation: Reducing Attack Surfaces in Modern Enterprise Security."

Alamri, B., Richardson, I., & Crowley, K. (2024). Cybersecuriy Risk Management and Evaluation Framework of Blockchain Identity Management Systems in HIoT: Experts Evaluation. *IEEE Access : Practical Innovations, Open Solutions*, *12*(September), 144652–144683. DOI: 10.1109/ACCESS.2024.3468379

Aledhari, M., Razzak, R., Qolomany, B., Al-Fuqaha, A., & Saeed, F. (2022). Biomedical IoT: Enabling Technologies, Architectural Elements, Challenges, and Future Directions. *IEEE Access : Practical Innovations, Open Solutions*, *10*, 31306–31339. DOI: 10.1109/ACCESS.2022.3159235

Al-Garadi, M. A., Mohamed, A., Al-Ali, A. K., Du, X., Ali, I., & Guizani, M. (2020). A Survey of Machine and Deep Learning Methods for Internet of Things (IoT) Security. *IEEE Communications Surveys and Tutorials*, *22*(3), 1646–1685. DOI: 10.1109/COMST.2020.2988293

Algfari, S. M., Alghamdi, A. S., Ali, E. I. A., Almuhaylib, A. M., Alzaher, M. A., Alshammry, M. M., Alharbi, A. T., Alharbi, S. H., & Alanazi, H. Al- waked, M. H., Alrashidi, A. A. M., Alrasheed, B. B., Alsarimi, F. A. H., Alotaibi, M. S. M., Alanazi, A. A., & Alumtairi, A. Z. (2020). Real-time health monitoring using iot devices for patients with chronic conditions. *International journal of health sciences.* https://api.semanticscholar. org/CorpusID:272628347

Ali, M., Naeem, F., Tariq, M., & Kaddoum, G. (2022). Federated Learning for Privacy Preservation in Smart Healthcare Systems: A Comprehensive Survey. *arXiv preprint*. https://arxiv.org/abs/2203.09702

Ali, S. Z., Ali, S. H., Javeed, A., Ullah, I., Memon, S. A., & Manzoor, S. (2024). Supervised Learning Approaches for Vibration Analysis and Anomaly Detection in Rotating Machines. *2024 3rd International Conference on Emerging Trends in Electrical, Control, and Telecommunication Engineering (ETECTE)*, 1-6. DOI: 10.1109/ETECTE63967.2024.10824020

Ali, T. E., et al. (2025). "Trends, prospects, challenges, and security in the healthcare internet of things." *Computing* 107.1-28.

Ali, M., Saleem, Y., Hina, S., & Shah, G. A. (2025). DDoSViT: IoT DDoS attack detection for fortifying firmware Over-The-Air (OTA) updates using vision transformer. *Internet of Things : Engineering Cyber Physical Human Systems*, *30*, 101527. Advance online publication. DOI: 10.1016/j.iot.2025.101527

Ali, T. E., Ali, F. I., Dakić, P., & Zoltan, A. D. (2025). Trends, prospects, challenges, and security in the healthcare internet of things. *Computing*, *107*(1), 1–29. DOI: 10.1007/s00607-024-01352-4

Alkan, G. O. (2023). The governance of healthcare internet: Understanding the impact on the workforce. *The European Proceedings of Social and Behavioural Sciences*. https: / / api . semanticscholar . org / CorpusID: 265230296

ALmojel, F., & Mishra, S.ALmojel. (2024). Advancing Hospital Cybersecurity Through IoT-Enabled Neural Network for Human Behavior Analysis and Anomaly Detection. *International Journal of Advanced Computer Science and Applications*, *15*(5). Advance online publication. DOI: 10.14569/IJACSA.2024.0150506

Almutairi, M., & Sheldon, F. T. (2025). IoT–Cloud Integration Security: A Survey of Challenges, Solutions, and Directions. *Electronics (Basel)*, *14*(7), 1394. Advance online publication. DOI: 10.3390/electronics14071394

Al-Na'amneh, Q., Hazaymih, R., Al-Harasis, T., Almaiah, M., Aljawarneh, M., Qadoumi, B., & Shah, S. M. (2025). Enhancing IoT security RPL attack detection using sine cosine algorithm with XGBoost. In *Cryptography* (pp. 1–28). Biometrics, and Anonymity in Cybersecurity Management., DOI: 10.4018/979-8-3693-8014-7.ch001

Al-Obeidat, F., & El-Alfy, E. M. (2019). Hybrid multicriteria fuzzy classification of network traffic patterns, anomalies, and protocols. *Personal and Ubiquitous Computing*, *23*(5), 777–791. DOI: 10.1007/s00779-017-1096-z

Al-Shargabi, B., & Abuarqoub, S. (2020). Iot-enabled healthcare: Benefits, is- sues and challenges. *Proceedings of the 4th International Conference on Future Networks and Distributed Systems*. https://api.semanticscholar. org/CorpusID:234487349

Alzahrani, A. I. A. (2025). Exploring AI and quantum computing synergies in holographic counterpart frameworks for IoT security and privacy. *The Journal of Supercomputing*, *81*(11), 1194. Advance online publication. DOI: 10.1007/s11227-025-07682-0

Annappa, B., Hegde, S., Abhijit, C. S., & Ambesange, S. (2024). Fedcure: A heterogeneity-aware personalized federated learning framework for intelligent healthcare applications in iomt environments. *IEEE Access*. https://ieeexplore.ieee.org/abstract/document/10412046/

Anthi, E., Williams, L., & Burnap, P. (2018). Pulse: An adaptive intrusion detection for the Internet of Things. In *Living in the Internet of Things: Cybersecurity of the IoT – 2018* (pp. 1–4). IET. DOI: 10.1049/cp.2018.0035

Arfi, W. B., Nasr, I. B., Khvatova, T., & Zaied, Y. B. (2020). Understanding acceptance of ehealthcare by iot natives and iot immigrants: An inte- grated model of utaut, perceived risk, and financial cost. *Technological Forecasting and Social Change*, *120437*, •••. https://api. semanticscholar. org/CorpusID:228829702

Arjunan, G. (2023). Optimizing Edge AI for real-time data processing in IoT devices: Challenges and solutions. [IJSRM]. *International Journal of Scientific Research and Management*, *11*(6), 944–953. DOI: 10.18535/ijsrm/v11i06.ec2

Article, O. (2024)... *Hybrid AI Models in Network Security : Combining ML, DL, and Rule-Based Systems*, *5*(4), 109–121.

Asghari, A., Bergantin, F., Forestiero, A., & Macrì, D. (2024, September). Anomalous behaviors detection of IoT devices through AI-based methodologies. In *2024 7th International Conference of Computer and Informatics Engineering (IC2IE)* (pp. 1-8). IEEE. DOI: 10.1109/IC2IE63342.2024.10748216

Asharf, J., Moustafa, N., Khurshid, H., Debie, E., Haider, W., & Wahab, A. (2020). A review of intrusion detection systems using machine and deep learning in internet of things: Challenges, solutions and future directions. *Electronics (Basel)*, *9*(7), 1177. Advance online publication. DOI: 10.3390/electronics9071177

Ashuro, T., Kant, S., & Adula, M. (2025). Multi-Stakeholder Collaboration Effect on Sustainable Supply Chain Optimization by Mediation of Vendor Managed Inventory in the Horn of Africa. In *Multi-Stakeholder Collaboration for Sustainable Supply Chain* (pp. 203–224). IGI Global Scientific Publishing. DOI: 10.4018/979-8-3693-8925-6.ch009

Attya, S. M., Jumaa, D. A., Hwezy, N. N., Sajid, W. A., Khaleefah, A. M., Zhyrov, G., & Ali, H. (2024). Harnessing Federated Learning for Secure Data Sharing in Healthcare Systems. *2024 36th Conference of Open Innovations Association (FRUCT)*, 390-399. DOI: 10.23919/FRUCT64283.2024.10749928

Avaji, G. M., & N, D. G. (2024). Iot innovations in healthcare: Enhancing pa- tient care and operational efficiency. *International Journal of Research Publication and Reviews*. https://api.semanticscholar.org/CorpusID: 270529020

Awan, U., Keprate, A., & Braathen, P. (2025). A Conceptual Framework of An Integrative Leadership for Cybersecurity Management and Designing Digital Road Map for Organizations. In *Digital Transformation* (pp. 47–59). Routledge India DOI: 10.4324/9781003626640-5

Baich, M., Hamim, T., Sael, N., & Chemlal, Y. (2022). Machine Learning for IoT based networks intrusion detection: A comparative study. *Procedia Computer Science*, *215*, 742–751. DOI: 10.1016/j.procs.2022.12.076

Balasubramanian, V., & Stranieri, A. (2014, December). A scalable cloud Platform for Active healthcare monitoring applications. In *2014 IEEE Conference on e-Learning, e-Management and e-Services (IC3e)* (pp. 93-98). IEEE. DOI: 10.1109/IC3e.2014.7081248

Balasubramanian, V., Stranieri, A., & Kaur, R. (2015, January). Appa: assistive patient monitoring cloud platform for active healthcare applications. In *Proceedings of the 9th International Conference on Ubiquitous Information Management and Communication* (pp. 1-8). DOI: 10.1145/2701126.2701224

Bao, F., Chen, I., Chang, M., & Cho, J. (2012). Hierarchical trust management for wireless sensor networks and its applications to trust-based routing and intrusion detection. *IEEE Transactions on Network and Service Management*, *9*(2), 169–183. DOI: 10.1109/TCOMM.2012.031912.110179

Baraneetharan, E. (2020). Role of Machine Learning Algorithms Intrusion Detection in WSNs: A Survey. *Journal of Information Technology and Digital World, 02*(03), 161–173. DOI: 10.36548/jitdw.2020.3.004

Bashir, A. K., Victor, N., Bhattacharya, S., Huynh-The, T., Chengoden, R., Yenduri, G., Praveen, K. R. M., Pham, Q.-V., Gadekallu, T. R., & Liyanage, M. (2023). A Survey on Federated Learning for the Healthcare Metaverse: Concepts, Applications, Challenges, and Future Directions. *arXiv preprint*. https://arxiv.org/abs/2304.00524

Beltramin, D., Lamas, E., & Bousquet, C. (2022). Ethical Issues in the Utilization of Black Boxes for Artificial Intelligence in Medicine. *Studies in Health Technology and Informatics*, *295*, 249–252. DOI: 10.3233/SHTI220709 PMID: 35773855

Benharref, A., & Serhani, M. A. (2013). Novel cloud and SOA-based framework for E-Health monitoring using wireless biosensors. *IEEE Journal of Biomedical and Health Informatics*, *18*(1), 46–55. DOI: 10.1109/JBHI.2013.2262659 PMID: 24403403

Berguiga, A., Harchay, A., & Massaoudi, A. (2025). HIDS-RPL: A Hybrid Deep Learning-Based Intrusion Detection System for RPL in Internet of Medical Things Network. *IEEE Access : Practical Innovations, Open Solutions*, *13*(February), 38404–38429. DOI: 10.1109/ACCESS.2025.3545918

Bhatia, M., & Rai, M. K. (2017). Identifying P2P traffic: A survey. *Peer-to-Peer Networking and Applications*, *10*(5), 1182–1203. DOI: 10.1007/s12083-016-0471-2

Boda, V. V. R., & Allam, H. (2021). Automating Compliance in Healthcare: Tools and Techniques You Need. *International Journal of Emerging Trends in Computer Science and Information Technology*, *2*(3), 38–48. DOI: 10.63282/3050-9246.IJETCSIT-V2I3P105

Bouman, R., & Heskes, T. (2025). Autoencoders for Anomaly Detection are Unreliable. *ArXiv, abs/2501.13864*. /arXiv.2501.13864DOI: 10.48550

Bovenzi, G., Aceto, G., Ciuonzo, D., Persico, V., & Pescape, A. (2020). A hierarchical hybrid intrusion detection approach in IoT scenarios. *Proceedings - IEEE Global Communications Conference, GLOBECOM, 2020-Janua*. DOI: 10.1109/GLOBECOM42002.2020.9348167

Brown, D. J., Suckow, B., & Wang, T. (2002). *A survey of intrusion detection systems. Technical Report*. Department of Computer Science, University of California.

Butt, S. A., Diaz-Martinez, J. L., Jamal, T., Ali, A., De-La-Hoz-Franco, E., & Shoaib, M. (2019, July). IoT smart health security threats. In *2019 19th International conference on computational science and its applications (ICCSA)* (pp. 26-31). IEEE. DOI: 10.1109/ICCSA.2019.000-8

Chakraborty, C., Banerjee, A., Garg, L., & Editors, • Joel J. P. C. Rodrigues. (2020). Cognitive Internet of Medical Things for Smart Healthcare. In *Springer* (Issue June). DOI: 10.1007/978-3-030-55833-8

Charyyev, B., Mansouri, M., & Gunes, M. H. (2021). Modeling the adoption of internet of things in healthcare: A systems approach. *2021 IEEE International Symposium on Systems Engineering (ISSE)*, 1–8. https: //api.semanticscholar.org/CorpusID:240156807

Chawki, M., & Schneier, B. (2021). Security and Privacy in the Era of Electronic Health Records (EHRs). DOI: 10.5281/zenodo.4782466

Chen, L., & Bate, I. (2016, June). Identifying usage anomalies for ECG-based sensor nodes. In *2016 IEEE 13th International Conference on Wearable and Implantable Body Sensor Networks (BSN)* (pp. 77-82). IEEE. DOI: 10.1109/BSN.2016 7516236

Chen, B., Qiao, S., Zhao, J., Liu, D., Shi, X., Lyu, M., Chen, H., Lu, H., & Zhai, Y. (2020). A security awareness and protection system for 5G smart healthcare based on zero-trust architecture. *IEEE Internet of Things Journal*, *8*(13), 10248–10263. DOI: 10.1109/JIOT.2020.3041042 PMID: 35783535

Chen, Y., & Kunz, T. (2016, April). Performance evaluation of IoT protocols under a constrained wireless access network. In *2016 International Conference on Selected Topics in Mobile & Wireless Networking (MoWNeT)* (pp. 1-7). IEEE. DOI 10.1109/MoWNet.2016.7496622

Cholakoska Cilakova, A., Pfitzner, B., Gjoreski, H., Rakovic, V., Arnrich, B., & Kalendar, M. (2021). Differentially Private Federated Learningfor Anomaly Detection in eHealth Networks. *Adjunct Proceedings of the 2021 ACM International Joint Conference on Pervasive and Ubiquitous Computing and Proceedings of the 2021 ACM International Symposium on Wearable Computers*. DOI 10.1145/3460418.3479365

Christy, A., Gandhi, G. M., & Vaithyasubramanian, S (2015). Cluster-based outlier detection algorithm for healthcare data. *Procedia Computer Science*, *50*, 209–215. DOI: 10.1016/j.procs.2015.04.058

Conti, M., Dehghantanha, A., Franke, K., & Watson, S. (2018). Internet of Things security and forensics: Challenges and opportunities. *Future Generation Computer Systems*, *78*, 544–546. DOI: 10.1016/j.future.2017.07 060

Copeland, S. (2018). Gathering basic information in support of medical network risk management. *Biomedical Instrumentation & Technology*, *52*(2), 112–119. DOI: 10.2345/0899-8205-52.2.112 PMID: 29558185

Cresswell, K., Williams, R., & Sheikh, A. (2021). Using cloud technology in health care during the COVID-19 pandemic. *The Lancet. Digital Health*, *3*(1), e4–e5. DOI: 10.1016/S2589-7500(20)30291-0 PMID: 33735067

Cvetkoska, V., Trpeski, P., Ivanovski, I., Peovski, F., İmrol, M. H., Babadoğan, B., Ecer, H., Görür, D. Z., Selvi, U., Hunde, A. B., Gemeda, F. T., Dubi, Y. B., Melnyk, S., Lytvynchuk, A., & Tereshchenko, H. (2025). Comparative Analysis of Skill Shortages, Skill Mismatches, and the Threats of Migration in Labor Markets: A Sectoral Approach in North Macedonia, Türkiye, Ethiopia, and Ukraine. *Social Sciences (Basel, Switzerland)*, *14*(5), 294. DOI: 10.3390/socsci14050294

Dang, V. A., Khanh, Q. V., Nguyen, V., Nguyen, T., & Nguyen, D. C. (2023). *Intelligent Healthcare : Integration of Emerging Technologies*.

Del-Valle-Soto, C., Briseño, R. A., Valdivia, L. J., & Nolazco-Flores, J. A. (2024). Unveiling wearables: Exploring the global landscape of biometric applications and vital signs and behavioral impact. *BioData Mining*, *17*(1), 15. DOI: 10.1186/s13040-024-00368-y PMID: 38863014

Deshpande, Y. D., & Rahman, S. (2023). *Edge-Based Real-Time Sensor Data Processing for Anomaly Detection in Industrial IoT Applications*. Research Journal of Computer Systems and Engineering., DOI: 10.52710/rjcse.71

Desingh, V., & R, B. (2021). Internet of things adoption barriers in the in- dian healthcare supply chain: An ism-fuzzy micmac approach. *The In- ternational journal of health planning and management*. https://api. semanticscholar.org/CorpusID: 238218586

Dey, S., Ye, Q., & Sampalli, S. (2019). A machine learning-based intrusion detection scheme for data fusion in mobile clouds involving heterogeneous client networks. *Information Fusion*, *49*, 205–215. DOI: 10.1016/j.inffus.2019.01.002

Dhillon, P. K., & Kalra, S. (2018). Multi-factor user authentication scheme for IoT-based healthcare services. *Journal of Reliable Intelligent Environments*, *4*(3), 141–160. DOI: 10.1007/s40860-018-0062-5

Diro, A. A., & Chilamkurti, N. (2018). Distributed attack detection scheme using deep learning approach for Internet of Things. *Future Generation Computer Systems*, *82*, 761–768. DOI: 10.1016/j.future.2017.08.043

Du, J., & Yu, B. (2023, November). Application of Isolation Forest Algorithm in Fraud Detection of Medical Insurance Big Data. In 2023 *8th International Conference on Intelligent Informatics and Biomedical Sciences (ICIIBMS)* (Vol. 8, pp. 504-509). IEEE. DOI: 10.1109/ICIIBMS60103.2023.10347658

Eappen, P., Gunn, V., Brar, H. S., & Stedman, I. (2025) Capitalizing on the transformative role of AI and human capital to strengthen cybersecurity in healthcare: Safeguarding patient data and advancing regulatory compliance. In *AI-Enabled Threat Intelligence and Cyber Risk Assessment* (pp. 112–125). CRC Press. DOI: 10.1201/9781003504979-7

Edo, O. C., Ang, D., Billakota, P., & Ho, J. C. (2024). A zero trust architecture for health information systems. *Health and Technology*, *14*(1), 189–199. DOI: 10.1007/s12553-023-00809-4

El Houda, Z. A., Brik, B., & Senouci, S. M. (2022). A Novel IoT-Based Explainable Deep Learning Framework for Intrusion Detection Systems. *IEEE Internet of Things Magazine*, *5*(2), 20–23. DOI: 10.1109/IOTM.005.2200028

Elbir, A. M., Soner, B., Coleri, S., Gunduz, D., & Bennis, M. (2022). Federated Learning in Vehicular Networks. *2022 IEEE International Mediterranean Conference on Communications and Networking, MeditCom 2022*, 72–77. DOI: 10.1109/MeditCom55741.2022.9928621

Elsisi, M., & Bergies, S. (2025). A robust IoT architecture for smart inverters in microgrids using hybrid deep learning and signal processing against adversarial attacks. *Internet of Things : Engineering Cyber Physical Human Systems*, *31*, 101576. Advance online publication. DOI: 10.1016/j.iot.2025.101576

Fadel, M. M., El-Ghamrawy, S. M., Ali-Eldin, A. M. T., Hassan, M. K., & El-Desoky, A. I. (2022). The proposed hybrid deep learning intrusion prediction IoT (HDLIP-IoT) framework. *PLoS ONE, 17*(7 July), 1–21. DOI: 10.1371/journal.pone.0271436

Fan, J., Yang, W., Liu, Z., Kang, J., Niyato, D., Lam, K. Y., & Du, H. (2023). Understanding security in smart city domains from the ant-centric perspective. *IEEE Internet of Things Journal*, *10*(13), 11199–11223. DOI: 10.1109/JIOT.2023.3252040

Fanucci, L., Saponara, S., Bacchillone, T., Donati, M., Barba, P., Sanchez-Tato, I., & Carmona, C. (2012). Sensing devices and sensor signal processing for remote monitoring of vital signs in CHF patients. *IEEE Transactions on Instrumentation and Measurement*, *62*(3), 553–569. DOI: 10.1109/TIM.2012.2218681

Freeman, R. L., Horner, R. H., & Reichle, J. (1999). Relation between heart rate and problem behaviors. *American Journal of Mental Retardation*, *104*(4), 330–345. DOI: 10.1352/0895-8017(1999)104<0330:RBHRAP>2.0.CO;2 PMID: 10450460

Gaikwad, P. S. V. (2024). Iot in healthcare domain. *International Journal for Research in Applied Science and Engineering Technology*. https://api. semanticscholar .org/CorpusID:267764216

García-Teodoro, P., Díaz-Verdejo, J., Maciá-Fernández, G., & Vázquez, E. (2009). Anomaly-based network intrusion detection: Techniques, systems, and challenges. *Computers & Security*, *28*(1–2), 18–28. DOI: 10.1016/j.cose.2008.08.003

Gebeyew, A. S., Zemene, W., Tilahun, B. C., Mengestie, N. D., Endehabtu, B. F., Wordofa, Z. R., Takillo, M. K., Ashagrie, G. B., & Sisay, M. M. (2025). Digital health data security practices among health professionals in low-resource settings: Cross-sectional study in Amhara Region, Ethiopia. *BMC Medical Informatics and Decision Making*, *25*(1), 60. DOI: 10.1186/s12911-025-02902-2 PMID: 39910558

Ghosh, A., Qin, S., Lee, J., & Wang, G. N. (2016). FBMTP: An automated fault and behavioral anomaly detection and isolation tool for PLC-controlled manufacturing systems. *IEEE Transactions on Systems, Man, and Cybernetics. Systems*, *47*(12), 3397–3417. DOI: 10.1109/TSMC.2016.2633392

Gopi, A., Aravinth, S. S., Charishma, N., Sravani, B., Gayatri, N., & Gowtham, K. (2024, April). A Holistic Approach with Behavioral Anomaly Detection (BAD) for Mitigating Insider Threats in Cloud Environments. In *2024 International Conference on Computing and Data Science (ICCDS)* (pp. 1-6). IEEE. DOI: 10.1109/ICCDS60734.2024.10560376

Govardanan, C. S., Murugan, R., Yenduri, G., Gurrammagari, D. R., Bhulakshmi, D., Kandati, D. R., ... & Jhaveri, R. H. (2024). The amalgamation of federated learning and explainable artificial intelligence for the internet of medical things: a review. Recent Advances in Computer Science and Communications (Formerly: Recent Patents on Computer Science), 17(4), 1-19.

Goyal, N. K. (2025). Security and Privacy in IoT, Fog, and Blockchain Networks. In Sathio, A., Rind, M., Awan, S., & Junejo, A. (Eds.), *Energy-Efficient Deep Learning Approaches in IoT, Fog, and Green Blockchain Revolution* (pp. 371–398). IGI Global Scientific Publishing., DOI: 10.4018/979-8-3373-0300-0.ch015

Goyal, N. K. (2025). Weaponizing Misinformation and Cyberattacks on Supply Chains. In Bukhari, S., & Zafar, I. (Eds.), *Mass Media and Impact of Fake News on Supply Chains* (pp. 177–210). IGI Global Scientific Publishing., DOI: 10.4018/979-8-3373-2175-2.ch007

Goyal, N. K., Dandotiya, M., Kumari, M., Kaloria, S., & Anushya, A. (2025). AI-Powered Haptic Devices for Patient Rehabilitation. In Mamodiya, U., Kalam, A., Bossoufi, B., Awad, M., & Somwanshi, D. (Eds.), *Integrating AI With Haptic Systems for Smarter Healthcare Solutions* (pp. 143–170). IGI Global Scientific Publishing., DOI: 10.4018/979-8-3373-2307-7.ch007

Goyal, N. K., Dandotiya, M., Kumari, M., Sheikh, M. F., & Sharma, S. (2025). Emerging Job Roles in the Tourism Sector Leveraging Artificial Intelligence. In Silic, M., Luthia, M., Ahmad, F., & Chakraborty, P. (Eds.), *Empowering Sustainable Performance and Competitive Advantage in Tourism* (pp. 89–126). IGI Global Scientific Publishing., DOI: 10.4018/979-8-3373-4546-8.ch004

Goyal, N. K., Dandotiya, M., Qurashi, J. A., Kumari, M., & Sharma, S. (2025). AI-Driven Predictive Analytics for Disease Management. In Ouaissa, M., Ouaissa, M., Imad, M., Qurashi, J., & Farooq, M. (Eds.), *Utilizing AI of Medical Things for Healthcare Security and Sustainability* (pp. 231–276). IGI Global Scientific Publishing., DOI: 10.4018/979-8-3373-0690-2.ch008

Goyal, N. K., Kumari, M., Kushwah, V., Dandotiya, M., & Vijay, A. (2025). Evaluating blockchain security: Trade offs in consensus mechanisms. *IET Conference Proceedings*, 2024(38), 80–88. DOI: 10.1049/icp.2025.0775

Gunupudi, R. K., Nimmala, M., Gugulothu, N., & Gali, S. R. (2017). CLAPP: A self constructing feature clustering approach for anomaly detection. *Future Generation Computer Systems*, *74*, 417–429. DOI: 10.1016/j.future.2016.12.040

Gupta, D., Gupta, M., Bhatt, S., & Tosun, A. S. (2021, August). Detecting anomalous user behavior in remote patient monitoring. In 2021 *IEEE 22nd International Conference on Information Reuse and Integration for Data Science (IRI) (pp. 33-40). IEEE.* DOI: 10.1109/IRI51335.2021.00011

Gupta, P., Yadav, L., & Tomar, D. S. (2022). Internet of Things: A Survey on Fused Machine Learning-Based Intrusion Detection Approaches. *Lecture Notes in Electrical Engineering*, *858*, 147–161. DOI: 10.1007/978-981-19-0840-8_11

Gupta, R., Saif, S., & Biswas, S. (2019). Implementation of cloud-assisted secure data transmission in WBAN for healthcare monitoring. In *Advanced Computational and Communication Paradigms* (pp. 665–674). Springer.

Hady, A. A., Ghubaish, A., Salman, T., Unal, D., & Jain, R. (2020). Intrusion detection system for healthcare systems using medical and network data: A comparison study. *IEEE Access : Practical Innovations, Open Solutions*, *8*, 106576–106584. DOI: 10.1109/ACCESS.2020.3000421

Hagemann, T., & Katsarou, K. (2020, December). A systematic review on anomaly detection for cloud computing environments. In *Proceedings of the 2020 3rd Artificial Intelligence and Cloud Computing Conference* (pp. 83-96). DOI 10.1145/3442536.3442550

Harb, H., Mansour, A., Nasser, A., Cruz, E. M., & de la Torre Diez, I. (2020). A sensor-based data analytics for patient monitoring in connected healthcare applications. *IEEE Sensors Journal*, *21*(2), 974–984. DOI: 10.1109/JSEN.2020.2977352

Hasan, M. K., Akhtaruzzaman, M., Kabir, S. R., Gadekallu, T. R., Islam, S., Magalingam, P., Hassan, R., Alazab, M., & Alazab, M. A. (2022). Evolution of Industry and Blockchain Era: Monitoring Price Hike and Corruption Using BIoT for Smart Government and Industry 4.0. *IEEE Transactions on Industrial Informatics*, *18*(12), 9153–9161. DOI: 10.1109/TII.2022.3164066

He, M., Petering, M. E., LaCasse, P. M., Otieno, W., & Maturana, F. P. (2023). Learning with supervised data for anomaly detection in smart manufacturing. *International Journal of Computer Integrated Manufacturing*, *36*(9), 1331–1344. DOI: 10.1080/0951192X.2023.2177747

Hernandez-Jaimes, M. L., Martinez-Cruz, A., Ramírez-Gutiérrez, K. A., & Morales-Reyes, A. (2025). Network traffic inspection to enhance anomaly detection in the Internet of Things using attention-driven Deep Learning. *Integration (Amsterdam)*, *103*, 102398. Advance online publication. DOI: 10.1016/j.vlsi.2025.102398

Hizal, S., Cavusoglu, U., & Akgun, D. (2024). A novel deep learning-based intrusion detection system for IoT DDoS security. *Internet of Things : Engineering Cyber Physical Human Systems*, *28*, 101336. Advance online publication. DOI: 10.1016/j.iot.2024.101336

Husnain, M., Hayat, K., Cambiaso, E., Fayyaz, U. U., Mongelli, M., Akram, H., Ghazanfar Abbas, S., & Shah, G. A. (2022). Preventing MQTT Vulnerabilities Using IoT-Enabled Intrusion Detection System. *Sensors (Basel)*, *22*(2), 567. Advance online publication. DOI: 10.3390/s22020567

Jaber, A. N., & Rehman, S. U. (2020). FCM–SVM based intrusion detection system for cloud computing environment. *Cluster Computing*, *23*(4), 3221–3231. DOI: 10.1007/s10586-020-03082-6

Jalali, N., Sahu, K. S., Oetomo, A., & Morita, P. P. (2020). Understanding user behavior through the use of unsupervised anomaly detection: Proof of concept using internet of things smart home thermostat data for improving public health surveillance. *JMIR mHealth and uHealth*, *8*(11), e21209. DOI: 10.2196/21209 PMID: 33185562

Jamaluddin, A. A., Alkathiri, I. A., Alghmadi, W. A., Khadawardi, H. A., & Alqahtani, A. Y. (2024). Overcoming iot implementation challenges in the saudi healthcare supply chain: An integrated ism-micmac analysis. *Proceedings of the International Conference on Industrial Engineer- ing and Operations Management*. https: // api . semanticscholar . org / CorpusID:270321417

Jamwal, Y., Kumari, P., Mishra, A., Goel, N., & Goswami, M. (2025). Security challenges and solutions in IoT: Analyzing threats, architectures, and policies. In *Hardware Security* (pp. 215–238). Challenges and Solutions., DOI: 10.1007/978-3-031-81213-2_10

Jio, W., & Kant, S. (2025). Market Mobility Effect on Gig Economy Adaptability by Mediation of Talent Management in the Horn of Africa. In *Sustainability and Adaptability of Gig Economies in Global Business* (pp. 205–230). IGI Global Scientific Publishing. DOI: 10.4018/979-8-3693-9385-7.ch008

Jose, A., Tortorella, G. L., Vassolo, R. S., Kumar, M. L, & Cawley, A. F. M. (2022). Professional competence and its effect on the implementation of healthcare 4.0 technologies: Scoping review and future research di- rections. *International Journal of Environmental Research and Public Health*, *20*(1), 478. https://api.semanticscholar .org/CorpusID:255252668. DOI: 10.3390/ijerph20010478 PMID: 36612799

Kadir, E. A., Putri, L. D., Rosa, S. L., Siswanto, A., Assidiqi, F., & Evizal, M. F. (2024, April). Anomaly Detection of Patient Data in Public Hospital used Internet of Things Sensors. In *2024 International Conference on Inventive Computation Technologies (ICICT)* (pp. 1734-1739). IEEE. DOI: 10.1109/ICICT60155.2024.10544697

Kant, S., Adula, M., Kaswan, K. S., Birhane, M., & Badi, S. (2025). Financial Innovations Effect on Smart Economy Through AI in the Horn of Africa. In *Economic and Political Consequences of AI: Managing Creative Destruction* (pp. 111-134). IGI Global Scientific Publishing. DOI: 10.4018/979-8-3693-7036-0.ch006

Kant, S., Terefe, A., & Adula, M. (2025). Transforming CRM: Effect on Service Sector Optimization by Mediation of AI Innovations in the Horn of Africa. In *AI Innovations for Customer Experience Optimization in the Service Sector* (pp. 179-202). IGI Global Scientific Publishing.

Kant, S., Adula, M., Nimbrain, N., & Kumari, M. (2025). Optimizing Resource Allocation for Green IT Future by Mediation of AI in the Horn of Africa. In *Sustainable Information Security in the Age of AI and Green Computing* (pp. 503–522). IGI Global Scientific Publishing. DOI: 10.4018/979-8-3693-8034-5.ch025

Kant, S., Balami, D. A., Alemu, Z. K., & Takaro, G. S. (2025). Digital Transformation in Accounting Effect on Public Sector Accountability Through Digital Innovations in the Public Sector in the Horn of Africa. In *Enhancing Public Sector Accountability and Services Through Digital Innovation* (pp. 237–264). IGI Global Scientific Publishing. DOI: 10.4018/979-8-3693-9251-5.ch007

Karunarathne, S. M., Saxena, N., & Khan, M. K. (2021). Security and Privacy in IoT Smart Healthcare. *IEEE Internet Computing*, *25*(4), 37–48. DOI: 10.1109/MIC.2021.3051675

Kasinathan, P., Pastrone, C., Spirito, M. A., & Vinkovits, M. (2013). Denial-of-service detection in 6LoWPAN-based Internet of Things. In 2013 IEEE 9th International Conference on Wireless and Mobile Computing, Networking and Communications (WiMob'13) (pp. 600–607). IEEE.

Kavitha, V. P., Theivanathan, G., Magesh, V., & G, J. (2024). A comprehen- sive survey of iot applications in remote patient monitoring, chronic disease management, and smart healthcare infrastructure. *2024 3rd In- ternational Conference on Sentiment Analysis and Deep Learning (IC- SADL)*, 689–696. https://api.semanticscholar.org/CorpusID:271463694

Kelly, J. T., Campbell, K. L., Gong, E., & Scuffham, P. A. (2020). The internet of things: Impact and implications for health care delivery. *Journal of Medical Internet Research, 22*. https: // api . semanticscholar . org / CorpusID:226298256

Khadidos, A.O., et al. (2022). "Healthcare data security using IoT sensors based on random hashing mechanism." *Journal of Sensors* 2022.1 8457116.

Khan, F. A., Haldar, N. A. H., Ali, A., Iftikhar, M., Zia, T. A., & Zomaya, A. Y. (2017). A continuous change detection mechanism to identify anomalies in ECG signals for WBAN-based healthcare environments. *IEEE Access : Practical Innovations, Open Solutions*, *5*, 13531–13544. DOI: 10.1109/ACCESS.2017.2714258

Khan, M. F. F., & Sakamura, K. (2020, December). A context-policy-based approach to access control for healthcare data protection. In *2020 International Computer Symposium (ICS)* (pp. 420-425). IEEE.

Khan, M. I., Naim, A., Khan, M. F., & Balqis, S. N. (2025). Leadership and Change Management for Sustainable Healthcare in the Digital Era. In *Fostering Economic Diversification and Sustainable Business Through Digital Intelligence* (pp. 257–282). IGI Global Scientific Publishing. DOI: 10.4018/979-8-3693-8492-3.ch013

Kierner, S., Kucharski, J., & Kierner, Z. (2023). Taxonomy of hybrid architectures involving rule-based reasoning and machine learning in clinical decision systems: A scoping review. *Journal of Biomedical Informatics, 144*, 104428. DOI: 10.1016/j.jbi.2023.104428 PMID: 37355025

Kim, K., & Aminanto, M. E. (2017). Deep learning in intrusion detection perspective: Overview and further challenges. *Proceedings - WBIS 2017: 2017 International Workshop on Big Data and Information Security, 2018-Janua*, 5–10. DOI: 10.1109/IWBIS.2017.8275095

Kim, S., Cai, H., Hua, C., Gu, P., Xu, W., & Park, J. (2020). Collaborative Anomaly Detection for Internet of Things based on Federated Learning. *2020 IEEE/CIC International Conference on Communications in China (ICCC)*, 623-628. DOI: 10.1109/ICCC49849.2020.9238913

Kishor Kumar Reddy, C., Kaza, V. S., Madana Mohana, R., Alhameed, M., Jeribi, F., Alam, S., & Shuaib, M. (2025). Detecting anomalies in smart wearables for hypertension: A deep learning mechanism. *Frontiers in Public Health, 12*, 1426168. DOI: 10.3389/fpubh.2024.1426168 PMID: 39850864

Kodali, R. K., Swamy, G., & Lakshmi, B. (2015). *"An implementation of IoT for healthcare." 2015 IEEE Recent Advances in Intelligent Computational Systems (RAICS)*. IEEE.

Kumar, M., et al. (2023). "Healthcare Internet of Things (H-IoT): Current trends, future prospects, applications, challenges, and security issues." *Electronics* 12.9 2050

Kumar, N., Kaushal, R. K., Panda, S. N., & Bhardwaj, S. (2022). Impact of the internet of things and clinical decision support system in healthcare. *IoT and WSN based Smart Cities*. https://api. semanticscholar. org/ CorpusID:249283542

Kumar, S., Pragya, e Fatima, S., & Nigam, R. (2025). Iot assisted optimization of resources for healthcare, mining and transportation industry. *Asian Journal of Research in Computer Science*. https://api.semanticscholar. org/CorpusID:277766059

Kumari, M., Gaikwad, M., & Chavan, S. A. (2025). A secure IoT-edge architecture with data-driven AI techniques for early detection of cyber threats in healthcare. *Discover Internet of Things, 5*(1), 54.

Kushwaha, N., Kushwaha, S. K. S., & Khare, S. (2025). An overview of artificial intelligence in healthcare system. *Current Artificial Intelligence*. https: //api .semanticscholar.org/CorpusID:276926641

Lau-Min, K. S., Asher, S. B., Chen, J., Domchek, S. M., Feldman, M., Joffe, S., Landgraf, J., Speare, V., Varughese, L. A., Tuteja, S., VanZandbergen, C., Ritchie, M. D., & Nathanson, K. L. (2021). Real-world integration of genomic data into the electronic health record: The PennChart Genomics Initiative. *Genetics in Medicine*, *23*(4), 603–605. DOI: 10.1038/s41436-020-01056-y PMID: 33299147

Lee, W., Kim, S., Jeon, H., & Kim, H. (2015, August). Detecting an abnormal traffic on healthcare network. In *2015 5th International Conference on IT Convergence and Security (ICITCS)* (pp. 1-4). IEEE. DOI: 10.1109/ICITCS.2015.7292970

Li, Z., & Zhang, X. (2024). An Enhanced Autoencoder-based Anomaly Detection Model for time series Data from Wearable Medical Devices. *IEEE journal of biomedical and health informatics, PP*. DOI: 10.1109/JBHI.2024.3434420

Li, J., Meng, Y., Ma, L., Du, S., Zhu, H., Pei, Q., & Shen, X. (2021). A federated learning based privacy-preserving smart healthcare system. *IEEE Transactions on Industrial Informatics, 18*(3), 2021–2031. Advance online publication. DOI: 10.1109/TII.2021.3098010

Li, J., Zhao, Z., Li, R., & Zhang, H. (2019). AI-based two-stage intrusion detection for software-defined IoT networks. *IEEE Internet of Things Journal, 6*(2), 2093–2102. DOI: 10.1109/JIOT.2018.2883344

Liu, D., Lung, C. H., Lambadaris, I., & Seddigh, N. (2013, May). Network traffic anomaly detection using clustering techniques and performance comparison. In 2013 *26th IEEE Canadian Conference on Electrical and Computer Engineering (CCECE)* (pp. 1-4). IEEE. DOI: 10.1109/CCECE.2013.6567739

Liu, H., & Lang, B. (2019). Machine learning and deep learning methods for intrusion detection systems: A survey. *Applied Sciences (Basel, Switzerland), 9*(20), 4396. Advance online publication. DOI: 10.3390/app9204396

Liu, L., Xu, B., Zhang, X., & Wu, X. (2018). An intrusion detection method for Internet of Things based on suppressed fuzzy clustering. *EURASIP Journal on Wireless Communications and Networking, 2018*(1), 1–12. DOI: 10.1186/s13638-018-1128-z

Liu, X., Liu, Y., Liu, A., & Yang, L. T. (2018). Defending ON–OFF attacks using light probing messages in smart sensors for industrial communication systems. *IEEE Transactions on Industrial Informatics, 14*(9), 3801–3811. DOI: 10.1109/TII.2018.2836150

Liu, X., Xie, L., Wang, Y., Zou, J., Xiong, J., Ying, Z., & Vasilakos, A. V. (2020). Privacy and security issues in deep learning: A survey. *IEEE Access : Practical Innovations, Open Solutions, 9*, 4566–4593. DOI: 10.1109/ACCESS.2020.3045078

Liu, Y., Zhang, L., Yang, Y., Zhou, L., Ren, L., Wang, F., Liu, R., Pang, Z., & Deen, M. J. (2019). A novel cloud-based framework for the elderly healthcare services using digital twin. *IEEE Access : Practical Innovations, Open Solutions*, *7*, 49088–49101. DOI: 10.1109/ACCESS.2019.2909828

Loftus, T. J., Ruppert, M. M., Shickel, B., Ozrazgat-Baslanti, T., Balch, J. A., Efron, P. A., Upchurch, G. R.Jr, Rashidi, P., Tignanelli, C. J., Bian, J., & Bihorac, A. (2022). Federated learning for preserving data privacy in collaborative healthcare research. *Digital Health*, *8*. Advance online publication. DOI: 10.1177/20552076221134455 PMID: 36325438

Lopez-Martin, M., Carro, B., Sanchez-Esguevillas, A., & Lloret, J. (2017). Conditional variational autoencoder for prediction and feature recovery applied to intrusion detection in iot. *Sensors (Basel)*, *17*(9), 1967. Advance online publication. DOI: 10.3390/s17091967

Ma, J., Nguyen, H., Mirza, F., & Neuland, O. (2017). Two way architecture between IoT sensors and cloud computing for remote health care monitoring applications. https://aisel.aisnet.org/ecis2017_rip/34

Madanian, S., Chinbat, T., Subasinghage, M., Airehrour, D., Hassandoust, F., & Yongchareon, S. (2024). Health iot threats: Survey of risks and vul- nerabilities. *Future Internet, 16*, 389. https://api.semanticscholar.org/ CorpusID:273582195

Maji, R., Gayen, B., & Saha, S. (2025). *A Robust IoT-Based Approach to Enhance Cybersecurity and Patient Trust in the Smart Health Care System: Zero-Trust Model*. Design and Forecasting Models for Disease Management. DOI: 10.1002/9781394234073.ch12

Maleh, Y., Ezzati, A., Qasmaoui, Y., & Mbida, M. (2015). A global hybrid intrusion detection system for wireless sensor networks. *Procedia Computer Science*, *52*, 1047–1052. DOI: 10.1016/j.procs.2015.05.108

Malhotra, P., Singh, Y., Anand, P., Bangotra, D. K., Singh, P. K., & Hong, W. C. (2021). Internet of things: Evolution, concerns and security challenges. *Sensors (Basel)*, *21*(5), 1–35. DOI: 10.3390/s21051809

Malik, K., Kant, S., Kaswan, K. S., Dhatterwal, J. S., & Panwar, A. (2025). Blockchain-Enabled Edge Computing for Cognitive IoT. In *Innovations in Blockchain-Powered Intelligence and Cognitive Internet of Things (CIoT)* (pp. 113–134). IGI Global Scientific Publishing.

Manogaran, G., et al. (2017). "Big data security intelligence for healthcare industry 4.0." Cybersecurity for Industry 4.0: Analysis for Design and Manufacturing. Cham: Springer international publishing, 103-126.

Maruthukannan, B., Karpagalakshmi, R. C., Lakshmi, D., Wise, D. J. W., & Srinivasan, C. (2024, May). IoT-Connected Telehealth Environments with Long Short-Term Memory Networks for Precise Time-Series Patient Behavior Analysis. In *2024 International Conference on Intelligent Systems for Cybersecurity (ISCS)* (pp. 1-6). IEEE. DOI: 10.1109/ISCS61804.2024.10581323

Mayani, M. B. (2025). The role of internet of things (iot) in healthcare: A revolutionary transformation. *International Scientific Journal of Engineering and Management, 277863219*(4), 1–8. https://api.semanticscholar.org/CorpusID. DOI: 10.55041/ISJEM00077

McDermott, C. D., Majdani, F., & Petrovski, A. V. (2018). Botnet Detection in the Internet of Things using Deep Learning Approaches. *Proceedings of the International Joint Conference on Neural Networks, 2018-July*. DOI: 10.1109/IJCNN.2018.8489489

Mehmood, T., & Rais, H. B. M. (2016). Machine learning algorithms in context of intrusion detection. *2016 3rd International Conference on Computer and Information Sciences, ICCOINS 2016 - Proceedings, April*, 369–373. DOI: 10.1109/ICCOINS.2016.7783243

Mehnaz, S., & Bertino, E. (2020, April). Privacy-preserving real-time anomaly detection using edge computing. In 2020 IEEE 36th International Conference on Data Engineering (ICDE) (pp. 469-480). IEEE. DOI: 10.1109/ICDE48307.2020.00047

Menachem, J. N., Golbus, J. R., Molina, M., Mazurek, J. A., Hornsby, N., Atluri, P., Fuller, S., Birati, E. Y., Kim, Y. Y., Goldberg, L. R., & Wald, J. W. (2017). Successful cardiac transplantation outcomes in patients with adult congenital heart disease. *Heart (British Cardiac Society), 103*(18), 1449–1454. DOI: 10.1136/heartjnl-2016-310933 PMID: 28258242

Menon, I. U., Babu Kumaravelu, V., Kumar, V. C., Rammohan, A., Chinnadurai, S., Venkatesan, R., Hai, H., & Selvaprabhu, P. (2025). AI-Powered IoT: A Survey on Integrating Artificial Intelligence With IoT for Enhanced Security, Efficiency, and Smart Applications. *IEEE Access : Practical Innovations, Open Solutions, 13*(February), 50296–50339. DOI: 10.1109/ACCESS.2025.3551750

Miao, X., Liu, Y., Zhao, H., & Li, C. (2018). Distributed online one-class support vector machine for anomaly detection over networks. *IEEE Transactions on Cybernetics, 49*(4), 1475–1488. DOI: 10.1109/TCYB.2018.2804940 PMID: 29994292

Mishra, T. K., Chinmay, A., & Pattanaik, A. (2023). Iot-enhanced healthcare infrastructure: Towards efficient resource management. *2023 2nd Inter- national Conference on Ambient Intelligence in Health Care (ICAIHC)*, 01–06. https://api.semanticscholar.org/CorpusID:267701212

Mishra, N., & Pandya, S. (2021). Internet of Things Applications, Security Challenges, Attacks, Intrusion Detection, and Future Visions: A Systematic Review. *IEEE Access : Practical Innovations, Open Solutions*, *9*, 59353–59377. DOI: 10.1109/ACCESS.2021.3073408

Mishra, P., Varadharajan, V., Tupakula, U., & Pilli, E. S. (2019). A detailed investigation and analysis of using machine learning techniques for intrusion detection. *IEEE Communications Surveys and Tutorials*, *21*(1), 686–728. DOI: 10.1109/COMST.2018.2847722

Mitchell, R., & Chen, R. (2014). Behavior rule specification-based intrusion detection for safety critical medical cyber physical systems. *IEEE Transactions on Dependable and Secure Computing*, *12*(1), 16–30. DOI: 10.1109/TDSC.2014.2312327

Mohammad, U., Sorour, S. M., & Hefeida (2020). Task Allocation for Mobile Federated and Offloaded Learning with Energy and Delay Constraints. *2020 IEEE International Conference on Communications Workshops (ICC Workshops)*. https://ieeexplore.ieee.org/document/9145450/

Moore, J. W., & Lu, H. (2020, November). Abnormal Activity Detection in Healthcare. In *2020 5th International Conference on Innovative Technologies in Intelligent Systems and Industrial Applications (CITISIA)* (pp. 1-7). IEEE. DOI: 10.1109/CITISIA50690.2020.9371790

Mosaiyebzadeh, F., Pouriyeh, S., Parizi, R. M., Sheng, Q. Z., Han, M., Zhao, L., & Batista, D. M. (2023). Privacy-enhancing technologies in federated learning for the internet of healthcare things: A survey. *Electronics (Basel)*, *12*(12), 2703.

Mrabet, H., et al. (2020). "A survey of IoT security based on a layered architecture of sensing and data analysis." *Sensors*20.13 3625.

Murugan, K., Shaheen, N., Prathyusha, P., Ashalatha, M., & Sahithi, A. (2024, December). IoT Enabled Diabetic Health Surveillance. In *2024 3rd International Conference on Automation, Computing and Renewable Systems (ICACRS)* (pp. 476-482). IEEE. https://10.0.4.85/ICACRS62842.2024.10841749

Murugan, T., & Singh, W. J. (Eds.). (2025). *Cybersecurity and Data Science Innovations for Sustainable Development of HEICC: Healthcare, Education, Industry, Cities, and Communities*. CRC Press.

Musthyala, R., Arawkar, S., & Gupta, M. (2021, June). Anomaly identification using multimodal physiological signals on the edge. In *Proceedings of the 2nd Workshop on Deep Learning for Wellbeing Applications Leveraging Mobile Devices and Edge Computing* (pp. 7-12). DOI: 10.1145/3469258.3469849

Nanayakkara, N. K. V., Halgamuge, M. N., & Syed, A. (2019). Security and privacy of internet of medical things (iomt) based healthcare applications: A review. https://api.semanticscholar.org/CorpusID:213987655

Nawaz, A., Khan, S. S., & Ahmad, A. (2024). Ensemble of autoencoders for anomaly detection in biomedical data: A narrative review. *IEEE Access : Practical Innovations, Open Solutions*, *12*, 17273–17289. DOI: 10.1109/ACCESS.2024.3360691

Nebbione, G., & Calzarossa, M. C. (2020). Security of IoT application layer protocols: Challenges and findings. *Future Internet*, *12*(3), 55.

Nguyen, D. C., Pham, Q. V., Pathirana, P. N., Ding, M., Seneviratne, A., Lin, Z., & Hwang, W. J. (2022). Federated learning for smart healthcare: A survey. *ACM Computing Surveys*, *55*(3), 1–37.

Niyaz, Q., Javaid, A. Y., Sun, W., & Alam, M. (2016). Deep learning approach for network intrusion detection system. In *ACM 9th EAI International Conference on Bio-inspired Information and Communications Technologies* (pp. 21–26).

Ouadrhiri, A. E., & Abdelhadi, A. M. (2022). Differential Privacy for Deep and Federated Learning: A Survey. *IEEE Access : Practical Innovations, Open Solutions*, *10*, 22359–22380. DOI: 10.1109/ACCESS.2022.3151670

Oyelade, J., Isewon, I., Oladipupo, O., Emebo, O., Omogbadegun, Z., Aromolaran, O., Uwoghiren, E., Olaniyan, D., & Olawole, O. (2019). Data Clustering: Algorithms and Its Applications. *Proceedings - 2019 19th International Conference on Computational Science and Its Applications, ICCSA 2019, January 2020*, 71–81. DOI: 10.1109/ICCSA.2019.000-1

Pakrooh, R., Jabbari, A., & Fung, C. (2024). Deep Learning-Assisted Security and Privacy Provisioning in the Internet of Medical Things Systems: A Survey on Recent Advances. *IEEE Access : Practical Innovations, Open Solutions*, *12*(February), 40610–40621. DOI: 10.1109/ACCESS.2024.3377561

Pandey, S., Bhushan, B., & Hameed, A. A. (2024). Securing Healthcare 5.0: Zero-Knowledge Proof (ZKP) and Post Quantum Cryptography (PQC) Solutions for Medical Data Security. In *Soft Computing in Industry 5.0 for Sustainability* (pp. 339–355). Springer Nature Switzerland. DOI: 10.1007/978-3-031-69336-6_15

Parvin, P. (2018, June). Real-time anomaly detection in elderly behavior. In *Proceedings of the ACM SIGCHI Symposium on Engineering Interactive Computing Systems* (pp. 1-6). DOI: 10.1145/3220134.3220145

Patel, V. A., Bhattacharya, P., Tanwar, S., Gupta, R., Sharma, G., Bokoro, P. N., & Sharma, R. (2022). Adoption of Federated Learning for Healthcare Informatics: Emerging Applications and Future Directions. *IEEE Access : Practical Innovations, Open Solutions*, *10*(July), 90792–90826. DOI: 10.1109/ACCESS.2022.3201876

Pathuri, K. (2025). Security and privacy vulnerabilities in iot-enabled medi- cal devices: Analyzing cleartext data leakage and metadata exposure. *World Journal of Advanced Engineering Technology and Sciences*. https: //api.semanticscholar .org/CorpusID:279386619

Pavithra, D., Parameswaran, T., Choudhry, M. D., Amrutha, S., Deepa, T., & Kiruthiga, R. (2024). Application of LSTM Networks for Continuous Patient Monitoring and Anomaly Detection in Wearable Health Devices. *Indian Journal of Science and Technology*, *17*(37), 3909–3921. Advance online publication. DOI: 10.17485/IJST/v17i37.2600

Prasad, D. S., & Das, B. C. (2009). Physical inactivity: a cardiovascular risk factor. http://hdl.handle.net/1807/55196

Provotar, O. I., Linder, Y. M., & Veres, M. M. (2019, December). Unsupervised anomaly detection in time series using lstm-based autoencoders. In 2019 *IEEE International Conference on Advanced Trends in Information Theory* (ATIT) (pp. 513-517). IEEE. DOI: 10.1109/ATIT49449.2019.9030505

Qadri, Y. A., Ali, R., Musaddiq, A., Al-Turjman, F., Kim, D. W., & Kim, S. W. (2020). The limitations in the state-of-the-art counter-measures against the security threats in H-IoT. *Cluster Computing*, *23*(3), 2047–2065. DOI: 10.1007/s10586-019-03036-7

Qadri, Y. A., Nauman, A., Zikria, Y., Vasilakos, A. V., & Kim, S. W. (2020). The Future of Healthcare Internet of Things: A Survey of Emerging Technologies. *IEEE Communications Surveys and Tutorials*, *22*(2), 1121–1167. DOI: 10.1109/COMST.2020.2973314

Racherla, S., Sripathi, P., Faruqui, N., Alamgir Kabir, M., Whaiduzzaman, M., & Aziz Shah, S. (2024). Deep-IDS: A Real-Time Intrusion Detector for IoT Nodes Using Deep Learning. *IEEE Access : Practical Innovations, Open Solutions*, *12*(May), 63584–63597. DOI: 10.1109/ACCESS.2024.3396451

Rački, D., Tomaževič, D., & Skočaj, D. (2023, July). Combining unsupervised and supervised deep learning approaches for surface anomaly detection. In *Sixteenth International Conference on Quality Control by Artificial Vision* (Vol. 12749, pp. 33-40). SPIE. DOI: 10.1117/12.2688559

Raghavan, S. (2025). Ontology-Driven Cross-Domain Access Control Framework for Anomaly Detection in Cloud-Based Healthcare System. DOI: 10.21203/rs.3.rs-6128795/v1

Rahman, F. (2024). Enhancing Medication Safety with ML-Enhanced Decision Support Systems: A Comparative Analysis of Prescription Error Detection. *Journal of Angiotherapy*, *8*(9), 1–6. DOI: 10.25163/angiotherapy.899870

Ramanathan, K. M., N., & P., A. S. (2021). Mitigating risks and barriers for promotion and implementation of technologies in e-healthcare. https: //api.semanticscholar .org/CorpusID:236696827

Ranjan, R., & Sahana, B. C. (2024). A Comprehensive Roadmap for Transforming Healthcare from Hospital-Centric to Patient-Centric through Healthcare Internet of Things (IoT). *Engineering and Science*, *30*, 1–16. DOI: 10.30919/es1175

Rashad, M., Hussein, D. L., Abdalkarim, H., & Azeez, R. (2022). Future IoT Software in Healthcare Also Exploring IoT Industry Application. *UHD Journal of Science and Technology*, *6*(1), 70–75. DOI: 10.21928/uhdjst.v6n1y2022.pp70-75

Rawat, R. S., Diwakar, M., Garg, U., & Srivastava, P. (2025). Developing an Intelligent System for Efficient Botnet Detection in IoT Environment. *International Journal of Mathematical. Engineering and Management Sciences*, *10*(2), 537–553. DOI: 10.33889/IJMEMS.2025.10.2.027

Rawindaran, N., Jayal, A., & Prakash, E. (2025). Cybersecurity Framework: Addressing Resiliency in Welsh SMEs for Digital Transformation and Industry 5.0. *Journal of Cybersecurity and Privacy*, *5*(2), 17. DOI: 10.3390/jcp5020017

Restuputri, D. P., Taheer, F. A., Masudin, I., & Nasyiah, T. (2025). The interconnection of human-technology interaction, transformational leadership and sustainable practice: Insights from the oil and gas industry using structural equation modelling and fuzzy-set qualitative comparative analysis. *Theoretical Issues in Ergonomics Science*, *26*(5), 1–36. DOI: 10.1080/1463922X.2025.2506421

Rondon, L. P., Babun, L., Aris, A., Akkaya, K., & Uluagac, A. S. (2022). Survey on Enterprise Internet-of-Things systems (E-IoT): A security perspective. *Ad Hoc Networks*, *125*, 1–33. DOI: 10.1016/j.adhoc.2021.102728

Saif, S., & Biswas, S. (2018). Secure data transmission beyond Tier 1 of medical body sensor network. In *International Ethical Hacking Conference* (pp. 405–417). Springer. https://doi.org/DOI: 10.1007/978-981-13-1544-2_33

Saif, S., & Biswas, S. (2020). On the implementation and performance evaluation of security algorithms for healthcare. In *2nd International Conference on Communication Devices and Computing* (pp. 629–640). Springer. DOI: 10.1007/978-981-15-0829-5_59

Salih, F. I., Abu Bakar, N. A., Hassan, N. H., Yahya, F., Kama, N., & Shah, J. (2019). IOT security risk management model for healthcare industry. *Malaysian Journal of Computer Science*, •••, 131–144. DOI: 10.22452/mjcs.sp2019no3.9

Sammartino, V., & Baiardi, F. (2024). Database Decomposition to satisfy the Least Privilege Principle in Healthcare. *ARIS2 : Advanced Research on Information Systems Security*, *4*(1), 47–69. DOI: 10.56394/aris2.v4i1.43

Saranya, T., Sridevi, S., Deisy, C., Chung, T. D., & Khan, M. K. A. A. (2020). Performance Analysis of Machine Learning Algorithms in Intrusion Detection System: A Review. *Procedia Computer Science, 171*(2019), 1251–1260. DOI: 10.1016/j.procs.2020.04.133

Sarker, I. H., Abushark, Y. B., Alsolami, F., & Khan, A. I. (2020). IntruDTree: A machine learning based cyber security intrusion detection model. *Symmetry*, *12*(5), 1–15. DOI: 10.3390/sym12050754

Saroja, S., Haseena, S., & Blessa, B. P. M. (2021). Data-driven decision making in iot healthcare systems—covid-19: A case study. *Smart Healthcare System Design*. https://api.semanticscholar.org/CorpusID:242668972

Sharma, N., & Shambharkar, P. G. (2025). Transforming security in internet of medical things with advanced deep learning-based intrusion detection frameworks. *Applied Soft Computing*, *180*, 113420. Advance online publication. DOI: 10.1016/j.asoc.2025.113420

Shelke, Y. (2020). Iomt and healthcare delivery in chronic diseases. https://api.semanticscholar.org/CorpusID:225941374

Shiny, M. L., Ramrao, N., & Murugan, K. (2023). A review on ongoing medical care observing framework for cardiovascular patients utilizing iot. *2023 7th International Conference on Computing Methodologies and Com- munication (ICCMC)*, 1310–1318. https: // api. semanticscholar. org / CorpusID:257959059

Shumba, A. T., Montanaro, T., Sergi, I., Fachechi, L., De Vittorio, M., & Patrono, L. (2022). Leveraging IoT-aware technologies and AI techniques for real-time critical healthcare applications. *Sensors (Basel)*, *22*(19), 7675. DOI: 10.3390/s22197675 PMID: 36236773

Singh, C., Mishra, R., Gupta, H. P., & Banga, G. (2023). A Federated Learning-Based Patient Monitoring System in Internet of Medical Things. *IEEE Transactions on Computational Social Systems*. https://ieeexplore.ieee.org/document/9994660/

Soldatos, J., Gusmeroli, S., Malo, P., & Di Orio, G. (2016). Internet of things applications in future manufacturing. *Digitising the Industry Internet of Things Connecting the Physical, Digital and Virtual Worlds*, 153–183. DOI: 10.1201/9781003337966-5

Somasundaram, R., & Thirugnanam, M. (2021). Review of security challenges in healthcare internet of things. *Wireless Networks*, *27*(8), 5503–5509. DOI: 10.1007/s11276-020-02340-0

Srivastava, S. K. (2025). Strengthening Cybersecurity: Strategies for National Governments. *Journal of Organizational Computing and Electronic Commerce*, •••, 1–19. DOI: 10.1080/10919392.2025.2470083

Su, H., Yao, L., Hou, D., Sun, M., Hou, J., Ying, J., & Hou, R. (2021, August). Cloud computing management architecture for digital health remote patient monitoring. In *2021 IEEE International Conference on Smart Computing (SMARTCOMP)* (pp. 209-214). IEEE. DOI: 10.1109/SMARTCOMP52413.2021.00049

Sukumar, S. R., & Aline, F. (2013). "Application of micro-segmentation algorithms to the healthcare market: A case study." *2013 Biomedical Sciences and Engineering Conference (BSEC)*. IEEE, DOI: 10.1109/BSEC.2013.6618489

Sultana, M., et al. (2020). "Towards developing a secure medical image sharing system based on zero trust principles and blockchain technology." *BMC Medical Informatics and Decision Making* 20.1 256.

Sultana, N., Chilamkurti, N., Peng, W., & Alhadad, R. (2019). Survey on SDN based network intrusion detection system using machine learning approaches. *Peer-to-Peer Networking and Applications*, *12*(2), 493–501. DOI: 10.1007/s12083-017-0630-0

Swamy, S. N., Jadhav, D., & Kulkarni, N. (2017). "Security threats in the application layer in IOT applications." *2017 International conference on i-SMAC (iot in social, mobile, analytics and cloud)(i-SMAC)*. IEEE, DOI: 10.1109/I-SMAC.2017.8058395

Tan, E. T., & Abdul Halim, Z. (2019). Health care monitoring system and analytics based on internet of things framework. *Journal of the Institution of Electronics and Telecommunication Engineers*, *65*(5), 653–660. DOI: 10.1080/03772063.2018.1447402

Tavallaee, M., Bagheri, E., Lu, W., & Ghorbani, A. (2009). A detailed analysis of the KDD CUP 99 data set. In Second IEEE Symposium on Computational Intelligence for Security and Defense Applications (CISDA). IEEE Ali, M. H., Fadlizolkipi, M., Firdaus, A., & Khidzir, N. Z. (2018). A hybrid particle swarm optimization–extreme learning machine approach for intrusion detection system. In 2018 IEEE Student Conference on Research and Development (SCOReD) (pp. 1–4). IEEE. DOI: 10.1109/CISDA.2009.5356528

Thakur, D., & Biswas, S. (2020). Smartphone-based human activity monitoring and recognition using ML and DL: A comprehensive survey. [Springer.]. *Journal of Ambient Intelligence and Humanized Computing*, *11*(5), 777–791. DOI: 10.1007/s12652-020-01899-y

Thamilarasu, G. (2016). iDetect: An intelligent intrusion detection system for wireless body area networks. *International Journal of Security and Networks*, *11*(2), 82–93. DOI: 10.1504/IJSN.2016.075074

Thamilarasu, G., Odesile, A., & Hoang, A. (2020). An intrusion detection system for Internet of Medical Things. *IEEE Access : Practical Innovations, Open Solutions*, *8*, 181560–181576. DOI: 10.1109/ACCESS.2020.3026260

Thirunavukkarasu, J., & Kumaratharan, D. N. (2012). Sensors Enabled Patient Monitoring System Using Cloud Computing Concepts. *IOSR Journal of Engineering*, *02*(2), 247–252. DOI: 10.9790/3021-0202247252

Tran, H. V., Kaddoum, G., Elgala, H., Abou-Rjeily, C., & Kaushal, H. (2020). Lightwave power transfer for federated learning-based wireless networks. *IEEE Communications Letters*, *24*(7), 1472–1476.

Tsiachri, R., & Sotiriadis, S. (2020). The Role of IoT and Cloud Computing in Health Monitoring Systems. DOI: 10.31224/osf.io/683ds

Ukil, A., Bandyoapdhyay, S., Puri, C., & Pal, A. (2016). IoT healthcare analytics: The importance of anomaly detection. In 2016 IEEE 30th International Conference on Advanced Information Networking and Applications (AINA) (pp. 994–997). IEEE.

Ullah, F., Naeem, H., Jabbar, S., Khalid, S., Latif, M. A., Al-Turjman, F., & Mostarda, L. (2019). Cyber security threats detection in internet of things using deep learning approach. *IEEE Access : Practical Innovations, Open Solutions*, *7*, 124379–124389. DOI: 10.1109/ACCESS.2019.2937347

Ursul, I., & Pereymybida, A. (2023, September). Unsupervised detection of anomalous running patterns using cluster analysis. In 2023 IEEE 13th International Conference on Electronics and Information Technologies (ELIT) (pp. 148-152). IEEE. DOI: 10.1109/ELIT61488.2023.10310751

Vatin, N. I., Pant, R., Mohan, C., Kumar, A., & Rajasekhar, N. (2024). Iot- enhanced healthcare: A patient care evaluation using the iot health- care test. *BIO Web of Conferences*. https://api.semanticscholar.org/ CorpusID:267186827

Vijayan, V., Connolly, J. P., Condell, J., McKelvey, N., & Gardiner, P. (2021). Review of wearable devices and data collection considerations for connected health. *Sensors (Basel)*, *21*(16), 5589. DOI: 10.3390/s21165589 PMID: 34451032

Waleed, M., Kamal, T., Um, T. W., Hafeez, A., Habib, B., & Skouby, K. E. (2023). Unlocking insights in iot-based patient monitoring: Methods for encompassing large-data challenges. *Sensors (Basel)*, *23*(15), 6760. DOI: 10.3390/s23156760 PMID: 37571543

Wang, B., Shi, X., Han, X., & Xiao, G. (2024). The digital transformation of nursing practice: An analysis of advanced iot technologies and smart nursing systems. *Frontiers in Medicine*, *11*, 1471527. https://api.semanticscholar. org/CorpusID:274404316. DOI: 10.3389/fmed.2024.1471527 PMID: 39678028

Wazid, M., Zeadally, S., Das, A. K., & Odely, V. (2016). Analysis of security protocols for mobile healthcare. [Springer.]. *Journal of Medical Systems*, *40*(4), 1–12. DOI: 10.1007/s10916-016-0596-0 PMID: 27640159

Williams, R., McMahon, E., Samtani, S., Patton, M., & Chen, H. (2017). Identifying vulnerabilities of consumer Internet of Things (IoT) devices: A scalable approach. *2017 IEEE International Conference on Intelligence and Security Informatics: Security and Big Data, ISI 2017, July*, 179–181. DOI: 10.1109/ISI.2017.8004904

Wyss, B. M. (2024). *CTC-SENTINEL-092024_cover-article-1*. 1–9.

Xiao, L., Wan, X., Lu, X., Zhang, Y., & Wu, D. (2018). *IoT Security Techniques Based on Machine Learning*. 1–20. https://arxiv.org/abs/1801.06275

Yew, H. T., Ng, M. F., Ping, S. Z., Chung, S. K., Chekima, A., & Dargham, J. A. (2020, February). Iot based real-time remote patient monitoring system. In *2020 16th IEEE international colloquium on signal processing & its applications (CSPA)* (pp. 176-179). IEEE. DOI: 10.1109/CSPA48992.2020.9068699

Yogi, K. S. V, D. G., B, M. K. S., R.Nithya, Begum, A., & Suganthi.N. (2024). Enhancing healthcare delivery through iot applications in remote pa- tient monitoring and telemedicine. *2024 IEEE North Karnataka Sub- section Flagship International Conference (NKCon)*, 1–8. https://api. semanticscholar.org/CorpusID:274541142

Zakerabasali, S., & Ayyoubzadeh, S. M. (2022). Internet of things and healthcare system: A systematic review of ethical issues. *Health Science Reports*, *5*(6), e863. https://api.semanticscholar.org/CorpusID:252709937. DOI: 10.1002/hsr2.863 PMID: 36210869

Zamini, M., & Hasheminejad, S. M. H. (2019). A comprehensive survey of anomaly detection in banking, wireless sensor networks, social networks, and healthcare. *Intelligent Decision Technologies*, *13*(2), 229–270. DOI: 10.3233/IDT-170155

Zhang, M., Qu, L., & Singh, P. (2022). Splitavg: A heterogeneity-aware federated deep learning method for medical imaging. https://ieeexplore.ieee.org/abstract/document/9806163/

Zhang, G., Hou, J., Wang, J., Yan, C., & Luo, J. (2020). Feature selection for microarray data classification using hybrid information gain and a modified binary krill herd algorithm. *Interdisciplinary Sciences, Computational Life Sciences*, *12*(3), 331–345. DOI: 10.1007/s12539-020-00372-w PMID: 32441000

Zhang, Y., Chen, Y., Wang, J., & Pan, Z. (2021). Unsupervised deep anomaly detection for multi-sensor time-series signals. *IEEE Transactions on Knowledge and Data Engineering*, *35*(2), 2118–2132. DOI: 10.1109/TKDE.2021.3102110 PMID: 36798878

Zheng, X., Shah, S. B. H., Ren, X., & Li, F. (2021). Mobile edge computing enabled efficient communication based on federated learning in internet of medical things. https://onlinelibrary.wiley.com/doi/abs/10.1155/2021/4410894

Zheng, Y., Li, Z., Xu, X., & Zhao, Q. (2022). Dynamic defenses in cyber security: Techniques, methods and challenges. *Digital Communications and Networks*, *8*(4), 422–435. DOI: 10.1016/j.dcan.2021.07.006

Ziani, I., Bendiab, G., Bouzenada, M., & Shiaeles, S. (2024). Video-Based Abnormal Human Behaviour Detection for Video Forensics. *2024 IEEE International Conference on Cyber Security and Resilience (CSR)*, 401-406. DOI: 10.1109/CSR61664.2024.10679423

# About the Contributors

**Chin-Shiuh Shieh** is a distinguished academic and researcher in the field of electronic engineering and computer science, currently serving as a Professor in the Department of Electronic Engineering at National Kaohsiung University of Science and Technology (NKUST), Taiwan. He received his Ph.D. in Computer Science and Engineering from the National Sun Yat-sen University, Taiwan, and has since dedicated his career to pioneering research and teaching in areas including computer networking, wireless communication, information security, computational intelligence, embedded systems, and medical informatics. With a career spanning several decades, Professor Shieh has made significant contributions to both academia and industry. In the past five years alone, he has authored or co-authored 28 journal papers, of which 24 are indexed in SCI (Science Citation Index), and 80 conference papers, encompassing 26 international and 54 domestic conferences. His editorial acumen is evident in his role as editor for two international academic conference proceedings. Professor Shieh has been actively engaged in various research initiatives, participating in 10 Ministry of Science and Technology (MOST) projects, leading five of them. He has also been involved in three Ministry of Education projects, one of which he led, and a campus research project. Furthermore, his strong industry collaboration is reflected in 10 industry-academia cooperation projects, eight of which he led. He has also contributed to one technology transfer authorization. As a recognized figure in the global research community, Professor Shieh is affiliated with four professional societies, and serves as a reviewer for 106 academic journals. He has participated as a committee member for 21 journals and 175 international conferences, underscoring his influence and expertise in his fields of specialization. Among his recent notable publications is the 2024 SCI-indexed paper titled "Open-set recognition in unknown DDoS attacks detection with reciprocal points learning" published in IEEE Access, which highlights his innovative work in cybersecurity and artificial intelligence. He has also played key editorial roles in conferences such as the International Conference on Genetic and Evolutionary Computing (ICGEC) and Intelligent Information Hiding and Multimedia Signal Processing (IIHMSP). His work has earned multiple accolades including Best Paper Awards and Excellent Paper Awards in international conferences. He has co-developed cutting-edge methods in machine learning, optimization algorithms, and adversarial defense mechanisms, particularly in the domain of cybersecurity threats such as DDoS attacks. His academic journey, prolific publication record, leadership in research projects, and commitment to interdisciplinary collaboration have established him as a leading voice in advancing electronic engineering and computing sciences in Taiwan and beyond.

**Mong-Fong Horng** received his B.S., Ms. and Ph.D degrees from National Chiao Tung University and National Cheng Kung University, Taiwan in 1989, 1991 and 2003, respectively. He now is a jointly-appointed professor with the department of Electronics Engineering at National Kaohsiung University of Science and Technology, and Kaohsiung Medical University, Taiwan. He served as the president of Taiwanese Association of Consumer Electronics (TACE), Chair of Tainan Chapter, IEEE Signal Processing Society. His research interest includes Internet of Things, machine learning, computer networks and medical informatics and related industrial cooperation.

***

**Bharti** is a Research Scholar in the Department of Management at Maharishi Markandeshwar (Deemed to be University), Mullana, Ambala, Haryana. She holds an MBA with dual specialization in Marketing and Finance. She has also earned a Master's degree in English from Kurukshetra University, Kurukshetra. Her academic journey began with a Bachelor of Arts degree. She has a strong interest in management research and interdisciplinary studies. Her work reflects a blend of business acumen and communication expertise. She is committed to contributing to the field of management through research and publications. With her diverse academic background, she aims to excel as an educator and researcher.

**Bhavanam Amarnath Reddy** is working as an Associate Professor, Department of FINANCE & MARKETING, VIGNANA JYOTHI INSTITUTE OF MANAGEMENT (VJIM) A Premium BusinessSchool, Hyderabad, Telangana, India. In his 16 years of teaching and research experience, he has served in an array of designations as Assistant Professor, Associate Professor and HOD of MBA Department, Head, Entrepreneurship Development Cell, President to Institution Innovation Council (IIC) and National Institutional Startup Policy (NISP) under MHRD Innovation Cell, also Mentor to various innovations under Innovation

Cell, MHRD Has authored 6 Text Books, published 31 patents, 82 National & International Paper Publications, presented papers in 34 International Conferences, Participated in more than 62 FDPs, 91 Webinars, Workshops, Refresher courses and has 24 Coursera Certifications, Won 6 International Awards, life time member in 6 International associations. Reviewer&Editor for 12 International Journals Has presented many Guest lectures and was Resource person for Workshops & Refresher Courses in several Universities, Engineering Colleges and Business Schools on a variety of topics. His research interests are Portfolio Management Services, Mutual Fund Investments, New Innovation Financial Methods, Marketing Administrative Reforms and Marketing Policy and Implementation. His teaching interests are Financial management, Financial accounting & analysis, Managerial Economics & Financial Analysis, Management Science, Security Analysis and Portfolio Management, Financial Institutions, Markets & Services, Strategic Management Accounting, International Financial Management, Strategic Investment and Financing Decisions, Financial Derivatives & Risk Management, Digital Marketing, Advertising and Sales Management,Consumer Behavior, Customer Relationship Management, Marketing of Services, Sales & Distribution Management.

**Malige Gangappa** is an Associate Professor in the Department of Computer Science and Engineering at VNR VJIET. He has been recognized by the institute multiple times for his excellence in teaching. With expertise in Machine Learning, R Programming, and Python Programming, he has delivered lectures at various organizations. Dr. Gangappa was honored with the Best Teaching Faculty and Best Researcher Award at the International Award Ceremony on Star Achievers in Engineering, Management, Arts, and Science (SAEMAS - 2022). Additionally, he is the author of books on Computer Architecture, and Object-Oriented Programming through Java. He has published numerous research papers in reputed national and international journals. His research interests include Deep Learning, Video Processing, and Soft Computing.

**Pawan Kr. Goel**, is a accomplished academician and researcher with 19.5 years of experience, is an Associate Professor at Raj Kumar Goel Institute of Technology, Ghaziabad. He holds a Ph.D. in Computer Science Engineering and is UGC NET qualified. His expertise spans various domains, including wireless sensor networks, cloud computing, and artificial intelligence. Dr. Goel has published extensively in prestigious journals and conferences, with notable papers on topics such as cybersecurity, IoT, and machine learning. He is an active member of numerous professional bodies, including the IEEE, Computer Society of India and the International Association of Engineers. Recognized for his contributions, he has received several awards and certificates of appreciation. Dr. Goel is dedicated to fostering industry-academia collaborations and has organized numerous workshops and seminars. He is also involved in various training programs, MOOCs, and NPTEL certifications, contributing significantly to the advancement of education and research in his field.

**K. Jyothsna** is serving as an Assistant Professor (Jr. G) in the Department of Data Science and Business Systems at SRM Institute of Science and Technology, Chennai. She has ten years of experience in the teaching field and two years of technical experience. She is currently pursuing a PhD degree with the Department of Networking and Communications at SRM Institute of Science and Technology, Kattankulathur, Chennai. Her research focuses on "Cyber Security" and "Deep Learning". She has presented research articles at various conferences and has published her research in reputed journals. Her area of expertise includes Cryptography, Data structures using C, Computer Architecture, Data warehousing and Big data Visualization. Her dedication to education and research has played a vital role in enhancing the institution's reputation in the field of engineering and technology

**Love Kumar**, Assistant Professor-II in the Department of Computer Engineering & Applications of the Mangalayatan University, Aligarh. . He received his B.Tech. Degree in Computer Science & Engineering from U.P. Technical University, Lucknow, U.P.; M.Tech in Computer Science Engineering from Aligarh Muslim University, Aligarh, U.P. Completed Ph.D. in 2025. He is having more than 15 years of teaching and one year industry experience. He has published 15 research papers which includes publications in International Journals, proceedings of International / National conferences along with two patents and five books in the field of Computer Science and Information Technology. His research interest is in the field of Internet of Things, RFID, E-learning, Digital Image Processing & Mobile Ad Hoc Networks. He has received two appreciations awards in the field of teaching and research. He was the member of Advisory Committee, Technical committee & program committee in various National & International conferences. He is the reviewer of two reputed journals. He is life time member of Professional Bodies namely Indian Science Congress Association.

**Dler Salih Hasan** is an Assistant Professor and Head of the Department of Computer Science and Information Technology at Salahaddin University-Erbil. He received his Ph.D. in Mechatronics and Robotics Engineering through a split-site program between Salahaddin University and the University of Florida (2017). With over two decades of academic service, he has taught courses in OOP, Robotics, Embedded Systems, Databases, and IoT at both undergraduate and postgraduate levels. His research focuses on robotics, IoT, AI applications, Sensors, and healthcare monitoring systems, with numerous international publications. He has supervised several MSc theses on robotics and IoT-based smart systems. Dr. Hasan has been actively involved in academic committees, conferences, and curriculum development at national and international levels.

**Binastya Anggara Sekti** has been a lecturer at the Faculty of Computer Science, Esa Unggul University, Jakarta, since 2016. He is actively involved in the Artificial Intelligence and Information Security Study Group. He holds a Bachelor's degree in Informatics Engineering from the Bandung Institute of Technology and a Master's degree in Information Systems Management from Trisakti University, Jakarta. Prior to entering academia, he accumulated over 25 years of professional experience as an IT practitioner in various companies across Jakarta. His work focused on developing data centers for internet service providers and delivering IT solutions for the manufacturing and oil & gas sectors. His research interests include artificial intelligence, cybersecurity, and the development of IT infrastructure.

**Varadharajan Bhoopathy** is a Professor at Sree Rama Engineering College He holds a Ph.D. in Information and Communication Engineering from Anna University and has over 16 years of academic experience. Specializing in wireless sensor networks and IoT, he has published numerous research papers and holds several international patents. Dr. Bhoopathy is a recipient of prestigious awards for his contributions to education and research. His commitment to academia continues to drive innovation and excellence in the field of computer science.

# Index

## I



## L



## M



## O



## P



## S



## T



## V



## W

www.ingramcontent.com/pod-product-compliance
Ingram Content Group UK Ltd.
Pitfield, Milton Keynes, MK11 3LW, UK
UKHW050844101026
15624UKWH00018B/559

9 798337 376103